COLOR ATLAS OF
COSMETIC
DERMATOLOGY

Marc R. Avram, MD
Clinical Associate Professor of Dermatology
Weill–Cornell Medical School
Private Practice—905 Fifth Avenue
New York, New York

Sandy Tsao, MD
Director of Procedural Dermatology
Harvard Medical School
Massachusetts General Hospital, Dermatology Laser and Cosmetic Center
Boston, Massachusetts

Zeina Tannous, MD
Director Mohs/Dermatologic Surgery, Boston VA Medical Center
Assistant in Dermatology, Massachusetts General Hospital, Dermatology, Laser and Cosmetic Center
Associate Program Director for Dermatopathology, Department of Dermatology, Harvard Medical School
Instructor in Dermatology, Harvard Medical School
Boston, Massachusetts

Mathew M. Avram, MD, JD
Director
Massachusetts General Hospital, Dermatology, Laser & Cosmetic Center
Instructor, Harvard Medical School
Boston, Massachusetts

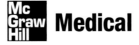

New York   Chicago   San Francisco   Lisbon   London   Madrid
Mexico City   Milan   New Delhi   San Juan   Seoul   Singapore   Sydney   Toronto

Color Atlas of Cosmetic Dermatology

Copyright © 2007 by The McGraw-Hill Companies, Inc. All rights reserved.
Printed in China. Except as permitted under the United States Copyright Act
of 1976, no part of this publication may be reproduced or distributed in any
form or by any means, or stored in a data base or retrieval system, without the
prior written permission of the publisher.

2 3 4 5 6 7 8 9 0 CTP/CTP 0 9 8

ISBN-13: 978-0-07-143761-5
ISBN-10: 0-07-143761-4

This book was set in Trade Gothic by TechBooks.
The editors were Anne M. Sydor and Christie R. Naglieri.
The production supervisor was Phil Galea.
The book designer was Alan Barnett.
The cover designer was Cathleen Elliott.
The indexer was Sara Lynn Eastler.
China Translation & Printing Services, Ltd., was printer and binder.

This book is printed on acid-free paper.
Printed in China

Library of Congress Cataloging-in-Publication Data

Color atlas of cosmetic dermatology
     p. cm.
   ISBN 0-07-143761-4
     1. Dermatology—Atlases.
RL87.C65 2006
616.5—dc22   2006046193

DEDICATION

I would like to dedicate this book to my loving wife Robin. Her beauty, charm and love make everyday exciting. I also want to thank my brothers Eric, Mathew, David, Louis and Harry and sister Rella for always being such good friends and teachers. To my parents Maria and Morrell and sons Robert and Jake—I love you.

Marc R. Avram, MD

To my husband, Hensin. You are my strength and inspiration. Your love, wisdom and encouragement help me realize anything is possible. You are a wonderful husband, father and best friend. I will love you always. To my sons, Sebastian and Hunter. Your unconditional love, enthusiasm and sense of adventure help me remember what is truly important. You brighten my days and fill my life with happiness and love.

Sandy Tsao, MD

I would like to dedicate this book to my beloved father Salem and my beloved mother Jeannette for their endless love and support. They are my inspiration. I would also like to thank my brothers Michel and Fadi and my sisters Fadia and Roula for always being there for me. They are my best friends.

Zeina Tannous, MD

To my parents, Morrell and Maria Avram, who have given me unconditional love and support my entire life. To Alison, Rachel and Alexander, who are my heart, soul and joy. Finally, Rella, Marc, Eric and David, you are my role models and best friends.

Mathew M. Avram, MD, JD

CONTENTS

PREFACE

There has been a revolution in the treatment of medical and cosmetic disorders of the skin. In large part, this is due to the availability of procedures and technologies that produce clear, cosmetic benefit with few side effects and little downtime. With the advent of lasers and light sources over the past 20 years, cosmetic improvement is a matter of quick, relatively painless procedures. Non-laser treatments such as soft tissue fillers, botulinum toxin injections, sclerotherapy, hair transplantation and others have also dramatically expanded the scope of this field. These procedures coincide with the busy lifestyle of many patients who seek an improvement in appearance that does not interfere with their professional, social or personal obligations.

These procedures, however, are not without potential side effects or complications. Physicians who perform these treatments in the absence of training or education are certain to encounter poor results, complications and irate patients. Because patients are pursuing elective treatments for cosmetic benefit, any worsening of appearance will understandably anger patients who undergo these procedures. The decision as to when *not* to treat a patient is perhaps the most important in this field.

With this in mind, *Color Atlas of Cosmetic Dermatology* seeks to provide a succinct yet broad overview of cosmetic therapy. There are a plethora illustrations and graphs to elucidate consultation, management, treatment and side effects of numerous cosmetic procedures. Its practical format is geared to the busy practitioner or trainee who seeks a quick, comprehensive reference for approaching the cosmetic patient. It also emphasizes pitfalls of treatment in order to educate the reader as to potential problems with certain treatments. It serves as an invaluable resource to both the experienced and novice.

Marc R. Avram, MD
Sandy Tsao, MD
Zeina Tannous, MD
Mathew M. Avram, MD, JD

ACKNOWLEDGMENTS

We would like to thank two people who provided significant help in the
production of this textbook, Dr. Rox Anderson and Dr. Gary Lask. In addition,
we would like to thank the office staff at the office of Dr. Marc Avram and the office
staff at the Massachusetts General Hospital Dermatology Laser & Cosmetic Center
for their hard work and dedication in obtaining high quality photographs.

Finally, we would like to thank the professional staff at McGraw Hill
for their great help and devotion in producing this book.
Thank you for pushing us to strive for the best possible Atlas.

SECTION ONE

Photoaging

CHAPTER 1 Analysis of the Aging Face

The face is the focal point of human beauty. Although various factors influence facial beauty, the aging process is the most common aspect prompting surgical intervention. Aging is a dynamic and continual process. Heredity and environmental factors (e.g., sun, wind, movement) are the main determinants of aging. In addition, cigarette smoking can accelerate the aging process. As one ages, changes can be observed in all facial anatomical compartments including the skin, subcutaneous fat, muscle, and bony structure. Use of a systematic approach in the analysis of the aging face will allow for the selection of appropriate, safe, and effective therapies.

ANATOMIC CONSIDERATIONS

Successful rejuvenation of the face requires a thorough understanding of age-related contour changes (underlying soft tissue aging) and textural changes (skin aging) (Tables 1.1-1.2). The youthful face can be divided into three facial zones: upper, middle, and lower zones, as well as the upper neck.

TABLE 1.1 ■ Age-Related Contour Changes

Malar crescent
Cheek depression
Nasolabial fold formation
Prejowl sulcus
Platysmal bands
Jowl formation

TABLE 1.2 ■ Age-Related Textural Changes

Superficial and deep rhytides
Pigmentary disturbances
Telangiectasia formation
Loss of skin elasticity
Actinic keratoses

The upper face includes the forehead, temple, and periorbital region. Aging results in a flattening of the brow arch, eyelid skin redundancy, pseudo fat herniation, and formation of dynamic rhytides at the lateral canthus. Horizontal forehead skin creases develop secondary to sustained contraction of the frontalis muscle in a subconscious attempt to elevate the sagging brows. A rim sulcus deformity develops between the cheek and the eyelid with upper cheek thinning. This sulcus is exacerbated by a preexisting tear trough deformity. Orbicularis oculi muscle ptosis can create a malar fullness referred to as a malar crescent.

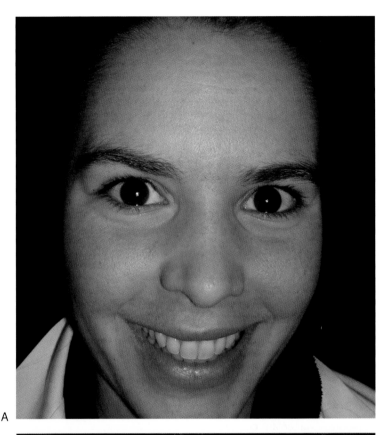

A

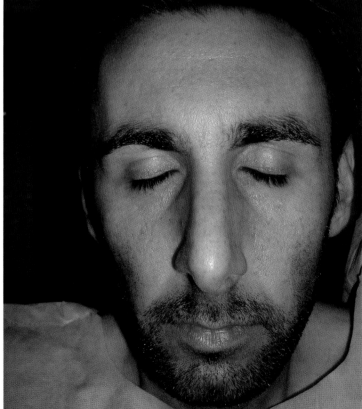

B

Figure 1.1 A&B *Glogau type 1 photoaging. Minimal signs of aging present*

The midface includes the cheekbones that form a smooth continuous convexity from the eyelid to the lip. The melolabial fold represents a flat, smooth junction between the lower cheek and the upper lip. The aging face results in a downward migration of the malar soft tissue, accentuating skeletonization of the orbital rim. Central cheek fat ptosis creates a fullness lateral to the melolabial fold, referred to as the nasolabial folds.

The lower face possesses a well-defined mandibular border and a well-defined cervicomental angle. With aging, platysmal muscle ptosis and cheek fat ptosis along the mandible produce "jowls" overlying the jawline. Soft tissue atrophy anterior to the jowls creates a "prejowl sulcus" which accentuates the skeletonized appearance. Platysmal ptosis of the upper neck blunts the cervicomental angle, creating platysmal bands, or a "turkey neck" deformity.

Facial textural changes include superficial and deep rhytides, pigmentary disturbances, telangiectasia formation, loss of skin elasticity, and actinic keratoses.

PREOPERATIVE EVALUATION

An individualized treatment plan designed to minimize surgical risk is essential. The goal is a youthful and natural postoperative result. The strategy should be formulated for each of the three facial zones, as each anatomic region requires a specific management.

A systematic evaluation should include the degree of photoaging, pigmentary changes, loss of subcutaneous fat, changes in facial musculature, cartilaginous and bony structures, and elasticity loss.

▦ Glogau Photoaging Classification— Wrinkle Scale

The Glogau Photoaging Classification has been devised which broadly defines the changes that may be seen at different ages with cumulative sun exposure.

Type 1—"no wrinkles" (Fig. 1.1)
- Early photoaging
  - Mild pigmentary change
  - No keratoses
  - Minimal wrinkles
- Patient age: twenties or thirties
- Minimal or no makeup use

Type 2—"wrinkles in motion" (Fig. 1.2)
- Early to moderate photoaging
  - Early senile lentigines visible
  - Keratoses palpable but not visible
  - Parallel smile lines beginning to appear
- Patient age: late thirties or forties
- Usually wears some foundation

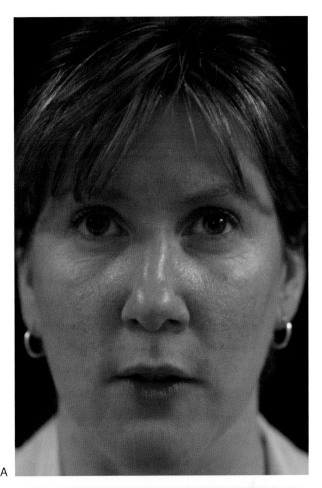

A

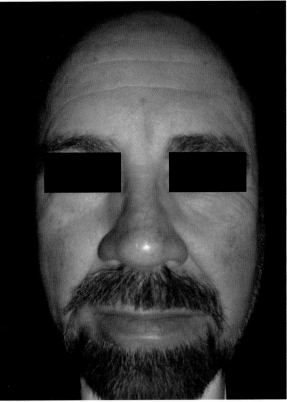

B

Figure 1.2 A&B *Glogau type 2 photoaging. Fine lines barely visible. Minimal pigmentary changes noted*

Type 3—"wrinkles at rest" (Fig. 1.3)

* Advanced photoaging
  - Obvious dyschromia, telangiectasia
  - Visible keratoses
  - Wrinkles even when not moving
* Patient age: fifties or older
* Always wears heavy foundation

Type 4—"only wrinkles" (Fig. 1.4)

* Severe photoaging
  - Yellow-gray [A3] color of skin
  - Prior skin malignancies
  - Wrinkled throughout, no normal skin
* Patient age: sixties or seventies
* Cannot wear makeup—"cakes and cracks"

■ Pigmentary Changes

A vital aspect of the patient evaluation is the determination of the patient's skin response to erythema-producing doses of ultraviolet light. Fitzpatrick's classification of skin types provides a strong indication of the potential for post-inflammatory hyperpigmentation and hypopigmentation and potential for dyschromia upon epidermal and/or papillary dermal injury (Table 1.3).

TABLE 1.3 ■ **Fitzpatrick's Classification of Skin Types**

Skin type	Color	Reaction to sun
I	Very white or freckled	Always burns
II	White	Usually burns
III	White to olive	Sometimes burns
IV	Brown	Rarely burns
V	Dark brown	Very rarely burns
VI	Black	Never burns

A patient's treatment response can be determined by assessing both the degree of photodamage present and the pigmentary skin type. A procedural risk–benefit ratio will differ depending on the patient's individual findings. In general, patients with Fitzpatrick skin types I–III can tolerate more epidermal and dermal injury with minimal risk of residual dyschromia. Patients with Fitzpatrick skin types IV–V have a high risk of residual dyschromia with increased skin injury that may preclude the use of many treatment modalities.

■ Subcutaneous Fat Atrophy

Aging results in a significant degree of loss or redistribution of subcutaneous fat, especially of the forehead, temporal fossae, perioral area, chin, and premalar areas. This leads to a skeletonized appearance. Restoration of volume loss results in the reshaping of the face for a fuller, rounder appearance.

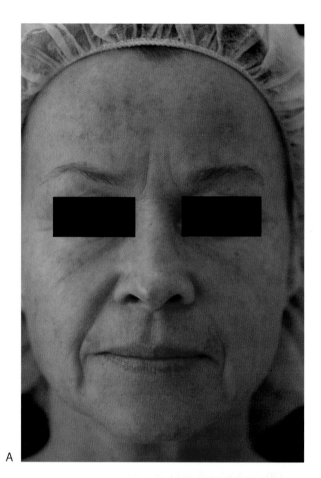

A

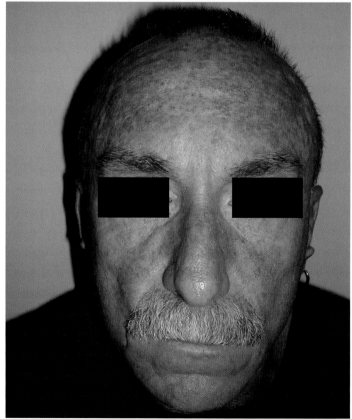

B

Figure 1.3 A&B *Glogau type 3 photoaging. Dyspigmentation and wrinkles are evident*

▣ Facial Musculature Changes

Aging also results in muscular atrophy, contributing to volume loss. As well, dynamic rhytides, which are muscular in origin, often create an angry, tired, or aged appearance. Selective chemical denervation provides marked relaxation of these lines.

▣ Changes in Cartilage, Bony Structures, and Underlying Supportive Structures

Aging results in sagging and loss of resiliency. Redraping, repositioning, and judicious removal of skin and soft tissue assist in the restoration of a youthful appearance.

Once a systemic approach has been followed, the four Rs of facial rejuvenation—relax, refill, redrape, and resurface—can be applied solely or in combination to help restore a more youthful appearance.

BIBLIOGRAPHY

Davis RE. Facelift and ancillary facial cosmetic surgery procedures. In: Nouri K, Leal-Nouri S, eds. *Techniques in Dermatologic Surgery*. London: Mosby; 2003:333–344.

Fitzpatrick T. The validity and practicality of sun-reactive skin types I through VI. *Arch Dermatol*. 1998;124:869–871.

Glogau R. Aesthetic and anatomic analysis of the aging skin. *Semin Cutan Med Surg*. September 1996;15(3):134–138.

Montagna W, Carlisle K, Kirchner S. *Epidermal and Dermal Histological Markers of Photodamaged Human Facial Skin*. Shelton, CT: Richardson-Vicks; 1988.

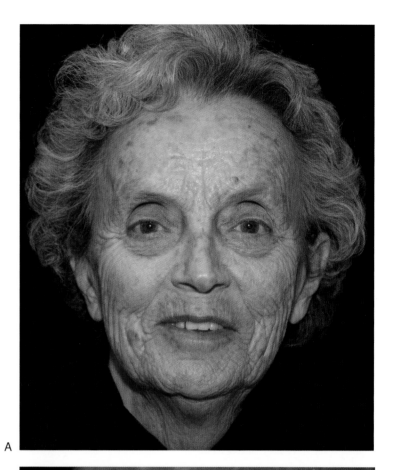

A

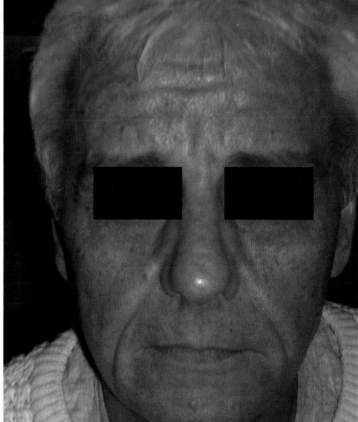

B

Figure 1.4 A&B *Glogau type 4 photoaging. Extensive wrinkles and prominent dyspigmentation*

CHAPTER 2 Dermatoheliosis

Dermatoheliosis results from excessive and/or prolonged exposure of the skin to ultraviolet radiation (UVR). Manifestations represent a polymorphic response of various skin components, especially the epidermis, dermis, and vascular system. The severity of dermatoheliosis is dependent on the duration and intensity of sun exposure, constitutive skin color (Fitzpatrick skin type), and the capacity to tan.

EPIDEMIOLOGY

Incidence: very common

Age: most frequently observed in persons over 40 years

Sex: slight male predominance

Race: most common in fair-skinned individuals (skin phototypes I and II); less commonly seen in darker skinned individuals (skin phototypes IV–VI)

Precipitating factors: chronic sun exposure including intentional sun exposure since youth and occupational exposure; trauma; chronological aging

PATHOGENESIS

UVB is the most damaging UVR, with high dose UVA contributing most significantly. In addition, visible and infrared radiation have been shown to augment the action of UVB.

Aberrant epidermal maturation with a loss of translucency results in the development of dry, rough skin, comedones, and actinic keratoses. Dermal elastin and collagen degeneration results in the appearance of wrinkles, creases, and folds. Disordered melanin production results in ephelides and lentigines. Melasma and post-inflammatory hyperpigmentation are aggravated. Irregularities in the papillary dermal flow result in telangiectasia formation. Loss of subcutaneous fat results in lipoatrophy.

PHYSICAL EXAMINATION

Variable clinical features can be present depending on the severity of findings.

- Epidermis: dry skin and skin fragility are common. Lentigines, dyspigmentation, and guttate hypomelanosis are observed. A leathery appearance may be noted. Exacerbation of melasma may occur. Actinic keratoses are common.

- Dermis: superficial and deep furrows that are present at rest (static rhytides) and with motion (dynamic rhytides) are prominent. Elastosis with skin creeping,

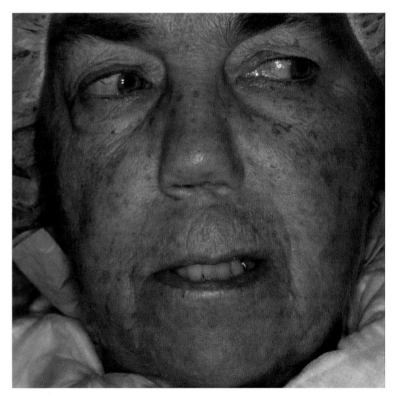

Figure 2.1 *Severe dermatoheliosis in a 65-year-old female. Superficial and deep furrows, dyspigmentation, telangiectasias, jowl formation, and lusterless skin are noted. Scor at nasal tip is the site of a prior skin cancer*

roughness, yellow papules, and plaques are seen. Prominent nasolabial and melolabial folds and jowl formation are seen. Telangiectasia and easy bruising are observed (Figs. 2.1-2.2).

- Pilosebaceous unit: periorbital comedones may develop (Favre–Racouchet).
- Subcutaneous fat: lip thinning, temporal wasting, flattened facies, inferior fat pad bulging, and a loss of the facial fullness and roundness are observed.

DIFFERENTIAL DIAGNOSIS

Xeroderma pigmentosum.

DERMATOPATHOLOGY

Epidermal acanthosis with flattening of the dermal–epidermal junction. Focal increase in epidermal basilar melanocytes; increased melanin formation. Dermal collagen and elastin breakdown with formation of amorphous masses and increase in glycosaminoglycans. Marked alteration in microcirculation.

COURSE

Chronic progressive course.

KEY CONSULTATIVE QUESTIONS

- Past medical history
- Medication use
- Occupation
- Sun exposure history
- Treatment goals
- Prior cosmetic and surgical procedures

MANAGEMENT

▪ Prevention

Strict sun avoidance is stressed. Patients with outdoor occupations, who participate in outdoor sports, or who will continue to spend extensive amounts of time in the sun after treatment should be advised as to the limited benefits to the treatments employed, given the continued sun exposure and subsequent sun damage.

TREATMENT

▪ Topical Therapy

- Topical sunscreen with UVB/UVA coverage
- Topical tretinoin applied nightly

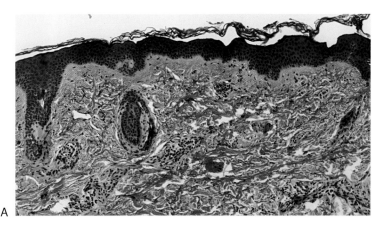

A

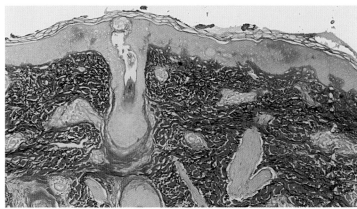

B

Figure 2.2 *Skin from the right cheek of a 65-year-old female.* **(A)** *H and E stain showing epidermis with normal pattern of rete ridges and no solar elastosis.* **(B)** *Elastic tissue stain showing fine elastic fibers in the dermis. Magnification: 100 × (photographs courtesy of Thomas Flotte, MD).*

- Topical α- or β-hydroxy acid applied daily
- Topical hydroquinone applied once or twice daily

Surgical Therapy

Combination therapy may be necessary to achieve the desired aesthetic effect.

- Volume loss/rhytides

  – Soft tissue augmentation: utilized in augmentation of static rhytides, for improvement of lipoatrophy, and as adjunctive treatment for dynamic rhytides.

  – Botulinum toxin: effective in improvement of dynamic rhytides and as adjunctive treatment for static rhytides.

  – Radiofrequency: utilized for skin tightening.

- Subcision: utilized to soften elevated bound-down scars.

- Photodamage

  – Nonablative resurfacing: utilized for fine lines, telangiectases, and dyspigmentation. Multiple treatments necessary with variable clinical efficacy.

  – Fraxel laser resurfacing: utilized for the reduction of fine lines and dyspigmentation. Applicable to patients with skin phototypes I–V.

  – Carbon dioxide (CO_2) laser resurfacing/erbium: utilized for the reduction of fine and deep rhytides, skin laxity, and scattered lentigines. Limited to individuals with skin phototypes I and II with limited associated dyspigmentation.

  – Dual-mode Er:YAG laser: utilized for the reduction of fine and deep rhytides, lentigines, and melasma. Treatment applicable for individuals with skin types I–III.

  – Chemical peels: utilized for reduction of dyspigmentation and static rhytides. Degree of clinical improvement dependent on the strength of the peel utilized.

  – Q-switched ruby and Q-switched Nd:YAG lasers: utilized for the reduction of lentigines. (Fig 2.3 A,B)

  – Dermabrasion: similar to CO_2 laser. Limited to individuals with skin phototypes I and II with limited associated dyspigmentation. The aerosolized particles produced during the procedure, the amount of procedural blood produced, and the existence of effective alternative treatments has reduced the use of this technique.

- Telangiectasia

  – Intense pulsed light: utilized for purpura-free treatment. Nonselective device. Most effective for fine telangiectasia. Multiple treatments generally required.

  – Pulsed dye laser: provides selective targeting of small and large facial vessels. Postoperative purpura lasting 12–14 days is undesirable for a majority of patients.

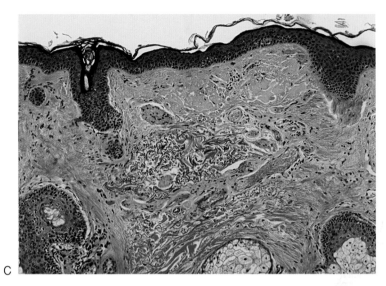

C

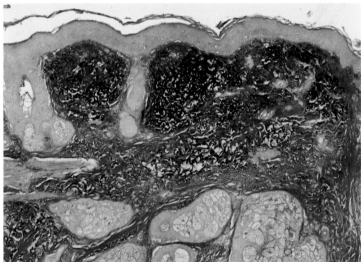

D

Figure 2.2 (*continued*) (C) *Skin from the right cheek of a 77-year-old male. H and E stain showing flattening of the rete ridges, solar elastosis in the superficial dermis, and prominent blood vessels.* **(D)** *Elastic tissue stain confirming the presence of nodular aggregates of elastotic material in the superficial dermis. Magnification: 100 × (photographs courtesy of Thomas Flotte, MD)*

– Photodynamic therapy: utilized for reduction of active keratoses, static rhytides and dyspigmentation (Fig 2.4 A, B).

– Electrocautery: can be employed to single lesions with efficacy. An increased risk of scar formation limits its application given the current alternate therapies.

PITFALLS TO AVOID

• Patients with extensive photodamage may require multiple treatments for the greatest treatment benefit. Addressing each patient's treatment goals and stressing possible treatment outcomes will result in patient satisfaction.

• Patients with extensive facial and truncal actinic damage may have significant dermarcation lines between treated and nontreated skin, which may appear more cosmetically bothersome to the patient than the actinic damage. Great care in patient and treatment selection will minimize this risk. Patients must be aware that some hypopigmentation may be observed when compared to untreated actinically damaged skin.

• Continued sun exposure after treatment may result in an expedient return of the dyspigmentation and actinic damage. Patients must be aware of this likelihood and the need for strict photoprotection.

BIBLIOGRAPHY

Alster TS. Cutaneous resurfacing with CO_2 and erbium:YAG lasers: preoperative, intraoperative and postoperative considerations. *Plast Reconstr Surg.* 1999;103: 619–634.

Alster T, Lupton J. Botulinum toxin type B for dynamic glabellar rhytides refractory to botulinum toxin type A. *Dermatol Surg.* 2003;29(5):516–518.

Anderson RR, Parrish JA. Selective photothermolysis: precise microsurgery by selective absorption of pulsed radiation. *Science.* 1983;220:524–527.

Blitzer A, Binder WJ, Aviv JE, et al. The management of hyperfunctional facial lines with botulinum toxin. A collaborative study of 210 injection sites in 162 patients. *Arch Otolaryngol Head Neck Surg.* 1997;123:389–392.

Brandt FS, Bellman B. Cosmetic use of botulinum A exotoxin for the aging neck. *Dermatol Surg.* 1998;24:1232–1234.

Brody HJ. Medium-depth chemical peeling of the skin: a variation of superficial chemosurgery. *Adv Dermatol.* 1988; 3:205–220.

Carruthers A, Carruthers J. Clinical indications and injection technique for the cosmetic use of botulinum A exotoxin. *Dermatol Surg.* 1998;2:1189–1194.

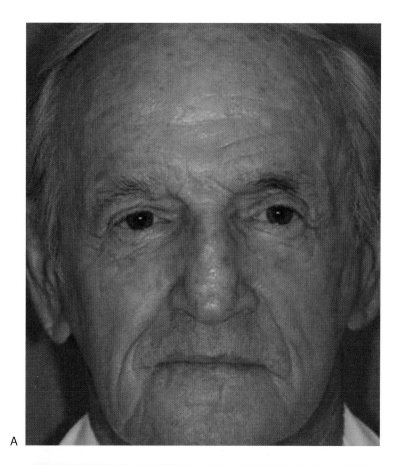

A

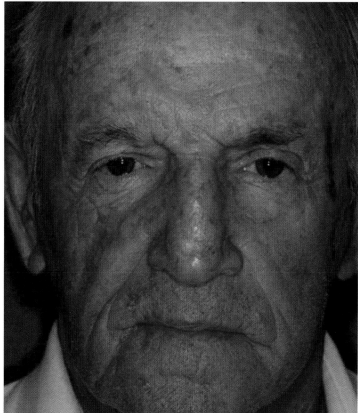

B

Figure 2.3 (A) *Lentigo pretreatment (note skin biopsy to confirm benign nature).* **(B)** *Lentigo immediately post-treatment*

Clark DP, Hanke CW, Swanson N. Dermal implants: safety of products injected for soft tissue augmentation. *J Am Acad Dermatol.* 1989;21:992–998.

Dover JS, Hruza GJ, Arndt KA. Lasers in skin resurfacing. *Semin Cutan Med Surg.* 1996;15:177–188.

Fitzpatrick R, Geronemus R, Goldberg D, et al. Multicenter study of noninvasive radiofrequency for periorbital tissue tightening. *Lasers Surg Med.* 2003;33:232–342.

Fitzpatrick RS, Goldman MP, Satur NM, Tope WD. Pulsed carbon dioxide laser resurfacing of photoaged facial skin. *Arch Dermatol.* 1996;132:395–402.

Fitzpatrick RE, Tope, WD, Goldman MP, et al. Pulsed carbon dioxide laser, trichloroacetic acid, Backer-Gordon phenol and dermabrasion: a comparative clinical and histologic study of cutaneous resurfacing in a porcine model. *Arch Dermatol.* 1996;132:469–471.

Klein AW. Indications and implantation techniques for the various formulations of injectable collagen. *J Dermatol Surg Oncol.* 1985;11:124.

Manstein D, Herron GS, Sink RK, Tanner H, Anderson RR. Fractional photothermolysis: a new concept for cutaneous remodeling using microscopic patterns of thermal injury. *Lasers Surg Med.* 2004;34(5):426–438.

Matarasso SL, Glogau RG. Chemical face peels. *Dermatol Clin.* 1991;9:131–150.

Monheit G. The Jessner's–trichloroacetic acid peel. *Dermatol Clin.* 1995;13(2):277–283.

Monheit GD. The Jessner's + TCA peel: a medium-depth chemical peel. *J Dematol Surg Oncol.* 1989;15:953–963.

Murad H, Shamban AT, Premo PS. The use of glycolic acid as a peeling agent. *Dermatol Clin.* 1995;13(2): 285–307.

Noninvasive rejuvenation of photodamaged skin using serial, full face intense pulsed light treatments. *Dermatol Surg.* 2000;26:835–842.

Orentreich D, et al. Subcutaneous incisionless (subcision) surgery for the correction of depressed scars and wrinkles. *Dermatol Surg.* 1995;21:543–549.

Schuller-Petrovic S. Improving the aesthetic aspect of soft tissue defects on the face using autologous fat transplantation. *Facial Plast Surg.* 1997;13(2):19–24.

Tannous ZS, Astner S. Utilizing fractional resurfacing in the treatment of therapy-resistant melasma. *J Cosmet Laser Ther.* 2005;7(1):39–43.

Treatment of essential telangiectasia with an intense pulsed light source (PhotoDerm VL) *Dermatol Surg.* October 1997; 23(10): 941–945.

Zimbler MS, Holds JB, Koloska MS, et al. Effect of botulinum toxin pretreatment on laser resurfacing results: a prospective, randomized, blinded trial. *Arch Facial Plast Surg.* 2001;3:165–169.

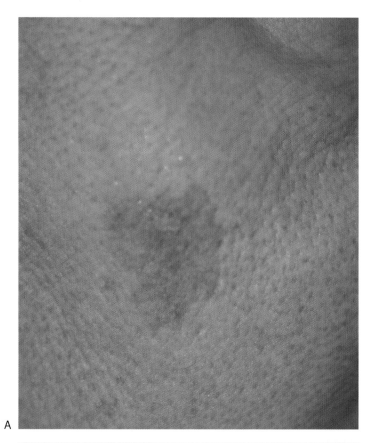

A

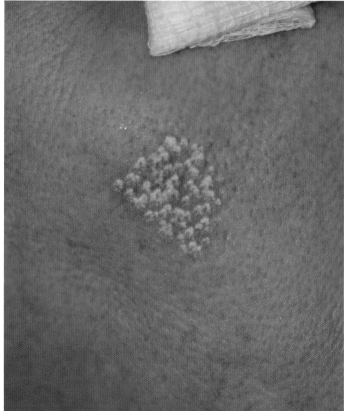

B

Figure 2.4 (A) *Chronic sun damage with diffuse wrinkles and dyspigmentation* **(B)** *Two days after photodynamic therapy treatment with typical aminolevulinic acid and pulsed dye laser. The swelling, redness, and crusting resolved within one week.*

CHAPTER 3 Dermatoheliosis, Soft Tissue Augmentation Options

MECHANISM OF ACTION

Use of a synthetic or biological product or surgical restructuring for the replacement of volume loss and enhancement of dermal, subcutaneous, and muscular deficiencies that result from trauma, surgical defects, lipoatrophic conditions, photoaging or chronological aging.

TABLE 3.1 ▪ Commonly Used Filling Agents

Name	Composition	FDA approval	Skin testing required	Longevity
Alloderm (Life Cell Corp., Branchburg, NJ; Obaji Medical, Chicago, IL)	Acellular processed human cadaveric dermal allograft	Yes	No	1–2 years
Artecoll (Canderm Pharma, Inc., Quebec, Canada; Medical International BV, Breda, The Netherlands)	Bovine collagen with poly(methyl methacrylate) beads	No	Yes	Permanent
Captique™ (Inamed Corp, Santa Monica, CA)	Non-animal-stabilized hyaluronic acid (NASHA) derived from plant	Yes	No	4–6 months
Cosmoderm™, Cosmoplast™ (Advanced Tissue Sciences, San Diego, CA; Inamed Corp., Santa Barbara, CA)	Recombinant human collagen	Yes	No	4–6 months
Cymetra Life Cell Corp., Branchburg, NJ; Obaji Medical, Chicago, IL	Acellular processed lyophilized human cadaveric tissue		No	4–6 months
Fascian (Fascia Biomaterials, Beverly Hills, CA)	Human cadaveric preserved particulate fascia lata		No	3–4 months
Fat, subcutaneous	Autologous	N/A	No	9–12 months
Hylaform® (Biomatrix Inc., Ridgefield, NJ; Inamed Corp., Santa Monica, CA)	Hyaluronic acid derived from domestic fowl coxcombs	Yes	No	4–6 months
Isolagen (Isolagen Inc., Houston, TX)	Autologous fibroblasts	Yes	No	1–2 years
Juvederm™ (Allergan, Inc., Irvine, CA)	Non-animal stabilized hyaluronic acid (NASHA) derived from bacterial fermentation	Yes	No	6–9 months
Restylane™ (Q-Med AB, Sweden; Medicis, Phoenix, AZ)	Non-animal-stabilized hyaluronic acid (NASHA) derived from bacterial fermentation	Yes	No	6–9 months
Silikone-1000, Adatosil-5000 (Dow-Corning, Midland, MI)	Silicone	No	No	Permanent
Softform (McGhan Medical, Santa Barbara, CA)	Goretex	N/A	No	Permanent
Sculptra™ (Biotech Industry, SA, Luxembourg; Dermik, Berwyn, PA)	Lyophilized poly-L-lactic acid	Yes	No	1–2 years
Zyderm®, Zyplast® (Inamed Corp., Santa Barbara, CA)	Bovine collagen	Yes	Yes	3–4 months

IDEAL FILLER (Table 3.1)

- Biocompatible
- Nonimmunogenic
- Noncarcinogenic, nonteratogenic
- Nonresorbable
- Nonmigratory
- Inexpensive
- Easily obtained and stored
- Easy to administer
- Provides reproducible cosmetically beneficial results
- FDA approved if not autologous
- Demonstrates multipurpose use
- No side effects

PREOPERATIVE EVALUATION

- Identify the appropriate patient and treatment region
  - Significant past medical history including history of bleeding or clotting disorders; keloid formation; existing drug allergies; immunocompromised state
  - Current medication use; past or current Isotretinoin use
  - Past surgical interventions, year and treatment response
  - Clinical evaluation to determine if the desired treatment areas are amenable to correction; outline baseline structural irregularities
  - Discuss medications to avoid 10 days preoperatively when medically safe including aspirin, nonsteroidal medications, Vitamin E supplements, St. John's Wort and other herbal medications that have an anticoagulative effect
- Discuss the risks and benefits of the treatment
  - Allergic reaction, localized versus systemic
  - Procedural and postoperative discomfort
  - Postoperative edema
  - Postoperative bruising
  - Scar formation
  - Infection
  - Incomplete augmentation
  - Irregular contour/texture
- Identify contraindications to treatment
  - Active infection at the treatment site
  - Nondistensible, rigid, or icepick scars
  - Extensive jowl formation, prominent folds, and furrows
  - Underlying connective tissue disorder
  - Immunologic disease
  - Prior allergic reaction to filler/related filler/positive skin test

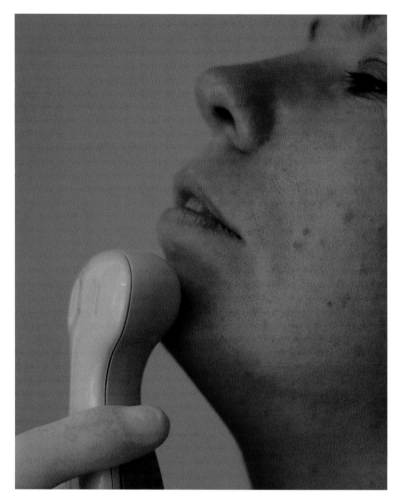

Figure 3.1 *Massager utilized during filler placement to minimize treatment discomfort*

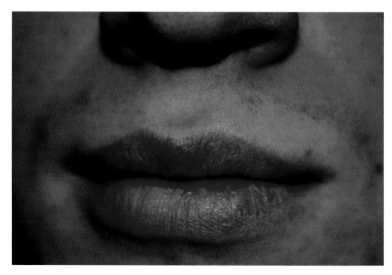

Figure 3.2 *Clinical findings after EMLA application to skin. Expected blanching lasts approximately 2-3 hours after application*

- Use of Isotretinoin within the preceding 6–12 months
- Pregnancy
- Unrealistic expectations
- Outline the predicted outcome and limitations to the treatment
  - Duration of correction
  - Postoperative recovery period
  - Tissue source
  - Expense

SKIN TESTING (WHEN APPLICABLE)

- Initial test dose—two skin tests recommended
  - Injected in tuberculin manner into volar forearm
  - Four-week observation period for first test
  - Repeat skin test placed in opposite forearm
  - Two-week observation period for second test
- Retest dose—single test recommended
  - For new patients who have received treatment by another physician or patients who have not received treatment for more than 1 year
  - Two-week observation period recommended
- Positive filler reaction
  - Swelling, induration, tenderness, or erythema that persists or occurs 6 h or longer after test implantation
  - A positive skin test is an absolute contraindication to filler use

ANESTHESIA

- "Talkesthesia," hand-holding, vibratory massager near the treatment site are useful for patient distraction (Fig. 3.1)
- Topical anesthesia can be utilized for small treatment areas. Commonly used agents include Betacaine Enhanced Gel" (Canderm, Quebec, Canada), Betacaine Plus" (Canderm, Quebec, Canada), L-M-X-4 and 5 (Ferndale Labs, Ferndale, MI), EMLA" (AstraZeneca, Boston, MA), and ice (Figure 3.2)
- Regional nerve blocks are easily administered prior to treatment
- Localized tumescent anesthesia is utilized for fat extraction with autologous fat transfer
- Infiltrative anesthesia is to be avoided to obviate tissue distortion of the treatment site

PROCEDURAL MEDICATIONS

- Valtrex 500 mg BID × 7 days initiated 1 day prior to the procedure for patients with a history of herpes simplex virus in or near the treatment site

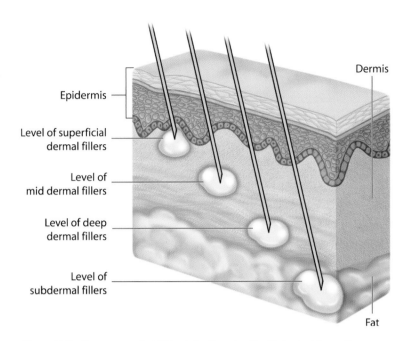

Figure 3.3 *Recommended filler injection depths (Adapted from Keyvan N, Susana L-K, eds. Techniques in Dermatologic Surgery. United Kingdom: Mosby; 2003)*

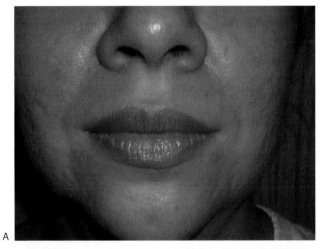

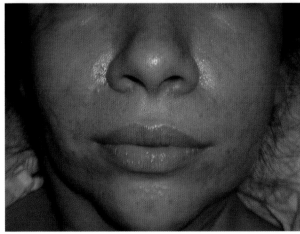

Figure 3.4 (A) *Prominent nasolabial folds and melolabial folds prior to autologous fat transfer.* **(B)** *Softening of folds after autologous fat transfer, total 20 cc placed into treatment sites*

• Keflex 500 mg BID × 7 days initiated 1 day prior to the procedure for patients undergoing autologous fat transfer or Goretex implantation

• Diazepam 5–10 mg can be offered to anxious patients 30 min prior to the procedure

LEVEL OF INJECTION (Fig. 3.3)

• Superficial dermis: fine lines; vermilion border lip augmentation

Zyderm I, II; Cosmoderm I, II; Restylane Fine Line; Hylaform Fine Line

• Mid to deep dermis: superficial to moderate rhytides, scars, and defects; lip augmentation

Zyderm II, Zyplast; Cosmoderm II, Cosmoplast; Restylane; Hylaform; Juvederm; Captique

• Deep dermis, subcutaneous fat, and muscle: deeper, more substantial defects and rhytides (Figure 3.4)

Perlane; Hylaform Plus; Sculptra; Autologous Fat Transfer; Goretex, Juvederm

• Combination dermal, subcutaneous, and muscle: defects with both a superficial and a deep component utilize both a superficial and deep fixer for optimal augmentation (Figure 3.5)

INJECTION TECHNIQUE (Fig. 3.8)

• Serial puncture: closely spaced punctures created along lines, folds (Fig. 3.6)

• Linear threading: withdrawal of filler along the length of the facial defect as a continuous thread of material (Fig. 3.7)

• Fanning: similar to linear threading. Needle direction is continually changed without withdrawing the needle tip. Useful for oral commissures, upper nasolabial folds

• Cross-hatching: similar to linear threading. Material is injected at right angles to the first injections. Use for shaping facial contours

DEGREE OF CORRECTION

Dependent on the filler used. In general, overcorrection is not recommended. The most common technique error is undercorrection.

DURATION OF CORRECTION

Dependent on the material implanted, implantation technique, and amount implanted, the type of defect and mechanical stresses at the implantation sites.

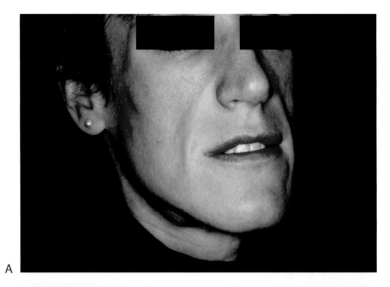

A

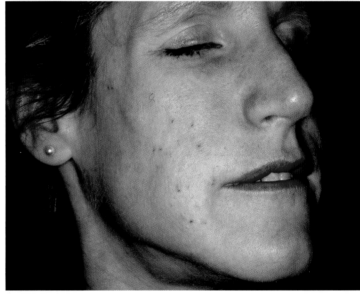

B

Figure 3.5 (A) *Facial lipoatrophy with "sunken cheek appearance" prior to Cymetra treatment.* **(B)** *Improvement of cheek volume after Cymetra treatment, 2.0 cc total volume*

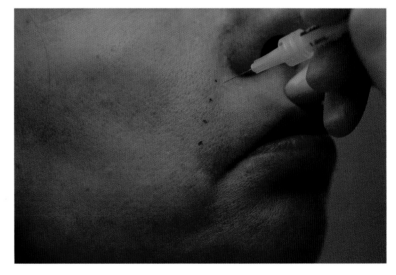

Figure 3.6 *Serial puncture method of injection*

ADVERSE REACTIONS

Hypersensitive

- Prolonged erythema and edema at injection sites
- Cyst/abscess formation—long-lasting; can persist for more than 2–3 years
- Granuloma formation
- Anaphylaxis

Nonhypersensitive

- Bruising
- Infection—includes reactivation of herpes simplex virus and bacterial infection
- Necrosis—due to vascular compromise at the treatment site
- Partial vision loss—due to vascular compromise at the treatment site
- Ulceration

Technique Complications

- Irregular texture—due to uneven placement
- Beading—due to too superficial placement (Figs. 3.9)
- Implant rejection—due to too superficial placement

PEARLS FOR TREATMENT SUCCESS

- With fillers, the affected treatment sites should be fully augmented to ensure an even, complete augmentation. Undercorrection will lead to an inadequate augmentation and patient dissatisfaction. With temporary fillers, this is obtained at the first treatment. Permanent fillers require repeat treatments for correction completion.

- With temporary fillers, patients must understand that the treatment response is variable and can last less than or greater than the average expected time. Repeat treatment will be required over time.

- Patient expectations must be tempered to minimize unrealistic expectations about filler benefits. Patients must be aware that the treatment endpoint is a softening of the affected areas.

- Postoperative beading is generally responsive to localized massage over 5–7 days. Persistent beading can be corrected by injecting 2 mg/mL of triamcinalone acetonide into the bead or by 11-blade incisional extraction of the filler material.

- A thorough preoperative evaluation is necessary to ensure there are no contraindications to filler use, especially when using permanent fillers.

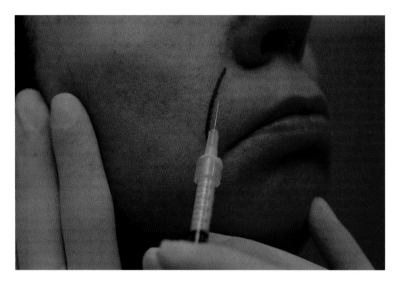

Figure 3.7 *Linear threading method of injection*

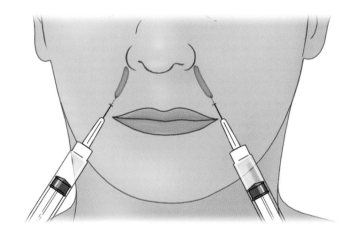

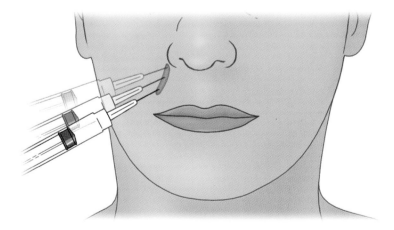

Figure 3.8 *Injection techniques A. Linear threading technique B. Serial puncture technique. (Adapted from Keyvan N, Susana L-K, eds. Techniques in Dermatologic Surgery. United Kingdom: Mosby; 2003)*

BIBLIOGRAPHY

Clark DP, Hanke CW, Swanson N. Dermal implants: safety of products injected for soft tissue augmentation. *J Am Acad Dermatol*. 1989;21:992–998.

Coleman SR. Facial recontouring with liposculpture. *Clin Plast Surg*. 1997;24(2): 347–367.

Jones RJ, Schwartz BM, Silverstein P. Use of a nonimmunogenic acellular dermal allograft for soft tissue augmentation: a preliminary report. *Aesthet Surg Q*. 1996;16:196–201.

Klein AW. Indications and implantation techniques for the various formulations of injectable collagen. *J Dermatol Surg Oncol*. 1985;11:124.

Schuller-Petrovic S. Improving the aesthetic aspect of soft tissue defects on the face using autologous fat transplantation. *Facial Plast Surg*. 1997;13(2):19–24.

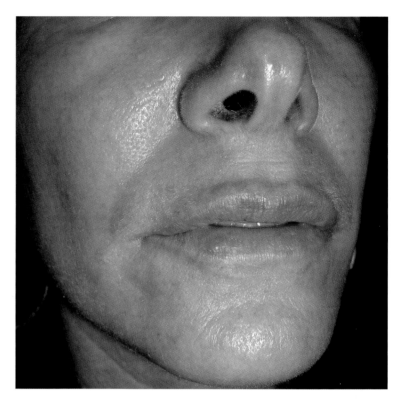

Figure 3.9 *Filler beading due to too superficial placement*

CHAPTER 4   Dermatoheliosis, Botulinum Toxin Options

PHARMACOLOGY

Toxin produced by the bacterium *Clostridium botulinum*. Seven serotypes exist, designated A, B, C, D, E, F, and G. Each is a protease with a light chain linked to a heavy chain by a disulfide bond.

Each is antigenically distinct. Botulinum toxin A (BTX-A), B (BTX-B) and F are the only serotypes currently available for clinical use (Table 4.1).

TABLE 4.1 ■ Botulinum Toxin Preparations

Type	Units toxin/bottle	Dosing equivalents	Dilution
Botox (Allergan Inc., Irvine, CA)—type A	100 U lyophilized powder	1 U Botox = 4 U Dysport	Average 1–4 mL in preservative-free or preserved saline
Dysport (Ipsen Limited, Berkshire, UK)—type A	500 U lyophilized powder	1 U Botox = 4 U Dysport	Average 2.5 mL in preservative-free or preserved saline
Myobloc (Elan Pharmaceuticals, San Francisco, CA)—type B	5000 U/mL aqueous solution	Not well established for cosmetic use	May be used as is or dilute with normal saline

MECHANISM OF ACTION

Inhibition of acetylcholine release at the neuromuscular junction resulting in muscular flaccid paralysis. Receptor site binding is mediated by the heavy chain portion of the toxin, is specific for the toxin serotype, and is irreversible. Once bound, the receptor–neurotoxin complex is internalized into the nerve terminal and the toxin light chain acts as a protease to cleave specific synaptic protein peptide bonds required for acetylcholine formation. The target of BTX-A is the synaptasome-associated protein of 25 kDa, SNAP-25. BTX-B and BTX-E cleave the vesicle-associated membrane protein, synaptobrevin.

DILUTION

BTX-A is stored in lyophilized vials. It can be reconstituted in preserved saline or preservative-free saline. Dilutions vary according to physician preference and experience with BTX. A dilution ranges from 1 mL (10 U/0.1 cc) to 4 mL (2.5 U/0.1 cc) on an average. Dysport diluted to 2.5 mL will attain a concentration of 20 U/0.1 cc. The injected volume must be sufficiently small to provide accurate toxin delivery without an excessive volume effect or delivery of toxin to surrounding muscles other than the targeted muscles. The volume must be sufficiently large to permit accurate injection into the targeted muscles.

CONTRAINDICATIONS

◼ Absolute

• Underlying neuromuscular condition
• Pregnancy/breast-feeding—pregnancy category C
• Unrealistic patient expectations

◼ Relative

• Calcium channel blockers use—may potentiate effect
• Aminoglycoside antibiotic use—may potentiate effect
• Patients who are dependent on facial expression for their livelihood (e.g., actors)
• Prominent eyelid ptosis or ectropion

PREOPERATIVE EVALUATION

• Patient expectations must be defined and matched with the expected treatment outcomes
• Patient medical history
• Past treatment history and outcome
• Clinical evaluation
• Determine location and extent of involvement of the treatment site
• Document asymmetries noted; present of ptosis/lid laxity

◼ Lower Eyelid "Snap Back" Test To Assess Lower Lid Laxity

The middle of the lower lid is grasped between the index finger and the thumb and pulsed forward and upward. The lid is then released and allowed to "snap" back against the globe. A quick return to its normal state indicates minimal laxity. Botox to this given can provide benefit. A slow U2 return indicates significant laxity. Botox should not be used in these patients, as it may accentnate the lines present

PROCEDURE

• Patient consent obtained
• Preoperative pictures taken, at rest and with targeted muscle groups contracted
• Patient placed upright
• Treatment areas wiped with alcohol
• Injections administered

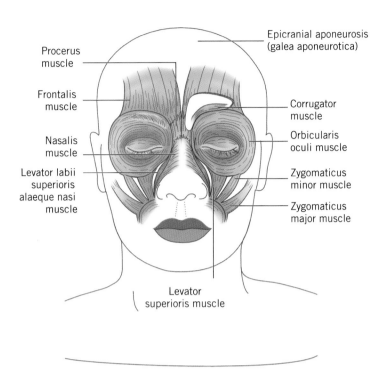

Figure 4.1 *Anatomical illustration of the upper and midfacial musculature*

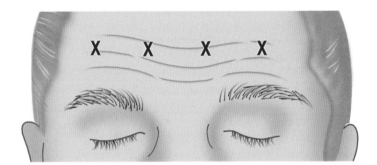

Figure 4.2 *Approximate injection sites for the forehead*

MUSCLE GROUPS

A thorough knowledge of the facial musculature and facial anatomy is required for the proper use and placement of botulinum toxin (Fig. 4.1).

■ Forehead—Frontalis Muscle (Figs. 4.2-4.3)

Insertion: Originates at frontal bone galea aponeurotica and inserts into fibers of the procerus, corrugator, and orbicularis oculi

Function: Opposes depressor muscles of the glabellar complex and brows to elevate the brow and forehead

Lines noted: Horizontal lines across the forehead

Injection technique: 2–3 units (U) added at 1.5-cm intervals across the mid-forehead, a minimum of 2 cm above the upper brow

Dose injected: Average 17.5–20 U

Avoid:

* Excess treatment of this muscle; unopposed depressor function will result in loss of upper facial expression, a "tired" appearance, brow ptosis, and risk of eyebrow ptosis

* Treatment of this muscle if the frontalis is supporting a ptotic upper eyelid

* Injection too close to the medial orbital rim; toxin diffusion through the orbital septum to the levator palpebrae superioris and orbicularis muscles may lead to diplopia

■ Glabellar Complex—The Corrugator Supercilii, the Procerus, Medial Orbicularis Oculi, and Frontalis Muscles (Figs. 4.4-4.5)

Insertion: Originates at the nasal process of the frontal bone and extends laterally and upward to insert into the middle third of the eyebrow

Function: Opposes elevator muscles of the frontalis for brow adduction and brow/skin downward and medial movement

Lines noted: Frown lines; "angry" or "worried" appearance

Injection technique: Females have arched eyebrows; males have flatter or horizontal eyebrows; technique tailored to match the brow shape. 5–10 U into the procerus; 4–6 U in the inferior and superior bellies of the corrugators; 2–3 U into the medial orbicularis oculi

Dose injected: 22–40 U (dependent on muscle mass)

Avoid:

* Undertreatment of this region

* Concurrent treatment of the forehead if a heavy brow is noted

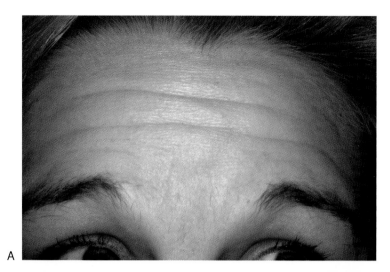

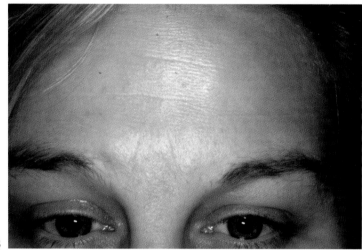

Figure 4.3 (A) *Forehead lines prior to BTX-A treatment.* **(B)** *Forehead lines 1 month following BTX-A treatment*

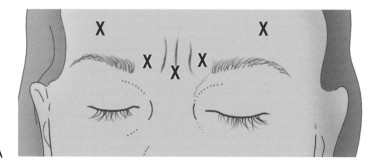

Figure 4.4 *Approximate injection sites for the glabellar frown lines.* **(A)** *Female brow.*

■ Periorbital Region—Orbicularis Oculi (Figs. 4.6-4.7)

Insertion: Encircles the periorbital region and inserts into the medial and lateral canthal tendons as well as into the fibers of the frontal, procerus, and corrugator supercilii muscles

Function: Forceful closure of the eyes and depression of the brows and eyelids

Lines noted: Lateral canthal lines; "crows feet"

Injection technique: 3–5 U are injected into three points in a vertical line 1 cm from the lateral canthus; if a strong snap test is noted, 2–4 U can be placed 3 cm below the midpupillary line

Dose injected: 22–38 U

Avoid:

- Injection of the infraorbital region if a delayed snap test is noted; ectropion of the injected eye may develop

- Overtreatment of this area; improper eye closure, brow ptosis, or lid ptosis may ensue

- An injection aimed too low at the lower periorbital wrinkles. Weakening of the levator labii superioris muscles with an upper lip droop and abnormal smile may be observed

■ Upper Nasal Root (Fig. 4.8)

Insertion: Encircles the periorbital region and inserts into the medial and lateral canthal tendons as well as into the fibers of the frontal, procerus, and corrugator supercilii muscles

Function: Nasal wrinkling

Lines noted: Upper nose fanning rhytides; "bunny lines"

Injection technique: 2–4 U is injected into each lateral nasal wall into the belly of the upper nasalis as it traverses the dorsum of the nose

Dose injected: 4–8 U

Avoid: Injection into the upper nasofacial groove may result in lip ptosis

Use of botulinum toxin in the lower face is minimally beneficial. Other treatment modalities are likely to be more beneficial with fewer potential side effects. A strong understanding of the lower face and neck anatomy is critical for injection placement. (Fig. 4.9)

■ Nasolabial Fold (Fig. 4.10)

It is key to weigh the limited benefit of BTX-A in this region compared to the increased risk of complications. Filling agents may provide greater benefit with fewer side effects.

Insertion: Result of skin laxity, gravitational ptosis, and subcutaneous fat loss overlying the cutaneous attachment

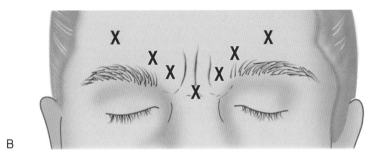

B

Figure 4.4 (*continued*) (B) *Male brow*

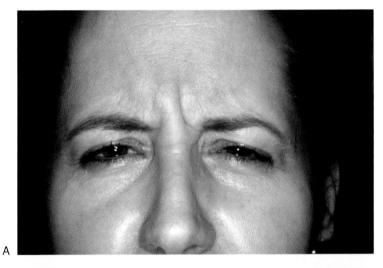

A

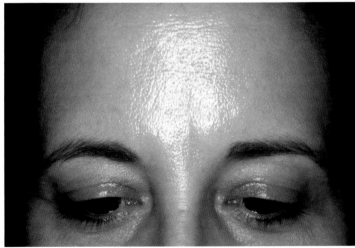

B

Figure 4.5 (A) *Glabellar complex before BTX-A injection and* **(B)** *3 weeks following BTX-A injection*

in the zygomaticus major and minor, levator labii superioris, and levator labii superioris alaeque nasi muscles

Function: Associated with mouth and lip movement

Lines noted: Prominent crease, medial cheek

Injection technique: 1–2 U injected into the upper aspect of the nasolabial fold 2–3 mm lateral to its insertion with the nose

Dose injected: 2–4 U

Avoid:

• Complete relaxation of this area; upper lip ptosis creating a sad appearance may occur

• Uneven paralysis; an asymmetric smile or disproportionate lip may be seen

▣ Perioral Region—Orbicularis Oris with Contributing Fibers from the Buccinator, Caninus, and Triangularis Muscles; Depressor Anguli Oris (DAO); Mentalis Muscle (Figs. 4.11-4.13)

Insertion: Orbicularis oris originates from the maxillary alveolar border running circumferentially around the mouth to the overlying cutaneous attachments; DAO arises from the mandibular oblique line, inserting into the angle of the mouth. It is continuous with the platysma muscle; mentalis muscle originates from the mandibular incisive fossa and descends to a cutaneous insertion

Function: Opposition and protrusion of the lips; mouth angle depression; lower lip protrusion and chin dimpling

Lines noted: Deep and superficial rhytides, upper and lower lip; prominent angular folds, "sad appearance"; chin wrinkling

Injection technique: 0.5–1.0 U injected 2–3 mm above the vermilion border in four areas each for the upper and lower lip; 1–2 U injected at the intersection of a line drawn from the nasolabial fold and an area 1 cm above the jawline angle; 5–10 U into the inferior midchin

Dose injected: 4–8 U for the upper and lower lips; 2–4 U for the DAO; 5–10 U for the mentalis muscle

Avoid:

• Overtreatment of this area; speech difficulties, an asymmetric smile, inability to close the mouth, and altered facial expressions may ensue

• Deep injections; increased risk of side effects

• Too high of an injection for the DAO; inability to raise the corner of the mouth may develop

▣ Neck—Platysma Muscle Complex (Fig. 4.14)

Insertion: Originates on the fascia of the upper pectoralis major and deltoid muscles and proceeds upward and

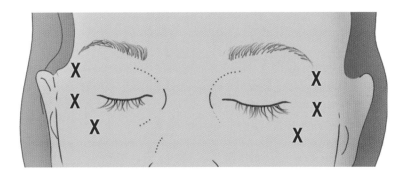

Figure 4.6 *Approximate injection sites for periorbital lines*

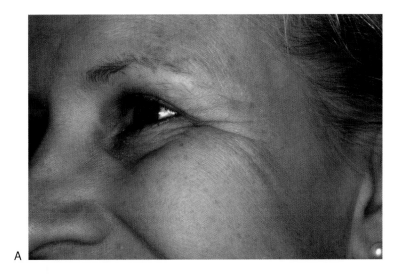

A

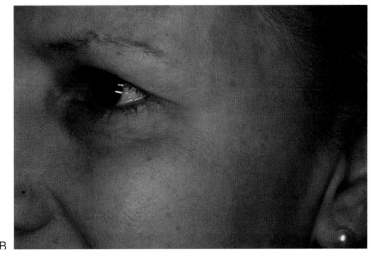

B

Figure 4.7 (A) *Periorbital lines prior to treatment with BTX-A.* **(B)** *Periorbital lines 6 weeks following BTX-A treatment*

medially along the sides of the neck. Fibers are inserted into the mandible, subcutaneous tissue of the lower face, perioral muscle, and skin

Function: Facial animation; lower jaw depression; lower lip depression

Lines noted: Neck wrinkling; central bands

Injection technique: 2–5 U injected from the superior to inferior portion of each platysmal band at 1–1.5 cm intervals with the patient's teeth clenched to contract the muscle during injection

Dose injected: 20–100 U

Avoid: Too deep an injection; neck weakness, laryngeal muscle weakness, or dysphagia may develop

COMPLICATIONS

- Eyelid ptosis
- Eyebrow ptosis
- Bruising
- Headache
- Incomplete or asymmetric chemical denervation
- Antibody resistance

TREATMENT BENEFITS

Recovery from BTX-A paralysis generally begins at 3–4 months after injection. Patients who routinely receive BTX-A may note the recovery time to extend to 4–6 months over time. Side effects including eyelid and eyebrow ptosis and bruising generally resolve within 2–3 weeks of onset.

PEARLS FOR TREATMENT SUCCESS

- Patients with known neutralizing antibodies against Botox-A may respond to Myobloc given the lack of significant cross-reactivity between the two toxins.
- Patients should be informed that the maximum benefit of Botox can take up to 4 weeks to develop.
- Deep furrows will only partially respond to botulinum treatment. Combination therapy with a filler substance may provide the best clinical endpoint.
- It should be emphasized to patients that a single botulinum treatment might not be completely effective in eliminating all lines and wrinkles. As well, it should be explained that complete muscular paralysis may not provide the greatest clinical improvement and that some residual muscular movement is the treatment endpoint.

BIBLIOGRAPHY

Alster T, Lupton, J. Botulinum toxin type B for dynamic glabellar rhytides refractory to botulinum toxin type A. *Dermatol Surg*. 2003;29(5):516–518.

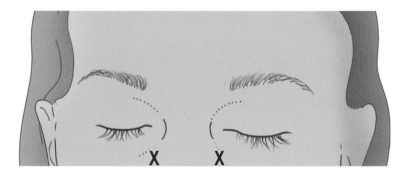

Figure 4.8 *Approximate injection sites for upper nasal root rhytides*

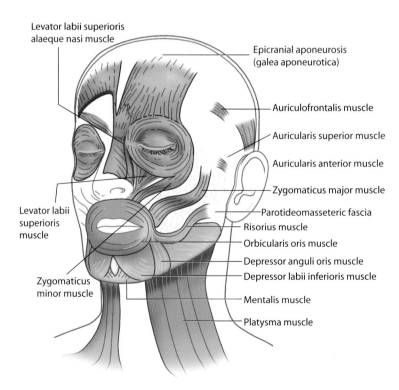

Figure 4.9 *Anatomical illustration of the musculature of the lower face and neck*

Blitzer A, Binder WJ, Aviv JE, et al. The management of hyperfunctional facial lines with botulinum toxin. A collaborative study of 210 injection sites in 162 patients. *Arch Otolaryngol Head Neck Surg.* 1997;123:389–392.

Blitzer A, Sulica L. Botulinum toxin: basic science and clinical uses in otolaryngology. *Laryngoscope.* 2001;111: 218–226,.

Brandt FS, Bellman B. Cosmetic use of botulinum A exotoxin for the aging neck. *Dermatol Surg.* 1998;24:1232–1234.

Carruthers A, Carruthers J. Clinical indications and injection techniques for the cosmetic use of botulinum A exotoxin. *Dermatol Surg.* 1998;24:1172–1174.

Carruthers A, Carruthers J. Clinical indications and injection technique for the cosmetic use of botulinum A exotoxin. *Dermatol Surg.* 1998;2:1189–1194.

Carruthers J, Carruthers A, Zelichowska A. The power of combined therapies: Botox and ablative laser resurfacing. *Am J Cosmetic Surg.* 2000;17:129–131.

Carruthers A, Kiene K, Carruthers J. Botulinum A exotoxin use in clinical dermatology. *J Am Acad Dermatol.* 1996;34:788–797.

LeLouarn C. Botulinum toxin A and facial lines: the variable concentration. *Aesth Plast Surg.* 2001;25:73–84.

Shaari C, Sanders I. Quantifying how location and dose of botulinum toxin injections affect muscle paralysis. *Muscle Nerve.* 1993;16:964-969.

Zimbler MS, Holds JB, Koloska MS, et al. Effect of botulinum toxin pretreatment on laser resurfacing results: a prospective, randomized, blinded trial. *Arch Facial Plast Surg.* 2001;3:165–169.

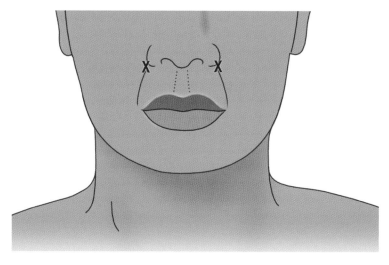

Figure 4.10 *Approximate injection sites for nasolabial folds*

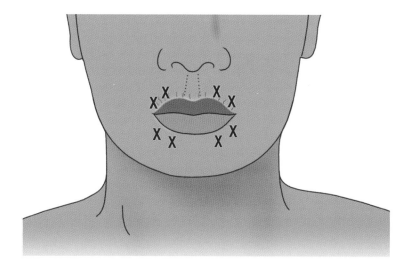

Figure 4.11 *Approximate injection sites for the perioral muscles*

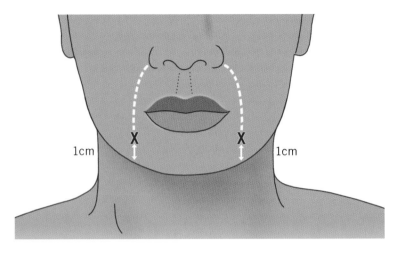

Figure 4.12 *Approximate injection sites for the depressor anguli oris muscle*

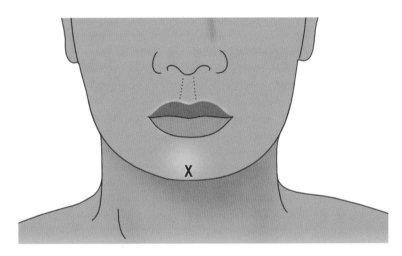

Figure 4.13 *Approximate injection site for the mentalis muscle*

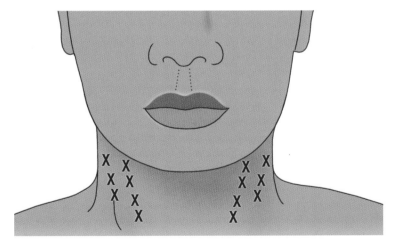

Figure 4.14 *Approximate injection sites for the platysma muscle complex*

CHAPTER 5 | Dermatoheliosis, Resurfacing Options

NONABLATIVE LASER RESURFACING

▦ Indications

To improve fine lines, reduce facial mottling and telangiectases, and improve skin texture. Ideal for patients who desire no "downtime" and cannot tolerate or do not desire ablative resurfacing.

▦ Mechanism of Action

Dermal wound created without epidermal damage. Resultant remodeling with increased collagen type I deposition and reorganization of collagen fibrils.

▦ Consultation

Patient motivations and expectations are key when utilizing a nonablative device (Table 5.1). The patient must be made aware of the variable benefits that will be achieved after multiple treatments.

TABLE 5.1 ▪ Commonly Utilized Nonablative Resurfacing Devices

Device	Wavelength	Cooling	Chromophore
V-Beam (Candela Corp., Wayland, MA)	595 nm pulsed dye laser	Dynamic cooling device	Hemoglobin
N-lite (ICN Pharmaceuticals, Costa Mesa, CA)	585 nm pulsed dye laser	None—ice may be applied	Hemoglobin
Softlight (Thermolase, London, UK)	1064 nm Nd:YAG laser	None	Water
Cooltouch (ICN Pharmaceuticals, Costa Mesa, CA)	1320 nm Nd:YAG laser	Dynamic cooling device	Water
Smoothbeam (Candela Corp, Wayland, MA)	1450 nm diode laser	Dynamic cooling device	Water
Aramis-Quantel (Quantel Medical, Clermont-Ferrand, France)	1540 nm Er:Glass laser	Cryo-sapphire-tipped handpiece	Water

▦ Contraindications

• Patients currently on or having taken isotretinoin in the past 6 months
• Patients with unrealistic expectations
• Pregnant women

▦ Treatment

• Preoperative written consent and pictures obtained
• Topical anesthetic applied 30–60 min prior to treatment
• Appropriate laser safety goggles for patient and staff utilized
• Treatment administered—parameters dependent on patient skin phototype and device utilized

- Postoperative lotion and ice applied

- Serial treatments employed every 2–3 weeks

▇ Postoperative Care

- No postoperative dressing necessary

- Makeup may be applied immediately after treatment

- Strict sun avoidance should be followed for a minimum of 4 weeks after treatment to minimize the risk of dyspigmentation

▇ Side Effects

Temporary erythema and edema lasting a few hours noted (Fig. 5.1). Purpura may be observed. Risk of temporary and permanent hyperpigmentation or hypopigmentation; scar formation; minimal to no benefit noted.

▇ Key Points for Treatment Success

- Careful patient selection is paramount. A realistic treatment endpoint must be clearly defined. If the patient has expectations greater than that the device can provide, patient dissatisfaction will be likely

- Multiple treatments are necessary to obtain the greatest benefit. These treatments are spaced 2–4 weeks apart

FRACTIONAL RESURFACING

▇ Mechanism of Action

Fractional resurfacing (FR) is a new concept of skin rejuvenation that can target both epidermal and dermal conditions. The light source for the FR laser system is an erbium-doped fiber laser at 1550 nm. FR produces a unique thermal damage pattern consisting of multiple columns of thermal damage, referred to as microthermal treatment zones (MTZs) (Fig. 5.2). FR characteristically spares the tissue surrounding each MTZ, thus allowing fast epidermal repair due to microscopic size of the wounds and short migratory distance for keratinocytes. The histology of an MTZ reveals homogenized columns of dermal matrix and the formation of microscopic epidermal necrotic debris (MEND) (Fig. 5.3). The process of MEND formation is thought to represent the elimination of the thermally damaged epidermis containing pigment.

FR can be helpful in the treatment of epidermal pigmentation such as melasma and lentigines due to the process of MEND formation. FR can also be helpful in improving rhytides and scarring due to the process of collagen remodeling and new collagen formation, induced by the dermal thermal damage.

▇ Indications

FR has been FDA approved for the treatment of periorbital fine rhytides and melasma. It has been employed in the treatment of melasma, lentigines, dyschromia, fine to

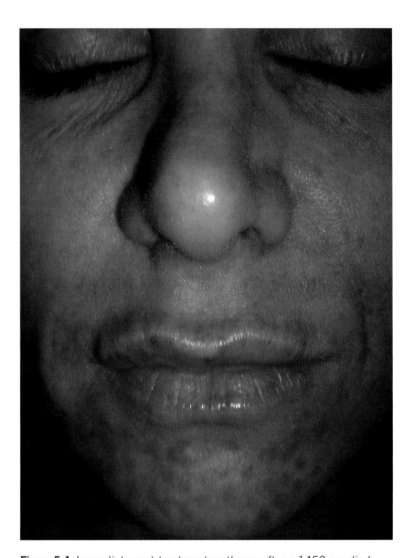

Figure 5.1 *Immediate post-treatment erythema after a 1450 nm diode laser treatment for chin acne scarring. This erythema generally lasts 2–3 h. This patient also underwent Restylane treatment for upper and lower lip rhytides with immediate swelling noted*

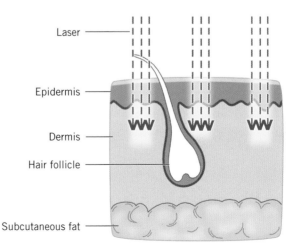

Figure 5.2 *Schematic of microscopic treatment zones (MTZ) created by Fraxel laser (note the characteristic sparing of the surrounding tissue between the treatment zones)*

moderate rhytides, striae, hypertrophic scars, boxcar acne scars, and atrophic scars with noted improvement.

■ Preoperative Evaluation

- Significant past medical history includes history of herpes labialis, keloid or hypertrophic scar formation, oral tretinoin intake (date last course completed), topical retinoid use, tobacco use, and known drug allergies including lidocaine allergy

- Significant past surgical history includes prior surgical treatments to the treatment sites, the dates of the procedures, the patient's response, and the associated side effects

- The patient should be aware of the following:
  - Procedural discomfort
  - Sunburn-like sensation for approximately 1 h after the procedure
  - Sunburn-like postoperative erythema that may persist for 3–7 days
  - Postoperative edema, generally mild, that usually resolves within 2–3 days
  - Postoperative bronzing that is generally noted on the third postoperative day and often persists for 3–4 days
  - Postoperative superficial peeling that is often mild and is noted to start on the third postoperative day and to persist for 3–4 days
  - Realistic expectations for the procedure: The patient should be aware that the treatment will improve fine to moderate wrinkles, pigmentation, and superficial scars but does not eliminate moderate to deep rhytides. A modest benefit may be noted for deeper wrinkles and scars
  - Procedural risks: Although these adverse events are uncommon and are much less frequent than those associated with ablative resurfacing, they still exist. They include laser nicks (Fig. 5.4), temporary or permanent hyperpigmentation (Fig. 5.5), hypo or depigmentation, herpes simplex reactivation, infection, delayed healing, and scarring. This is in addition to the predictable side effects that include procedural discomfort, postoperative erythema, bronzing, and edema. Unlike ablative resurfacing, there is usually no associated oozing or crusting unless very high energies and/or high densities are utilized

- The ideal candidate is a fair skin patient (Fitzpatrick phototypes I–III). However, FR has been noted to be much safer in darker skin types (Fitzpatrick phototypes IV and V) than ablative resurfacing. It is also safe to use on nonfacial areas including the neck, trunk, and extremities provided that decreased fluences and densities are utilized

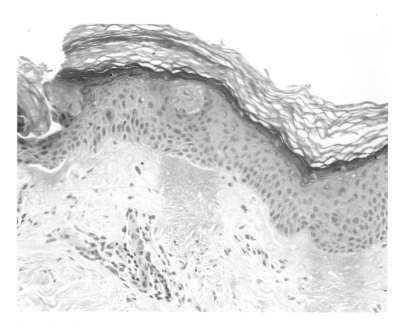

Figure 5.3 *H & E histology of microthermal treatment zone (MTZ) 1 day after fractional resurfacing treatment (note the microscopic epidermal necrotic debris (MEND) overlying a column of homogenized dermis)*

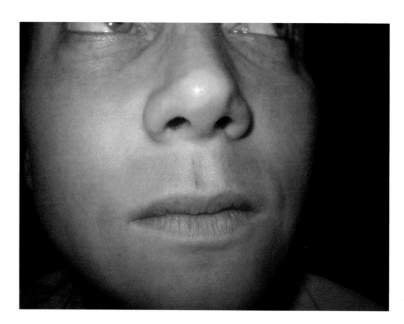

Figure 5.4 *Laser nicking observed 2 days following fractional resurfacing treatment*

▄ Contraindications

- Oral tretinoin use within 6 months to 1 year of surgery
- Active cutaneous infection
- Unrealistic patient expectations
- Pregnant or lactating woman

▄ Medications

- Antibacterial therapy: prophylactic antibiotics are generally not required
- Antiviral therapy
  - FR may trigger reactivation of herpes simplex that can spread to the treatment sites
  - Prophylactic antiviral medications are initiated 1 day prior to the procedure. Valacyclovir 500 mg PO BID or acyclovir 400 mg PO TID for 7–14 days is usually recommended
- Tretinoin: it is advised to discontinue tretinoin cream at least 2 weeks before FR to prevent skin irritation at the treatment sites

▄ Anesthesia

- Cold-air cooling (Zimmer) is very effective in decreasing the procedural discomfort.
- Topical anesthesia (oil or cream base) applied 1 h before the procedure is generally adequate, especially in combination with cold-air cooling (Zimmer).
- Regional nerve blocks can be effective to reduce the discomfort for patients with low pain thresholds, especially when utilizing higher fluences and densities. Infraorbital and mental blocks are very helpful when treating perioral wrinkles.

▄ Preoperative Preparation

- Explain the risks and benefits of the procedure
- Obtain the patient's written consent
- Wash the area to be treated with soap and water
- Obtain preoperative pictures
- Wipe with gauze soaked in 70% isopropyl alcohol to degrease the treatment site
- Apply a thick layer of topical anesthetic in an oil or cream base to the treatment site
- Wait 30–60 min to achieve optimal anesthetic effect
- Wipe off the topical anesthetic with a damp cloth
- Place seven to ten drops of OptiGuide Blue (FD&C #1, water-soluble blue tint) on a gauze pad and apply evenly over the entire treatment area. The FR laser (Fraxel Laser; Reliant technologies, San Diego, CA) will only treat areas coated with OptiGuide Blue. Allow the dye to dry (Fig. 5.6)

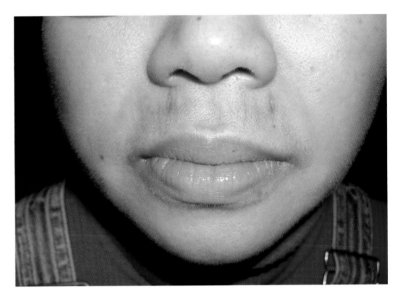

Figure 5.5 *Post-inflammatory hyperpigmentation 2 weeks following fractional resurfacing treatment to the upper lip with some crusting observed after treatment*

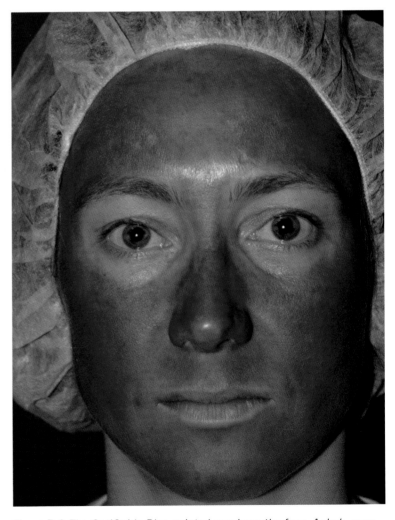

Figure 5.6 *The OptiGuide Blue painted evenly on the face. A dark, even application is critical for treatment success. The laser will not fire without adequate blue dye present*

• Apply a thin layer of lipid-based anesthetic or aquaphor ointment to the skin (Fig. 5.7)

▓ Procedure

1. The choice of laser parameters varies depending on the clinical situation

   • Higher fluences (10–20 mJ) are needed when targeting deeper processes such as wrinkles or scarring. It is advised that you use the lower density setting (125 MTZ/cm^2) when using higher fluences to avoid excess tissue heating and help reduce the potential of adverse side effects such as blistering and possibly scarring. Lower density settings can be compensated by delivering more passes. Always allow some time between the passes especially when treating smaller areas. Do not stack pulse your treatments.

   • Lower fluences (6–10 mJ) are adequate when targeting epidermal processes such as melasma, lentigines, and dyschromia. Density setting of 250 MTZ/cm^2 and eight passes are usually employ to a total density of 2000 MTZ/cm^2.

2. When treating the full face, divide the face into five treatment areas

   a) Right cheek

   b) Left cheek

   c) Right forehead

   d) Left forehead

   e) Nose, upper lip, and chin

3. Treatment

   a) Place the handpiece in contact with the skin, then depress the foot pedal and begin treatment (Fig. 5.8)

   b) Use a double pass, 50% overlap technique to treat

      i. Start treating away from your body, deliver one pass, come to a complete stop, then pull back towards your body to deliver the second pass with 100% overlap

      ii. Move the handpiece laterally by 50% and repeat step (i)

   c) Use the topical anesthetic ointment to help you track the treated areas

   d) Gently flatten treatment areas as needed

   e) You can change the tip size from 15 mm to 7 mm to treat smaller areas such as around the eyes and nose

   f) Always remember to come to a complete stop before changing direction

   g) Maintain the handpiece perpendicular and in full contact with the skin at all times. Tilting or lifting the handpiece can cause laser nicks

   h) Guide the handpiece over the treatment site as evenly as possible. If you move the handpiece too fast, the green indicator light will change to orange.

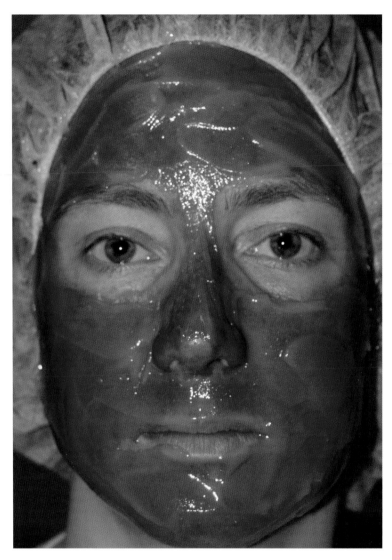

Figure 5.7 *A thick layer of lipid-based topical anesthetic is applied above the OptiGuide Blue*

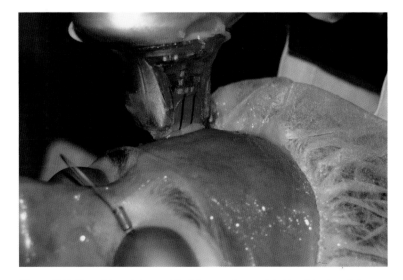

Figure 5.8 *Fraxel handpiece with 15 mm disposable tip. The handpiece should be perpendicular and in full contact with the skin throughout the treatment*

Fast movement of the handpiece will create unnecessary patient discomfort and the laser will deliver fewer MTZs than desired

i) Avoid bulk heating especially when treating smaller areas such as the upper lip and nose

    i. Wait a few minutes between the passes to allow the skin to cool down

    ii. When treating the upper lip, alternate the treatment between the right side and the left side, and start each pass from the same point

j) After treatment, the patient will wash off the OptiGuide Blue using a gentle cleanser (Fig. 5.9)

Postoperative Care

- Postoperative discomfort is generally mild and transient. The patient will experience a sunburn sensation for approximately 1 h.
- Patients may apply makeup immediately after the treatment.
- Patients are encouraged to use mild moisturizers for several days after the procedure.
- Postoperative edema is usually minimal but can be controlled with ice packs and head elevation. In rare instances of marked swelling, oral prednisone can be prescribed for 3–7 days.
- Sun avoidance is maintained for 6–12 months after the procedure to minimize the risk of post-inflammatory hyperpigmentation. Sunscreens with a minimum spf of 30 are recommended.
- Typically, patients can return to work on the first postoperative day.

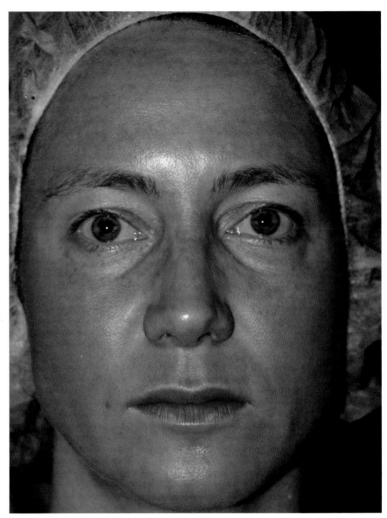

Figure 5.9 *Mild sunburn-like erythema immediately following Fraxel laser treatment with 6–8 mJ, 250 MTZ/cm², eight passes. This erythema may persist for 3–7 days.*

Pearls for Treatment Success

- Patient selection is key. Treating rhytides or scars that are too deep will prove disappointing to the patient and physician. The patient must be aware of the need for multiple treatments to obtain the desired clinical benefit (Fig. 5.10).
- Fraxel is an ablative device with similar clinical characteristics and side effect profile when used at high fluences. Great caution should be taken to stay within the recommended parameters to avoid potential complications.
- Elevating the handpiece during active treatment may result in a superficial burn with subsequent crusting. Hand movements should be from side to side when moving to a new treatment location.
- The long-lasting benefits of Fraxel are unknown at present. Patients must be aware that benefits may be short-lasting and may require maintenance treatments for continued clinical benefit.

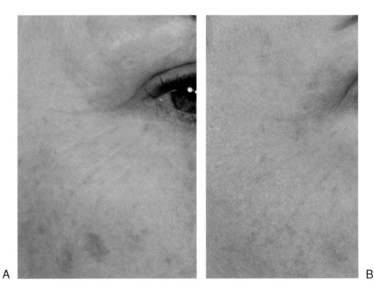

Figure 5.10 *Periorbital rhytides (**A**) following one fractional resurfacing treatment and (**B**) following four fractional resurfacing treatments. An appreciable softening is noted (photographs courtesy of R. Fitzpatrick, MD)*

• Effective Fraxel treatment in patients with skin photo-types III–V can be achieved. An increased incidence of temporary post-inflammatory hyperpigmentation is generally noted. Patients must be aware of the possibility of a short-lived increase in pigmentation with each treatment.

ABLATIVE LASER RESURFACING

■ Mechanism of Action

Utilizing the principles of selective photothermolysis, ablative removal of skin in a precisely controlled fashion with resultant minimal surrounding thermal damage is achieved. The depth of tissue penetration is dependent on selective absorption of water. Immediate tissue effects are dependent on the spot size and power utilized as well as the speed of treatment administration. The time of laser–tissue interaction is the critical factor for residual thermal damage. Epidermal obliteration and/or partial ablation or coagulation of the upper dermis is the endpoint. Reepithelialization results from the migration of cells that arise from surrounding follicular adnexae. Normal compact collagen and elastic fibers replace the amorphous elastotic dermal components and normal, well-organized epithelial cells replace the disorganized photodamaged epidermis. Collagen remodeling is noted both intraoperatively via thermal shrinkage and contraction and postoperatively within the remodeling phase of wound healing.

Carbon dioxide laser (CO$_2$)

Continuous wave (10,600 nm), super-pulsed, and scanned CO$_2$ lasers are utilized for resurfacing. A relatively bloodless surgery with reduced swelling is achieved via the photocoagulative effect on blood vessels and lymphatics. The risk of scarring, unpredictable level of thermal damage, and delayed healing of the continuous wave laser limits its clinical use. The scanned and pulsed CO$_2$ lasers deliver high peak fluences in less than 0.001 s to achieve tissue vaporization of 20–30 μm per pass. Approximately 40–120 μm of residual thermal damage is noted per pass (Fig. 5.11).

Erbium:yttrium-aluminum garnet laser (Er:YAG)

A laser of wavelength 2490 nm is utilized for more superficial resurfacing. It is 16× more selectively absorbed by water. It achieves tissue vaporization of 1–5 μm per pass. It results in a narrower zone of residual thermal damage (5–30 μm). As a zone of thermal damage of 50 μm or greater is required for photocoagulation, Er:YAG treatment results in a slightly bloody surgical field. The thermal damage is also insufficient to produce immediate collagen contraction. Long-term collagen remodeling is limited (Fig. 5.12).

■ Indications

Ablative lasers have been utilized as a cutting tool and vaporizing tool to treat epidermal and superficial dermal lesions.

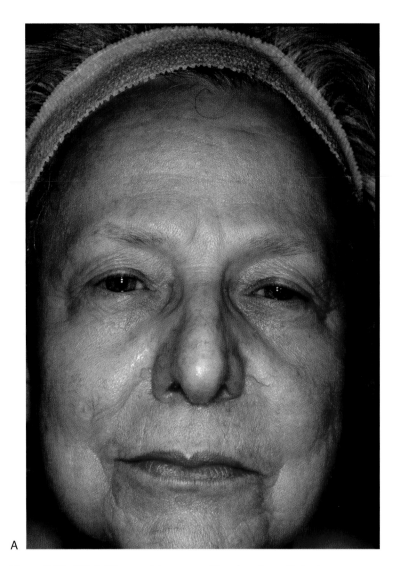

A

Figure 5.11 (A) *A 58-year-old woman with extensive actinic damage*

- Cutting tool: Keloids, acne keloidalis nuchae, cyst removal, basal carcinoma, burn, and ulcer debridement; hair transplantation; blepharoplasty; other incisional surgeries where controlled hemostasis is desired or where epinephrine is contraindicated or a pacer precludes use of electrosurgery.

- Vaporizing tool: Treatment of numerous conditions including static and dynamic rhytides, boxcar, crateriform and hypertrophic acne scars, pox scars, warts, lentigines, adenoma sebaceum, angiokeratomas, pyogenic granuloma, lymphangioma circumscriptum, Bowen's disease, erythroplasia of Queyrat, oral florid papillomatosis, actinic cheilitis, actinic keratoses, epidermal nevi, syringomas, granuloma faciale, neurofibromas, xanthelasma, and tattoos.

- Not indicated for the treatment of ice-pick acne scars.

■ Preoperative Evaluation

Significant past medical history includes a history of herpes labialis; underlying autoimmune disease or immune deficiency; underlying koebnerizing/infectious conditions including psoriasis, verrucae, and molluscum; history of keloid or hypertrophic scar formation; underlying cardiac or pulmonary conditions that may be exacerbated by the use of anesthetic medications; existing drug allergies; tobacco use; active acne vulgaris.

Significant past surgical history includes prior surgical treatments to the treatment sites, surgical dates, and patient response.

The patient must be aware of the lengthy recovery period that will require extensive hands-on patient care for optimal treatment results. Reepithelialization requires 7–10 days with associated pain, edema, and erythema. Postoperative erythema resolves over an average period of 3–5 months. Strict sun avoidance must be followed for a minimum of 1 year postoperatively to avoid pigmentary changes and photosensitivity. Realistic expectations are the most important determinants of treatment success. The patient must be aware that the treatment will improve but does not eliminate all or even most rhytides or scars and that dynamic rhytides are likely to recur within a few months postoperatively.

Procedural risks to emphasize include temporary and/or permanent hyperpigmentation and depigmentation, infection (viral, bacterial, yeast), and scar (atrophic, hypertrophic, keloidal) formation; acne flare; eczema lasting 1–2 months. Predictable side effects include procedural and postoperative discomfort; edema, oozing, and crusting lasting 1–2 weeks; erythema, skin tightness, and pruritus lasting up to 3–4 months.

- Ideal laser candidate: Fair skin type (Fitzpatrick phototypes I–III); laser-amenable lesions; minimal associated dyspigmentation of neck and chest; able to tolerate extended period of convalescence postoperatively; able to follow and execute necessary postoperative skin care regimen

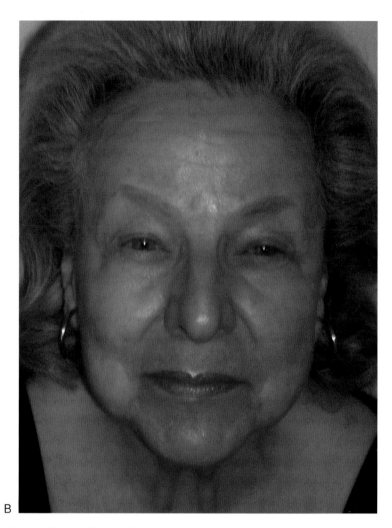

B

Figure 5.11 (*continued*) (**B**) *A marked reduction in rhytides and dyspigmentation is noted 2 months after full-face carbon dioxide resurfacing*

- Less ideal laser candidate: Darker skin type (Fitzpatrick phototypes IV and V); treat with caution, due to significant risk of temporary and permanent pigmentary alterations; moderate associated dyspigmentation of neck and chest; unable to follow and execute necessary postoperative skin care regimen; prior surgical procedures performed

▨ Contraindications

- Laboratory screening is generally not required
- Absolute
  - Use of oral tretinoin within 1 year of surgery
  - Active cutaneous infection
  - Preexisting ectropion (for infraorbital resurfacing)
  - Poor patient compliance
  - Unrealistic patient expectations
- Relative
  - Extensive underlying dyspigmentation
  - Underlying connective tissue; koebnerizing condition or immunologic disease
  - Previous lower lid blepharoplasty (for infraorbital resurfacing)
  - Previous ablative resurfacing, dermabrasion, cryosurgery; facelift or phenol peel
  - History of facial radiation treatment

▨ Medications

- Antibacterial therapy: to avoid impetiginization and bacterial infection of the treatment sites, prophylactic antibiotics are initiated 1 day preoperatively. Dicloxacillin 500 mg PO BID or Keflex 500 mg PO BID for 10–14 days is prescribed. In penicillin-allergic individuals, azithromycin 500 mg PO × 1 followed by 250 mg daily for 5 days or clindamycin 150 mg PO QID for 5 days is recommended.

- Antiviral therapy: laser resurfacing may trigger a herpes simplex outbreak that can spread to the treatment sites with an increased risk of scarring. Prophylactic antiviral medications are initiated 1 day preoperatively. Valacyclovir 500 mg PO BID for 14 days or acyclovir 400 mg PO TID for 14 days is recommended.

- Tretinoin: use of tretinoin prior to CO_2 laser resurfacing has been shown clinically and via biochemical analysis to not provide enhanced collagen formation, accelerated reepithelialization, or quicker resolution of postoperative erythema. Use of this modality is optional.

- Bleaching creams: no published, controlled trials have demonstrated the benefits of preoperative bleaching creams to reduce the risk of post-inflammatory hyperpigmentation. To possibly reduce this risk, patients with skin phototypes III and IV are prescribed a bleaching cream to be applied twice daily for 6–7 weeks prior to treatment. As well, strict sun avoidance is mandatory.

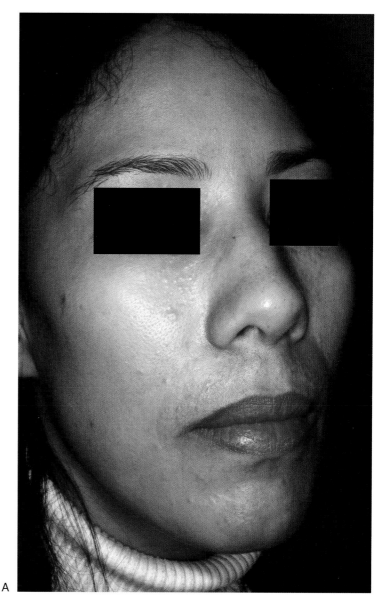

A

Figure 5.12 (A) *A 45-year-old woman with facial photoaging and mild acne scarring*

■ Anesthesia

- Cold-air cooling (Zimmer) may be adequate for localized or single-pass CO_2 treatment or Er:YAG treatment.

- Topical anesthesia may be adequate for localized or single-pass CO_2 treatment or Er:YAG treatment.

- Regional nerve blocks with supplemental infiltrative anesthesia are generally administered for multiple-pass CO_2 treatment. Site-dependent blocks include supraorbital, supratrochlear, infraorbital, and mental blocks. Lidocaine (1%) with 1:100,000 or 1:200,000 epinephrine, a total of 0.5–1.0 mL is administered per site. Supplemental infiltrative anesthesia consisting of an equal mixture of 1% lidocaine, 0.5% bupivacaine, and 1:10 sodium bicarbonate is generally required, especially for the jawline, upper eyelids, and temples. Hyaluronidase (Wydase) 75 U for tissue diffusion may be added to the infiltrative anesthesia. Treatment is delayed 10–15 min to allow for complete anesthetic effect.

- Conscious intravenous sedation and general anesthesia have been employed by trained physicians in certified facilities in patients unable to tolerate the injections or for larger procedures.

■ Safety Measures

- Eye protection

  - One or two drops of 0.05% topical proparacaine (Alcaine) or 0.05% topical tetracaine (Pontocaine) are placed into each patient eye, followed by the application of topical erythromycin ointment or ophthalmic lubricant (e.g., Lacri-Lube) and nonreflective metallic ocular shields (e.g., Byron Medical, Tucson, AZ; Oculo-Plastik, Montreal, Canada).

  - All personnel must wear clear plastic safety glasses to avoid inadvertent corneal damage.

- Operative field

  - All reflective surfaces and windows must be covered to avoid inadvertent treatment of a reflective surface.

  - The treatment room door must be labeled properly to warn others not to enter during laser treatment.

  - All flammable materials and anesthetic gases must be kept away from the operative field.

  - Wet drapes and sponges are placed around the surgical site to prevent accidental irradiation of surrounding skin and to minimize potential fire.

  - A nonflammable ointment (e.g., Surgilube; KY Jelly) must be placed over the exposed hairline and eyebrows to avoid hair singeing. Surgilube should not be used over the eyelashes to avoid the risk of corneal keratitis.

  - All surgical tools utilized must possess a nonreflective or roughened black coating to prevent laser beam deflection.

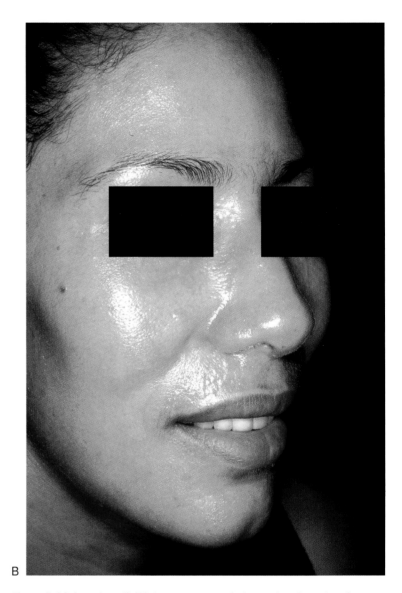

B

Figure 5.12 (*continued*) (B) *Improvement of photoaging 3 weeks after full-face erbium treatment*

- A laser smoke evacuator that filters particles as small as 0.12 m in diameter and laser-grade surgical masks must be used to reduce potential spread of infectious particles in the laser plume.

- Use of Hibiclens, isopropyl alcohol, and acetone is prohibited due to their flammable nature.

- All makeup and hairspray are to be removed, as they are potentially flammable.

- The laser should be kept in the standby mode at all times other than active treatment to avoid accidental firing.

- Oxygen should be avoided or be used only in conjunction with a closed gas system that includes either endotracheal intubation of laryngeal mask airway.

■ Procedure

- A thorough review of the risks and benefits is performed.

- Patient written consent is obtained.

- Representative preoperative pictures are obtained.

- The choice of laser and laser parameters varies depending on the clinical situation. The CO_2 laser is preferable for deeper lines and scarring processes. The Er:YAG laser is suitable for superficial lines and dyspigmentation. The patient's postoperative considerations also affect the choice of laser.

- In general, treatment of a cosmetic unit or full face is best to minimize the risk of textural mismatch between nontreated and treated areas. In an isolated treatment, one must treat the entire lesion or line to their end rather than remain within a cosmetic unit.

- The vermilion border can be treated conservatively to minimize lipstick "bleeding".

- Treatment should extend beyond the anatomical unit being treated, with a feathering technique (decreased fluence) employed to blend into the untreated skin.

- For depressed scars, additional passes with a smaller spot size on the defect edge allows for more significant flattening of the surface.

- Scar contraction will occur with healing. To avoid atrophic scar formation, administer treatment to the level of near normal adjacent skin only.

- Ablative resurfacing of dynamic rhytides provides only temporary benefit. Consideration of combination therapy with botulinum toxin or a filler substance should be entertained to achieve maximum benefit.

- Minimal mechanical trauma technique: fewer CO_2 passes performed with retainment of the last pass eshcar to expedite healing and minimize scar risk and pigmentary changes. This technique is optimal for younger patients with more superficial lesions and for darker skin types.

- With any treatment modality, the presence of larger collagen bundles herald entry into the deep reticular dermis

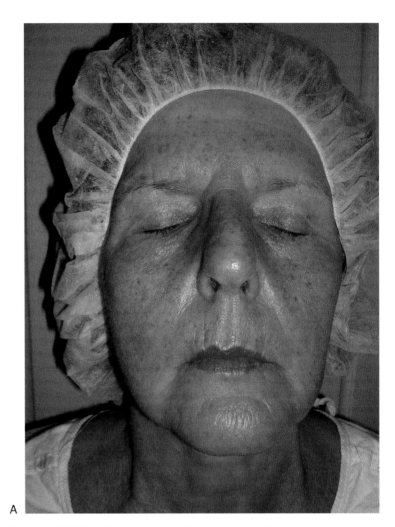

A

Figure 5.13 (A) *A 53-year-old female who was most bothered by her perioral rhytides, but was also noted to have moderate dermatoheliosis with numerous lentigines and actinic damage of the remainder of her face.* **(B)** *Same patient immediately after perioral carbon dioxide laser resurfacing and a Jessner/35% trichloroacetic acid peel to the remainder of her face.* **(C)** *Same patient 8 weeks following her treatment. A marked reduction in both her rhytides and dyspigmentation is appreciated*

and warn of the possibility of scar formation. Treatment should be discontinued immediately.

- Resurfacing of nonfacial rhytides is associated with a high risk for textural and pigmentary changes due to the reduction in adnexal structures and poor vascularity in comparison to the face. The CO_2 laser should not be utilized for the treatment of nonfacial rhytides. The Er:YAG laser should be utilized with extreme caution.

- Combination therapies of carbon dioxide resurfacing and chemical peels, botulinum toxin, or soft tissue augmentation may provide the greatest benefit (Fig. 5.13).

Postoperative Care

- An open wound technique or closed technique may be followed.

- Postoperative discomfort is characterized by moderate burning within the first 24 h. This is minimized with the use of an occlusive dressing. It can generally be controlled with ice packs, cold compresses, and acetaminophen, as well as frequent wound care.

- Postoperative edema develops 24–48 h postoperatively and can be controlled with ice packs and head elevation. Oral steroids are employed when marked swelling develops intraoperatively or immediately postoperatively.

- Reepithelialization occurs within 3–10 days and is dependent on the laser utilized, the number of laser passes executed, and the surgical candidate. Younger patients, patients who undergo Er:YAG treatment and fewer passes show faster healing. Delayed healing is observed in older patients, smokers, and increased laser passes.

- Topical antibiotics and Aquaphor Healing Ointment should be avoided due to the risk of allergic contact dermatitis (Fig. 5.14).

- Close follow-up is mandatory to ensure proper care and healing of the treated sites (Figs. 5.15-5.16).

- Prophylactic antibiotics and antiviral medications are continued for 10–14 days postoperatively.

- Strict sun avoidance is maintained for 1 year postoperatively to avoid photosensitivity and to minimize the risk of post-inflammatory hyperpigmentation.

Pearls for Treatment Success

- Preoperative wound care instructions are critical for treatment success. The patient and significant others must be prepared for the extensive care that will be required for expedient and safe healing. Patients should be shown postoperative pictures to prepare them for how they will appear. Postoperative supplies, including wound care supplies and desired camouflage foundation should be obtained prior to the treatment date. Patients with younger children must prepare

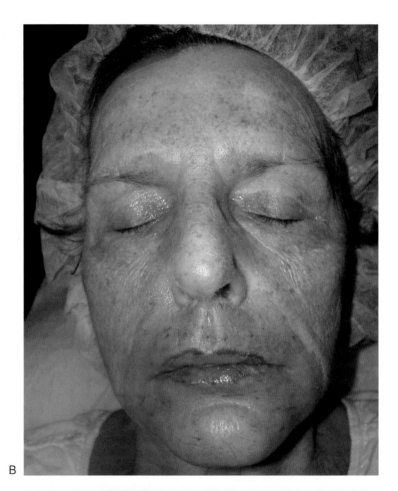

B

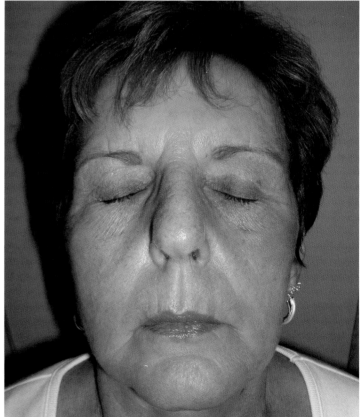

C

Figure 5.13 (*continued***)**

them for the significant changes that will be noted during the healing period. Any postoperative assistance the patient may require should be arranged prior to treatment if possible.

- Patients require frequent postoperative evaluation for the first 14 days to ensure proper wound care is being employed, predicted healing is noted, and no side effects such as scar formation or infection occur. Patients should be evaluated on post-op day 2, post-op day 5–7, and post-op day 10–14 and anytime the patient expresses a concern of need for evaluation.

- Patient expectations must be tailored to the expected benefits. Patients should be informed that the greatest benefits will not be appreciated for 6–12 months postoperatively.

- Strict photoprotection and sun protection are critical in reducing the occurrence of post-inflammatory hyperpigmentation and sunburn and should be followed for a minimum of 1 year after treatment.

- Treated skin is sensitive to a majority of facial products, perfumes, and topical medications for an average of 12 weeks post-treatment. Bland products including a sun block are recommended during this healing time.

- Persistent areas of erythema should raise concern regarding scar formation or infection. A culture is recommended to rule out bacterial or yeast infection. Use of a potent topical corticosteroid is crucial with close follow-up to ensure resolution.

CHEMICAL PEELS (Tables 5.2-5.3)

▥ Mechanism of Action

The application of a wounding agent to induce epidermal and/or dermal sloughing.

▥ Indications

- Epidermal defects—ephelides, melasma
- Epidermal and dermal defects—melasma, lentigines, post-inflammatory hyperpigmentation, actinic keratoses, superficial rhytides, acne vulgaris
- Dermal defects —deep rhytides, acne scarring, scars

▥ Preoperative Evaluation

Peeling agents are selected based on the patient's lifestyle, defect depth, skin characteristics, and defect location (Table 5.4).

- Past medical history
  - Past radiation history—decreased adnexal structures likely
  - History of oral herpes simplex virus—reactivation may occur

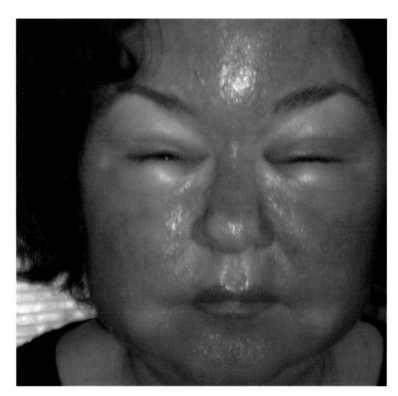

Figure 5.14 *Contact dermatitis secondary to Aquaphor Healing Ointment application. Subsequent patch testing revealed a hypersensitivity to lanolin in the ointment*

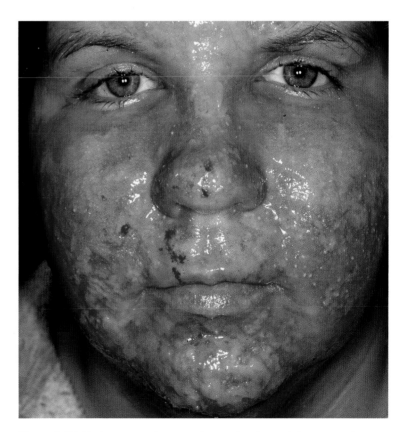

Figure 5.15 *Under aggressive wound care. A substantial amount of crusting is observed. Proper wound care was demonstrated in-office and with repeat written instructions reviewed*

- Pregnancy—peels contraindicated with the exception of glycolic acid
- History of keloid formation—moderate and deep-depth peels should be avoided
- Past surgical history
  - Prior cosmetic procedures—prior face lift, blepharoplasty, carbon dioxide resurfacing, or dermabrasion may affect peel outcome. Increased ectropion risk present
- Medication use
  - Previous isotretinoin use and year
  - Topical medications such as tretinoin and α-hydroxy acids may potentiate peel penetration
  - Coumadin use
- Fitzpatrick skin phototype
  - Skin phototypes I–III patients respond to all peel types
  - Skin phototypes IV and V patients also respond to all peel types, but the risk of post-treatment dyspigmentation is greater
  - A test site may be warranted for darker skin types to evaluate peel outcome
- Degree of actinic damage and photoaging
  - A white line of demarcation between peeled and unpeeled skin may be prominent in the presence of moderate to severe dermatoheliosis

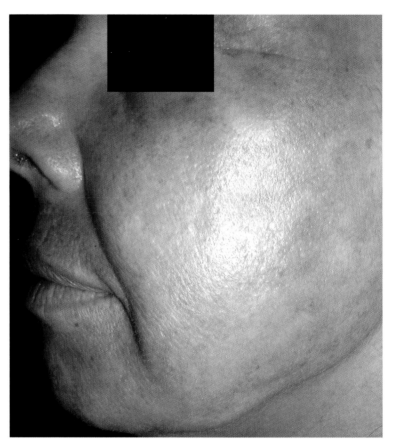

Figure 5.16 *Post-inflammatory hyperpigmentation 6 weeks after perioral carbon dioxide resurfacing. This pigmentation resolved with the use of 4% hydroquinone twice daily for 2 months*

TABLE 5.2 ■ Clinical Indications and Peel Types

Indication	Peel type	Peel depth/treatment endpoint
Acne vulgaris	Superficial when active	Localized epidermal peeling required; lesional improvement
Ephelides; lentigines	Superficial or medium	Total epidermal peeling required for complete removal; lightening with superficial application
Post-inflammatory inflammation	Superficial or medium	Total epidermal peeling required; lightening with either strength
Melasma	Superficial or medium	Total epidermal peeling required; lightening with either strength; inconsistent response
Superficial rhytides	Superficial	Localized epidermal peeling required; softening
Moderate rhytides	Medium or deep	Total epidermal and papillary dermal peeling required; softening
Deep rhytides	Deep	Total epidermal to reticular dermal peel required; softening
Actinic keratoses	Medium	Total epidermal to papillary dermal peeling required; lesional clearance
Depressed scars	Medium or deep	Lesional edges targeted; total epidermal and partial dermal peeling required; lesional flattening; variable response

TABLE 5.3 ■ Wounding Depth of Superficial, Medium-Depth, and Deep-Depth Strength Peels

Superficial peel	Medium-depth peel	Deep peel
α-hydroxy acid	Glycolic acid and TCA	Baker's Gordon phenol, unoccluded
Modified Unna's resorcinol paste	Jessner's and TCA	Baker's Gordon phenol, occluded
Jessner's	Solid carbon dioxide and TCA	
Salicylic acid	50% TCA	
Solid carbon dioxide slush	Pyruvic acid	
Tretinoin	88% full-strength phenol	
10–25% TCA; 35% variable		

TABLE 5.4 ■ Peeling Agent Characteristics

Peel type	Color endpoint	Application	Healing time	Safe for
Glycolic acid	Confluent erythema	1–2 coats	1–2 h	All skin types
Jessner	Pale white	Coats are applied singly and endpoint monitored for 3–4 min prior to repeat application	4–5 days; mild epidermal desquamation noted	All skin types
TCA (30% or greater)	Solid white	Single even application; localized applications for lighter white areas may be considered	10–14 days; severe sunburn-like peeling observed	I and II; caution with III and IV
Phenol	Gray white	Single even application; can be conservatively reapplied	10–14 days; superficial burn appearance	I and II

- Wood's lamp evaluation
  - Helpful in ascertaining pigmentation type present
  - Epidermal origin: lesional color enhancement
  - Dermal or mixed origin: no lesional color enhancement
  - Examination does not predict clinical peel response
  - Epidermal pigment may respond better to peeling agents
- Medical clearance
  - A recent electrocardiogram is necessary to serve as a baseline for phenol peels in event of cardiotoxicity
  - Liver function and renal function tests should be evaluated to ensure adequate hepatorenal function for phenol peels

■ Ideal Candidate

- Skin phototype I or II
- Actinic damaged skin
- Static rhytides associated with sun exposure

■ Less Ideal Candidate

- Dynamic rhytides—achieved benefits are temporary in nature

- Extensive gravitational folds and furrows—likely to require surgical intervention in conjunction with chemical peels
- Deep rhytides
- Boxcar acne or moderate depth atrophic scarring

Contraindications

- Unrealistic patient expectations
- Patient unable to perform necessary postoperative care
- Patients with ice-pick scars or deep atrophic scars
- Patients with dilated, large pore size
- History of oral iretinoin use within 1 year prior to procedure
- History of keloid formation
- Patient with underlying cardiac arrhythmias (for deep peels)
- Coumadin use (for deep peels)
- Skin phototypes III–VI (for deep peels)

Medications

- Preoperative antiviral medications are recommended. Valtrex 500 mg BID or Acyclovir 400 mg TID initiated the day of procedure and continued for 7–14 days is administered
- Topical retinoic acid and α-hydroxy acid products are discontinued 48 h prior to a glycolic acid peel and 1 week prior to a deeper peel and not reinitiated for one week post treatment

Wound Depth

Determined by multiple factors.

- Anatomic considerations

Facial skin differs from nonfacial skin in the relative number of pilosebaceous units per cosmetic unit and thickness. Prominent adnexal structures are required to promote reepithelialization post treatment.

- The nose and forehead have more sebaceous glands than do the cheeks or temples
- The face has more sebaceous glands than the nonfacial areas including the neck
- More actinically damaged skin is thinner with fewer pilosebaceous units present

Body location and presence of actinically damaged skin significant affects the selection of the wounding agent. The peeling agent may be more destructive in areas with fewer adnexal structures and thinner skin; therefore a less aggressive peeling agent should be utilized in these areas.

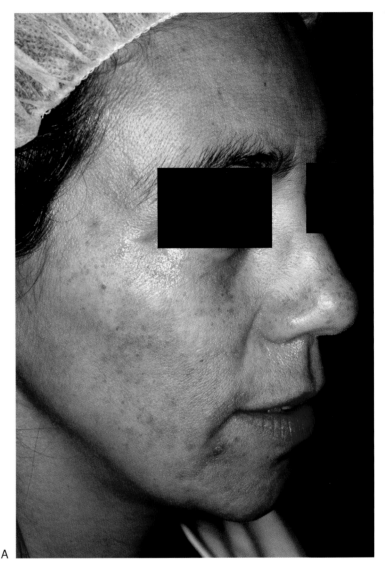

A

Figure 5.17 (A) *Epidermal melasma unresponsive to topical bleaching creams.*

- Prepeel skin defatting—use of acetone to defat the treatment area results in a deeper penetrating peel
- Wounding agent strength—an increased strength will result in deeper skin peeling
- Amount of agent applied—deeper skin penetration with each peel layer applied

Peel Types

- Superficial peels—partial or complete epidermal injury; may extend into the papillary dermis (Fig. 5.17)
- Medium-depth peels—injury extends into the papillary to upper reticular dermis (Fig. 5.18)
- Deep peels—injury extends into the midreticular dermis

Procedure

- Preoperative written consent obtained
- Preoperative pictures taken
- Patient makeup removed and face cleansed with an antiseptic wash (e.g., chlorhexidine)
- Scrub the treatment area with acetone on cotton gauze for 2–3 min
- The peeling agent should be poured into a glass cup
- The peeling agent is applied to the treatment site
  - A paintbrush or cotton ball may be used to apply glycolic acid
  - A sable brush is recommended for Jessner peel for increased penetration
  - Cotton-tipped applicators or cotton gauze may be used to apply TCA peeling agents
  - One or two small cotton-tipped applicators are used for phenol application
  - A round toothpick or wooden portion of a broken cotton-tipped applicator may be used to treat individual rhytides and ice-pick acne scars
  - The number of applicators used and the pressure applied to the treatment site with agent application will affect solution delivery and depth of penetration (Figs. 5.19-5.20)
- A fan is required to help reduce the associated patient discomfort
- Pretreatment with Jessner or glycolic acid prior to a TCA peel allows for deeper peel penetration
- Feathering into the hairline and at the jawline conceals the possible line of demarcation. Feathering should also be performed when the perioral area is treated alone to prevent lines of demarcation (Fig. 5.21)
- The periorbital tissue should be treated first with TCA peels, followed by the nose, cheeks, perioral area, and

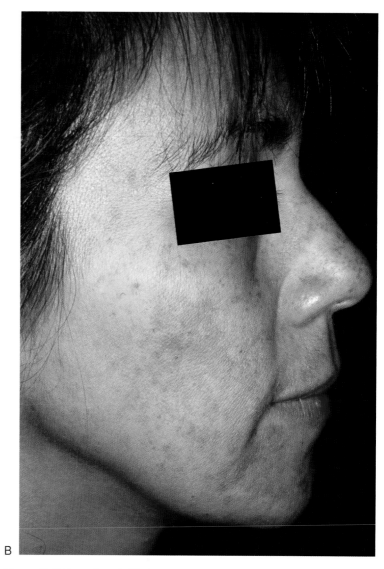

B

Figure 5.17 (*continued*) (B) *Mild improvement noted following two 50% glycolic acid peels*

forehead for best patient tolerance The upper and lower eyelids may be treated. Extension 2–3 mm onto the perioral vermillion is beneficial for rhytides reduction

• A saline syringe should be available in the case of inadvertent introduction of the peeling agent into the eye

• The applicator should be wrung out and semi-dried to prevent dripping. The glass container should be held away from the patient to avoid direct spilling onto the patient

• Jessner peel, TCA, and phenol peels are self-neutralizing. Glycolic acid peels must be neutralized with water or bicarbonate solution

• Cool washcloth is applied to the treated areas

• Vaseline is applied to the treatment site for Jessner, TCA, and phenol peels. Glycolic acid peels require a light moisturizer

• Deep peels have inherent cardiac, renal, and hepatic toxicities. Full-face application require intravenous fluids, sedation, cardiac monitoring, pulse oximeter, and blood pressure monitoring

▣ Complications

• Greater depth of peel provided than expected (Fig. 5.22)

• Infection—viral, bacterial, fungal

• Temporary or permanent hyperpigmentation or depigmentation

• Prolonged erythema

• Scarring—atrophic, hypertrophic, keloidal; ectropion, delayed healing

• Contact dermatitis

• Textural changes

• Acne

• Milia

• Cardiac arrythmias (deep phenol peel)

• Laryngeal edema (deep phenol peel)

▣ Postoperative Care

• A light moisturizer is applied twice daily for glycolic acid peels

• Vaseline is kept on round the clock with twice daily cleansing soap and water, Jessner, TCA, and phenol peels

• Strict photoprotection is stressed for a minimum of 1 month after a glycolic acid peel and 2–3 months for remainder of peels

• Patients are instructed to allow natural sloughing of the treated skin. The skin must not be manually removed

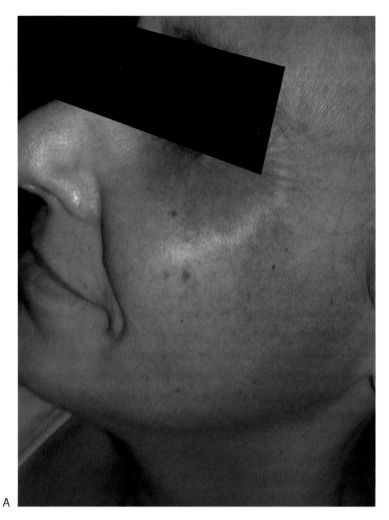

A

Figure 5.18 (A) *Pseudoochronosis. The pigmentary changes persisted despite discontinuation of the inciting medication.*

■ Pearls for Treatment Success

• Careful patient selection and peel selection are necessary for treatment success. It is best to undertreat with a less potent peeling agent in nonfacial areas to minimize the risk of scar formation.

• Patients must be aware of the expected recovery time with each chemical peel and the necessary postoperative wound care they will need to perform to expedite healing. Although one deep peel may provide the greatest benefit, lifestyle or work constraints make serial superficial or medium-depth peels a better long-term goal.

• The margin of safety is much narrower and the risk of complications much greater with increased peel strengths.

• Patients with skin phototypes III and IV have a greater risk of developing PIH after a chemical peel. Consideration of a test site is warranted for medium-depth peels.

• Chemical peels will not alter pore size and may in fact increase their size.

BIBLIOGRAPHY

Alster TS. Cutaneous resurfacing with CO_2 and erbium:YAG lasers: preoperative, intraoperative and postoperative considerations. *Plast Reconstr Surg.* 1999;103: 619–634.

Anderson RR, Parrish JA. Selective photothermolysis: precise microsurgery by selective absorption of pulsed radiation. *Science.* 1983;220:524–527.

Baker TJ, Gordon HL, Mosienko P, et al. Long-term histological study of skin after chemical facial peeling. *Plast Reconstr Surg.* 1974;53:522–525.

Brody HJ. Medium-depth chemical peeling of the skin: a variation of superficial chemosurgery. *Adv Dermatol.* 1988;3:205–220.

Carruthers J, Carruthers A, Zelichowska A. The power of combined therapies: Botox and ablative laser resurfacing. *Am J Cosmet Surg.* 2000;17:129–131.

David I, Ruiz-Esparza J. Fast healing after laser skin resurfacing. The minimal mechanical trauma technique. *Dermatol Surg.* 1997;23:359–361.

Dover JS, Hruza GJ, Arndt KA. Lasers in skin resurfacing. *Semin Cutan Med Surg* 1996;15:177–188.

Duke D, Grevelink JM. Care before and after laser skin resurfacing. A survey and review of the literature. *Dermatol Surg.* 1998;24:201–206.

Fitzpatrick RS, Goldman MP, Satur NM, Tope WD. Pulsed carbon dioxide laser resurfacing of photoaged facial skin. *Arch Dermatol.* 1996;132:395–402.

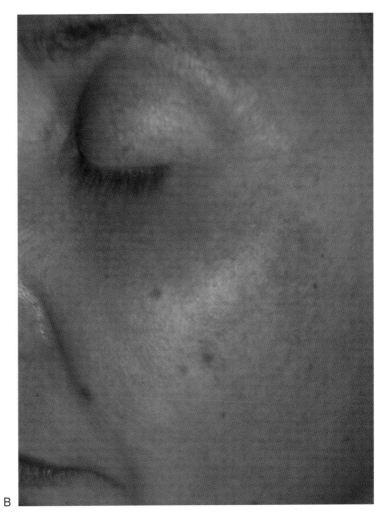

B

Figure 5.18 (*continued*) (B) *Marked pigment lightening after three Jessner/35% TCA peels*

Fitzpatrick RE, Tope WD, Goldman MP, et al. Pulsed carbon dioxide laser, trichloroacetic acid, Backer–Gordon phenol and dermabrasion: a comparative clinical and histologic study of cutaneous resurfacing in a porcine model. *Arch Dermatol.* 1996;132:469–471.

Grimes PE: Melasma: etiologic and therapeutic considerations. *Arch Dermatol.* 1997;131:1453–1457.

Gross D. Cardiac arrhythmia during phenol face peeling. *Plast Reconstr Surg.* 1984;73:590–594.

Kligman AM, Baker TJ, Gordon HL. Long-term histologic follow-up of phenol face peels. *Plast Reconstr Surg.* 1985;75:652–659.

Lanzame RJ, Naim JO, Rogers DW, et al. Comparisons of continuous-wave, chop-wave and super-pulse laser wounds. *Lasers Surg Med.* 1988;8:108–118.

MacKee GM, Karp FL. The treatment of post-acne scars with phenol. *Br J Dermatol.* 1952;64:456–459.

Manstein D, Herron GS, Sink RK, Tanner H, Anderson RR. Fractional photothermolysis: a new concept for cutaneous remodeling using microscopic patterns of thermal injury. *Lasers Surg Med.* 2004;34(5):426–438.

Matarasso SL, Glogau RG. Chemical face peels. *Dermatol Clin.* 1991;9:131–150.

Monheit G. The Jessner's-trichloroacetic acid peel. *Dermatol Clin.* 1995;13(2):277–283.

Monheit GD. The Jessner's + TCA peel: a medium-depth chemical peel. *J Dermatol Surg Oncol.* 1989;15:953–963.

Murad H, Shamban AT, Premo PS. The use of glycolic acid as a peeling agent. *Dermatol Clin.* 1995;13(2):285–307.

Nanni CA, Alster TS. Complications of carbon dioxide laser resurfacing: an evaluation of 500 patients. *Dermatol Surg.* 1998;24:315–320.

Bitter, PH. Noninvasive rejuvenation of photodamaged skin using serial, full face intense pulsed light treatments. *Dermatol Surg.* 2000;26:835–842.

Orentreich D, et al. Subcutaneous incisionless (subcision) surgery for the correction of depressed scars and wrinkles. *Dermatol Surg.* 1995;21:543–549.

Orringer JS, Kang S, Johnson TM, et al. Tretinoin treatment before carbon-dioxide laser resurfacing: a clinical and biochemical analysis. *J Am Acad Dermatol.* December 2004;51(6):940–946.

Raulin C, Grema H. Single-pass carbon dioxide laser skin resurfacing combined with cold-air cooling: efficacy and patient satisfaction of a prospective side-by-side study. *Arch Dermatol.* 2004;140(11):1333–1336.

Ruiz-Esparza J, Barba Gomez JM, Gomez de la Torre OL. Wound care after laser skin resurfacing. A combination of open and closed methods using a new polyethylene mask. *Dermatol Surg.* 1998;24:79–81.

Szczchowicz EH, Wright WK. Delayed healing after full-face chemical peels. *Facial Plast Surg.* 1989;6(1):6–13.

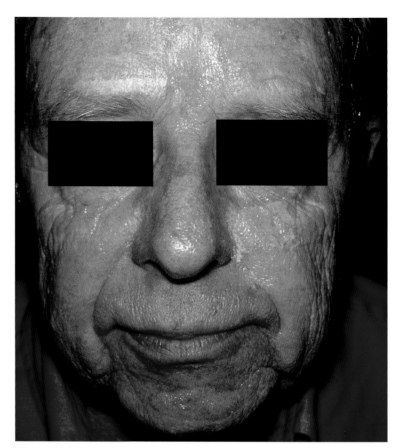

Figure 5.19 *Pale white color immediately following a Jessner peel*

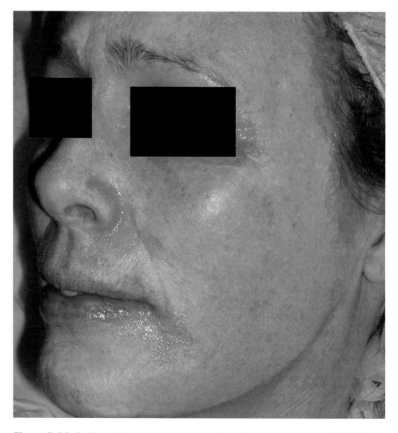

Figure 5.20 *Solid white color immediately following a Jessner/35% TCA peel*

Tannous ZS, Astner S. Utilizing fractional resurfacing in the treatment of therapy-resistant melasma. *J Cosmet Laser Ther.* 2005;7(1):39–43.

Zukowski ML, Mossie RD, Roth SI, et al. Pilot study analysis of the histologic and bacteriologic effects of occlusive dressings in chemosurgical peel using a minipig model. *Aesthetic Plast Surg.* 1993;17:53–59.

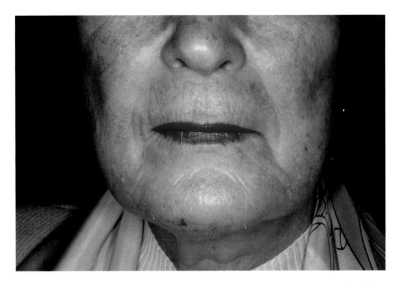

Figure 5.21 *Patient with line of demarcation between the Jessner/35% TCA peel treated perioral area and untreated skin. Patient appears hypopigmented in the treatment site. A subsequent medium-depth peel to the remainder of the face resulted in a more even facial appearance*

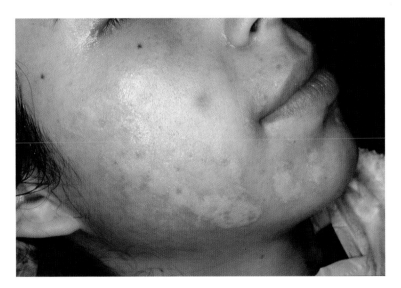

Figure 5.22 *Localized frosting following application of a 50% glycolic acid peel. The localized peel resulted in some mild desquamation for 3 days*

CHAPTER 6 | Dermatoheliosis, Treatment Management

OCCLUSIVE DRESSINGS

▣ Open Technique (Fig. 6.1)

Application of a hydrophilic ointment or cream directly to the treated areas of skin without an overlying textile dressing.

- Cream or ointment applied immediately after treatment administered
- Soak the treated sites with normal saline, 0.25% acetic acid or cool tap water, a clean washcloth or gauze for 10–15 min
- Gently remove the excess crusting/scabbing with a water-soaked Q-tip
- Re-apply the topical salve, 1/2-in. thick over the treatment site
- Repeat every 3–4 h during waking hours while healing

Advantages: Decreased bacterial colonization; easy wound monitoring; less expensive

Disadvantages: Labor intensive; increased patient compliance required; slightly increased patient discomfort while healing

Examples: Petrolatum, Complex C-3 ointment (Procyte, Redmond, Washington), Aquaphor (Beiersdorf–Jobst, Charlette, NC)

Avoid: Topical antibiotic application—increased risk of development of contact dermatitis

▣ Closed Technique (Fig 6.2)

Application of a textile dressing to treated skin.

- Apply immediately after treatment completed. Use of concomitant cream/ointment is dressing dependent
- Two days and 5 days postoperatively the patient is evaluated, dressing changed, treatment site cleaned, and new dressing applied

Advantages: Minimal patient compliance required; expedited wound healing

Disadvantages: Increased bacterial colonization; increased expense

Examples: Flexzan (composite foam); Second Skin (hydrogel); Silon-TSR (polymer film); Mepitel (polymer mesh)

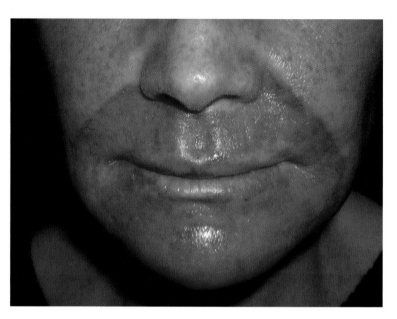

Figure 6.1 *Patient utilizing an open technique for healing 4 days following carbon dioxide resurfacing*

LOCAL ANESTHESIA

■ Mechanism of Action

Interruption of nerve conduction via sodium channel disruption and actual blockage of the sodium channel preventing sodium influx. The solubility, lipophilicity, and capacity to block sodium channels determine the relative anesthetic properties. Anesthetic selection is based on the possibility of adverse reactions, requirements for the time of onset of action, and duration of the anesthesia required. Two classes are defined: (1) ester anesthetics (procaine, tetracaine, benzocaine, cocaine, and chloroprocaine) are metabolized through plasma pseudocholinesterases into PABA metabolites and cleared by renal excretion. Cocaine differs from other esters by being partially metabolized in the liver and excreted unchanged in the urine and (2) amide anesthetics (lidocaine, etidocaine, mepivacaine, dibucaine, and prilocaine) are metabolized through dealkylation and hydrolysis by hepatic microsomal enzymes and cleared by renal excretion.

■ Topical (Table 6.1)

Effective for achieving anesthesia for superficial laser surgery, shave biopsies, soft tissue augmentation, and painless needle insertion.

Examples: Creams; ointments; gels; patches; cryoanesthesia (refrigerant sprays such as dichlorotetraflouroethane and ethyl chloride; ice cube application; cryogen spray; cold glass window, forced cool air); iontophoresis.

Judicious use of EMLA as a topical anesthetic in children must be followed in order to avoid the possibility of methemoglobinemia (Tables 6.2-6.3).

■ Local Infiltration

Injection of an anesthetic solution into the region in which the nerve endings that supply the treatment site are located. Injection is directed intradermally for a fast onset and longer duration of activity and into the subcutaneous fat for larger procedures.

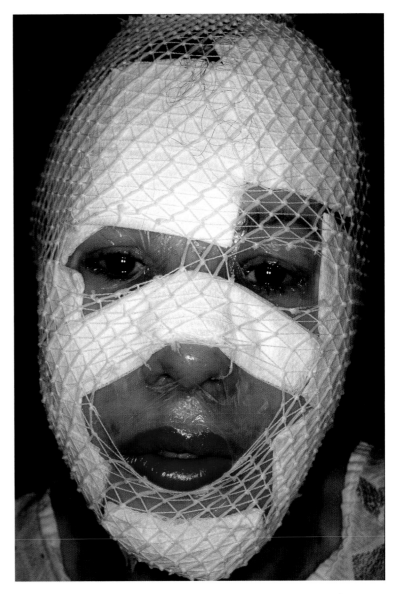

Figure 6.2 *Silon TSR dressing in place immediately following full-face carbon dioxide resurfacing*

TABLE 6.1 ■ Common Topical Anesthetics for Dermatologic Surgery

Topical agent	Composition	Occlusive required	Duration of occlusion (min)
EMLA (Astra Zeneca, Wayne, PA)	5% eutectic mix of lidocaine and prilocaine in an oil-in-water emulsion	Yes	60–90
LMX-4, LMX-5 (Ferndale Laboratories, Ferndale, MI)	4 or 5% lidocaine in liposomal vehicle	No	15–30
Betacaine-LA	Lidocaine, betacaine, and vasoconstrictor in liquid paraffin ointment	No	30–45
Tetracaine gel	4% tetracaine in a lethacin gel	Yes	30
Topicaine	4% lidocaine	Yes	60

TABLE 6.2 ▪ Recommended EMLA Dosing on Intact Skin for Infants and Children

Age	Body weight (kg)	Max total dose EMLA (gm)	Max application area (cm^2)
1–3 months	<5	1	10
4–12 months	5–10	2	20
1–6 years	>10–20	10	100
7–12 years	>20	20	200

Maximum recommended doses of lidocaine are 5 mg/kg plain, 7 mg/kg with epinephrine using 1–2% concentrations.

▪ Field Block

Injection of a ring of anesthetic around the proposed surgical site. It is useful for anesthetizing large areas while minimizing the amount of anesthetic used. This achieves anesthesia with minimal hemostasis. This is most frequently used on the scalp, nose, ear pinna, and truncal and extremities prior to the infiltration inside the ring block.

▪ Nerve Block

Injection of anesthetic near the region of a nerve to anesthetize a large area with minimal amounts of anesthetic. Anesthetic is injected near and not within a nerve or foramen to minimize the risk of nerve injury and subsequent dysesthesia. If a patient feels a sharp pain radiating along a nerve during injection, the needle must be withdrawn and repositioned to avoid injury. Care is also taken to avoid intravascular injection. Lidocaine (1%) with 1:100,000 epinephrine and bicarbonate is adequate in a majority of cases. A 30-gauge ½ inch or 1 inch needle is utilized with a 1–3 mL syringe. Alternatively, a 30-gauge, 13/16 short dental needle with a Septocaine cartridge (4% articaine hydrochloride with 1:100,000 epinephrine; Septodont, Inc.) may be used. Approximately 1 mL of anesthetic is generally sufficient per nerve block. Anesthetic effect may take 20–25 min. Topical anesthetic jelly can be applied to the buccal groove prior to the use of intraoral injections to minimize injection discomfort.

• Facial nerve blocks

 – Supraorbital nerve—Anesthetic injected perpendicularly into the skin immediately above the periosteum at the orbital rim in the mid-pupillary line (Fig. 6.3).

 – Supratrochlear nerve—Anesthetic injected perpendicularly into the skin above the periosteum at the superomedial orbital rim at the junction of the glabella and medial eyebrow (Fig. 6.4).

 – Infraorbital nerve—Two methods. Can be injected perpendicularly into the skin above the periosteum 1 cm inferior to the orbital rim in the mid-pupillary line.

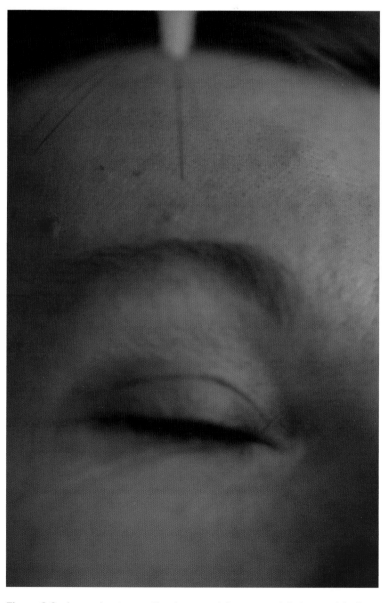

Figure 6.3 *Approximate needle placement for supraorbital nerve block*

TABLE 6.3 ■ **Local Anesthetics for Infiltrative Anesthesia**

Generic name	Onset (min)	Duration Plain (h)
Amides		
Bupivacaine	2–10	3–10
Etidocaine	3–5	3–10
Lidocaine	3–5	3–5
Mepivacaine	3–20	2–3
Prilocaine	5–6	0.5–2
Esters		
Benzocaine	Rapid	Short
Chloroprocaine	5–6	0.5–2
Cocaine	2–10	1–3
Procaine	5	1–1.5
Tetracaine	7	2–3

Can also be injected through an intraoral approach, with the needle being inserted between the first and second premolars, moving upward along the periosteum to 1 cm below the orbital rim. The needle is withdrawn as the anesthetic is deposited (Fig. 6.5).

– Intratrochlear nerve—Anesthetic injected perpendicular into the skin above the periosteum at the inferomedial orbital rim at the nasal–cheek junction.

– Anterior ethmoidal nerve—Anesthetic injected perpendicular into the skin within the perichondrial component of the lateral nasal tip.

– Mental nerve—Two methods. Can be injected perpendicular into the skin above the periosteum in the mid-pupillary line halfway above the mandible. Can also be injected through an intraoral approach, between the first and second premolars caudally along the periosteum to a halfway point down the mandible (Fig. 6.6).

– An additional 0.25 mL anesthetic is added at the base of the upper labial frenulum to completely numb the philthrum and Cupid's bow. An additional 0.1 mL is injected directly into each lateral oral commissure in a medial position to achieve complete lip anesthesia (Fig. 6.7).

• Digital nerve blocks: Two methods; similar for fingers and toes. Should be performed without epinephrine with small volumes (limited to less than 1.5 mL) to minimize the risk of ischemia due to mechanical compression of the blood supply.

– Anesthetic injected perpendicular to the digit near the base in the horizontal plane above the bone, positioned dorsally with injection followed by needle placement ventrally with additional anesthetic placed. Process repeated on other side of the digit.

– Anesthetic injected dorsally between the metacarpal/metatarsal bones with anesthetic administered while needle is advanced ventrally. Process repeated on the other side of the digit.

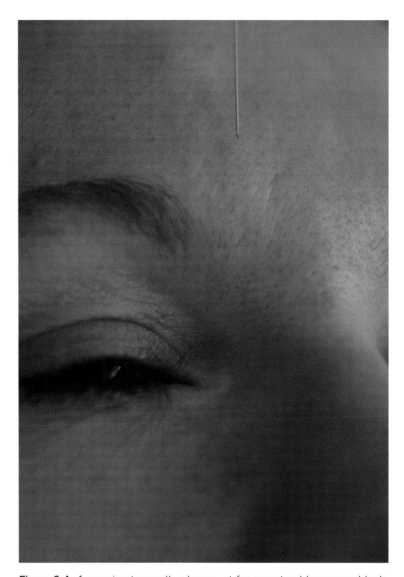

Figure 6.4 *Approximate needle placement for supratrochlear nerve block*

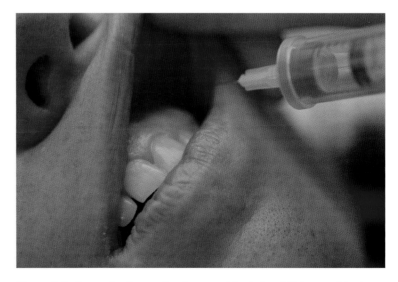

Figure 6.5 *Approximate needle placement for infraorbital nerve block—intraoral approach*

• Hand nerve block

  – Median nerve (palmar surface of first three and half fingers and two-thirds palmar surface)—Appose the thumb and fifth finger with slight wrist flexion to locate the palmaris longus tendon. Anesthetic injected into the first wrist crease immediately medial to the tendon, with advancement into the carpal tunnel.

  – Ulnar nerve (half of fourth finger, fifth finger, and one-third palmar surface—Arm flexed at the elbow. Anesthetic injected between the olecranon process and the humerus epicondyle.

• Foot nerve block: Anesthesia of the plantar surface requires nerve blocks of the tibial, sural, superficial peroneal, saphenous, and deep peroneal nerves. Patient placed in prone position. Anesthetic first injected immediately lateral to the palpable tibial artery between the medial malleolus and the Achilles tendon. Patient then placed in supine position and anesthetic injected from malleolus to malleolus on the dorsal surface of the foot. The patient foot is slightly dorsiflexed and the extensor hallucis longus tendon located. Anesthetic is injected lateral to the tendon.

Tumescent anesthesia (Tables 6.4-6.5)

Subcutaneous infiltration of large amounts of 0.05–0.1% lidocaine with 1:1,000,000 epinephrine through the use of long 18–20 gauge spinal needles or multiport cannulas

TABLE 6.4 ▪ **Tumescent Anesthesia Formula (for 1 L)**

Ingredient	Quantity (mL)
Lidocaine (1%)	50–100
Epinephrine (1:1000)	1
Sodium bicarbonate (8.4%)	10
Triamcinalone acetonide (40 mg/mL) (optional)	0.25
Normal saline (0.9%)	900–950

TABLE 6.5 ▪ **Contraindications to Local Anesthetics**

Absolute	Relative
Uncontrolled hyperthyroidism	End stage liver disease
Pheochromocytoma	Severe cardiac dysfunction; angina
Pseudocholinesterase deficiency (ester use contraindicated)	Pregnancy
Allergy to PABA related compounds	Nonselective beta-blockers
Allergy to antioxidants (metabisulfite, sodium bisulfite)	Injection site infection or inflammation

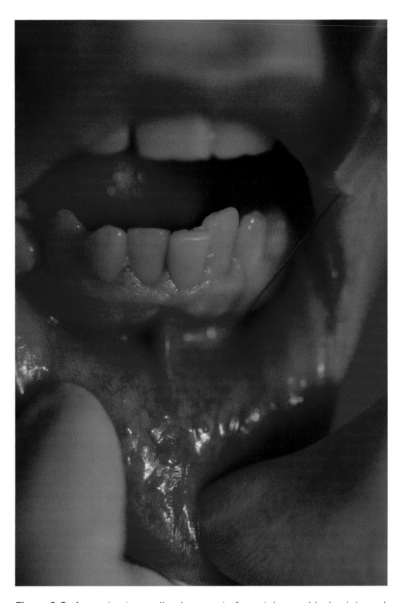

Figure 6.6 *Approximate needle placement of mental nerve block—intraoral approach*

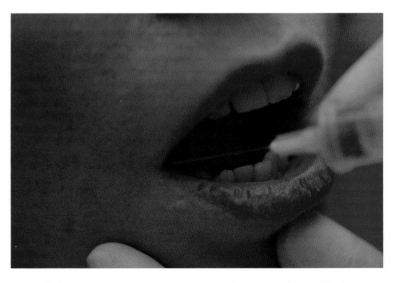

Figure 6.7 *Approximate needle placement for a commissure block*

via a pump. The deep subcutaneous tissue is infiltrated followed by the superficial fat component to achieve firm tissue tumescence. Anesthesia and epinephrine-induced hemostasis are achieved within about 20 min and last for several hours.

Maximum recommended dose: 35–50 mg/kg of 0.05–0.1% tumescent lidocaine with dilute epinephrine concentrations.

Overdosage

Symptoms are directly related to serum blood level. Central nervous symptoms start with circumoral and digital numbness and tingling, followed by lightheadedness, tinnitus, visual disturbances, slurred speech, muscle twitching, and finally seizures and coma. Cardiovascular symptoms develop at higher doses and include hypotension, arrhythmias, respiratory arrest, and cardiac arrest. Bupivacaine has a greater risk of cardiac toxicity than lidocaine. Prilocaine is metabolized to ortho-toluidine, an oxidizing agent capable of converting hemoglobin to methemoglobin, which is significant in infants or with the use of doses of more than 500 mg.

PEARLS FOR TREATMENT SUCCESS

- Addition of 8.4% sodium bicarbonate to 1–2% lidocaine with 1:100,000 epinephrine in a 1:10 ratio (1 mL 8.4% lidocaine for every 9 mL lidocaine) reduces the acidity of the solution for a reduction of injection pain.

- Injection discomfort can be reduced by using smaller gauge needles (e.g., 30 gauge) and injecting with smaller syringes (e.g., 1–3 mL), both of which can reduce tissue pressure.

- Most adverse reactions to anesthetic agents are vasovagal in nature and can be minimized by performing the procedure in a supine position and managed by placing patient in a Trendelenburg position with cool compresses.

- For patients with allergic reactions (e.g., hypersensitivity to methylparabens or sodium metabisulfite), possible agents to use in a controlled environment include ester-class anesthetics or paraben-free lidocaine.

- Epinephrine is usually avoided in patients with a history of cardiac arrythmias, in pregnant women and used with caution in patients on beta-blockers or digital lesions.

BIBLIOGRAPHY

Alster TS. Cutaneous resurfacing with CO_2 and erbium: YAG lasers: preoperative, intraoperative and postoperative considerations. *Plast Reconstr Surg*. 1999;103: 619–634.

Arpey CJ, Lynch WS. Advances in local anesthesia. *Dermatol Clin*. 1992;10:275–283.

Auletta MJ. Local anesthesia for dermatologic surgery. *Semin Dermatol*. 1994;13:35–42.

David L, Ruiz-Esparza J. Fast healing after laser skin resurfacing. The minimal mechanical trauma technique. *Dermatol Surg.* 1997;23:359–361.

Dover JS, Hruza GJ, Arndt KA. Lasers in skin resurfacing. *Semin Cutan Med Surg.* 1996;15:177–188.

Duke D, Grevelink JM. Care before and after laser skin resurfacing. A survey and review of the literature. *Dermatol Surg.* 1998;24:201–206.

Friedman PM, Fogelman JP, Nouri K, et al. Comparative study of the efficacy of four topical anesthetics. *Dermatol Surg.* 1999;25:950–954.

Nanni CA, Alster TS. Complications of carbon dioxide laser resurfacing: an evaluation of 500 patients. *Dermatol Surg.* 1998;24:315–320.

Ruiz-Esparza J, Barba Gomez JM, Gomez de la Torre OL. Wound care after laser skin resurfacing. A combination of open and closed methods using a new polyethylene mask. *Dermatol Surg.* 1998;24:79–81.

Szzchowicz EH, Wright WK. Delayed healing after full-face chemical peels. *Facial Plast Surg.* 1989;6(1):6–13.

Van der Hove J, Decroix J, Tennstedt D, et al. Allergic contact dermatitis from prilocaine, one of the local anesthetics in EMLA cream. *Contact Dermat.* 1994;30(4):239.

Zukowski ML, Mossie RD, Roth SI, et al. Pilot study analysis of the histologic and bacteriologic effects of occlusive dressings in chemosurgical peel using a minipig model. *Aesthetic Plast Surg.* 1993;17:53–59.

CHAPTER 7 Actinic Keratosis

Single or multiple discrete, scaly lesions, found most frequently in habitually sun-exposed skin of adults.

EPIDEMIOLOGY

Age: most commonly noted in middle age; rarely occurs in patients under 30

Sex: more common in males

Incidence: very common; in Australia 1:1000 persons

Race: skin phototypes I–III; rarely seen in skin phototypes IV–VI

Occupation: outdoor workers (e.g., farmer, rancher, sailor) and outdoor sports (golf, tennis, sailing)

PATHOGENESIS

Prolonged and repeated sun exposure in susceptible persons results in cumulative keratinocyte damage. Principle sun damage secondary to UVB (290–320 nm) light.

PHYSICAL EXAMINATION

Single or multiple skin-colored, erythematous, or brown scaly patches. Predilection for sun-exposed areas including the face, ears, neck, forearms, dorsal hands. May become thickened, forming a cutaneous horn. More easily palpated than seen. Generally asymptomatic but may be tender or pruritic. Actinic cheilitis develops on the vermilion border as diffuse scaling or dryness. Associated telangiectasia, solar elastosis, and lentigines frequently observed.

DERMATOPATHOLOGY

Epidermal proliferation; mild to moderate basilar keratinocyte pleomorphism, parakeratosis, dyskeratotic keratinocytes. Cytologically atypical keratinocytes confined to the epidermal basal layer.

DIFFERENTIAL DIAGNOSIS

- Discoid lupus erythematosus
- Eczematous dermatitis
- Extramammary Paget's

COURSE

Keratoses can self-resolve, but generally are persistent in nature. Progression to skin cancer within preexisting keratoses unknown but estimated at less than 1% of individual lesions. Biopsy warranted for pigmented keratosis (superficial pigmented actinic keratosis) or nodular keratosis.

KEY CONSULTATIVE QUESTIONS

- Duration of lesion(s)
- Lesional rate of growth
- Prior treatment for lesions and response
- Personal and family history of prior skin cancers
- History of prior radiation treatment to the area
- Current medical history
- Medication use
- Evidence of immunosuppression
- Predisposing syndromes

MANAGEMENT

Assessment of the number, size, location, frequency of development and any underlying immunosuppressed state should be obtained. A biopsy should be obtained of any lesion that is suspicious for skin cancers. Consideration may then be given to treatment of individual or multiple lesions, prophylactic therapy, and determination of the need for clinical follow-up.

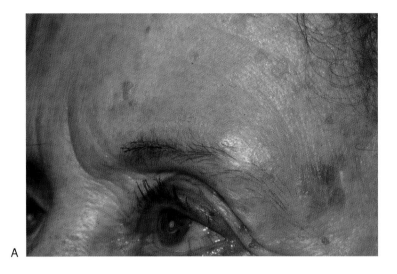

A

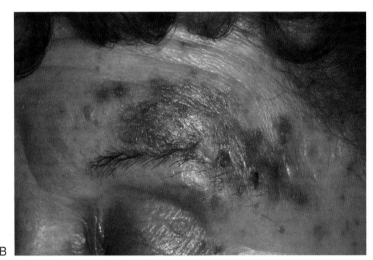

B

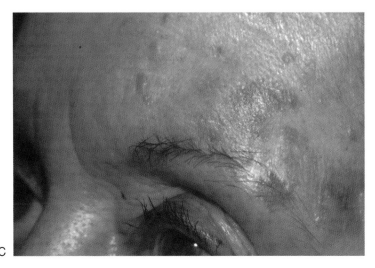

C

Figure 7.1 **(A)** *Numerous facial actinic keratoses pre-Aldara treatment.* **(B)** *Expected erythema and crusting during Aldara treatment.* **(C)** *Facial actinic keratoses post-Aldara treatment applied twice weekly for 4 weeks (Photographs courtesy of Richard Johnson, MD)*

TREATMENT

- Prevention

    - Application of daily sunscreen with UVA/UVB protection

    - Topical tretinoin applied nightly

- Topical

    - Once daily (Carac) or twice daily (Efudex) application of 5% 5-fluorouracil for 3–4 weeks

    - Twice weekly or every third day application of imiquinod (Aldara 3m St. Paul mn) for 4 weeks (Fig 7.1)

    - Diclofenac (Solaraze) 3% sodium topical gel twice daily for 2–3 months

    - Gentle cryosurgery with a single freeze–thaw cycle. Blister formation possible. Repeat treatment may be required. Risk of temporary and permanent pigmentary changes must be addressed to the patient. Best for isolated number of lesions

- Systemic

    - Long-term low-dose oral retinoid has been used; requires close follow-up to avoid potential side effects. Beneficial only while on medication

    - Oral vitamin A has been used; requires close follow-up to avoid potential side effects. Beneficial only while on medication

- Surgical

    - Photodynamic therapy with topical aminolevulinic acid (Lerulen, Dusa, pharmaceutis, Wilmington, MA) has been successfully utilized. Multiple treatments required. Topical levulan applied 1 h prior to light treatment may be used. Photosensitivity post-treatment prominent

    - Chemical peels—serial medium-depth peels including Jessner/10–35% trichloroacetic acid peels are highly beneficial in reducing lesion count. Postoperative peeling may last up to 2 weeks depending on the strength utilized

    - Pulsed carbon dioxide laser—highly effective in management of actinic cheilitis (Fig. 7.2). The vermilion border is outlined prior to the administration of mental block and/or localized infiltrative anesthesia with 1% lidocaine with 1:100,000 epinephrine. Ultrapulse CO_2, 3-mm collimated handpiece, 500 mJ/pulse, nonoverlapping pulses utilized or CPG, density 6, 60 W, and 300 mJ/pulse or Sharplan Feathertouch, 36 W, 200-mm handpiece, and 6-mm scan size can provide benefit. Passes are performed until removal of epidermis is observed. Area wiped with saline soaked sponges between the passes. Postoperative care requires soaking the treatment site with water and a clean washcloth to remove any crusting and application of vaseline 3–4 times/day. Risk of scar formation and infection must be considered

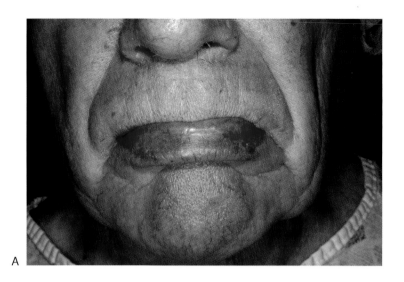

A

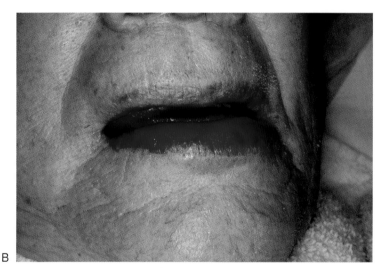

B

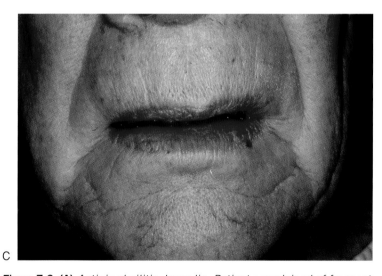

C

Figure 7.2 (A) *Actinic cheilitis, lower lip. Patient complained of frequent peeling that was poorly responsive to cryosurgery.* **(B)** *Lower lip confluent erythema immediately following carbon dioxide resurfacing.* **(C)** *Reduction in actinic damage 12 weeks following carbon dioxide resurfacing. Patient reported complete resolution of peeling*

PITFALLS TO AVOID

- With actinic cheilitis, it is essential to avoid vaporization of the vermilion border to prevent scarring. Delineating the border prior to administration of anesthesia is helpful.

- Patients must be aware that any treatment administered does not eliminate the development of future premalignant and malignant growths. Strict photoprotection and sun avoidance is mandatory.

- Patients utilizing topical treatments must be made aware of the expected erythema, crusting, and discomfort that will persist for the duration of treatment and for 1–2 weeks post-treatment. A mild topical corticosteroid may be prescribed post-treatment completion to assist in the resolution of these findings.

BIBLIOGRAPHY

Alberts D, Ranger-Moore J, Einspahr J, et al. Safety and efficacy of dose-intensive oral vitamin A in subjects with sun-damaged skin. *Clin Cancer Res.* March 15, 2004;10(6):1875–1880.

Cartmel B, Moon TE, Levine N. Effects of long-term intake of retinal on selected clinical and laboratory indexes. *Am J Clin Nutr.* 1999;67:937–943.

Ericson MB, Sandberg C, Stenquist B, et al. Photodynamic therapy of actinic keratosis at varying fluence rates: assessment of photobleaching, pain and primary clinical outcome. *Br J Dermatol.* December 2004;151(6):1204–1212.

Glogau RG. The risk of progression to invasive disease. *J Am Acad Dermatol.* 2000;42:S23–S24.

Jorizzo JL, Carney PS, Ko WT, et al. Fluorouracil 5% and 0.5% creams for the treatment of actinic keratosis: equivalent efficacy with a lower concentration and more convenient dosing schedule. *Cutis.* December 2004;74(suppl 6):18–23.

Lysa B, Tatler U, Wolf R, et al. Gene expression in actinic keratoses: pharmacological modulation by imiquinod. *Br J Dermatol.* December 2004;151(6):1150–1159.

Nelson C, Rigel D, Smith S, et al. Phase IV, open-label assessment of the treatment of actinic keratosis with 3.0% diclofenac sodium topical gel (Solaraze). *J Drugs Dermatol.* July–August 2004;3(4);401–407.

Szeimies RM, Gerritsen MJ, Gupta G, et al. Imiquimod 5% cream for the treatment of actinic keratosis: results from a phase IAII, randomized, double-blind, vehicle-controlled, clinical trial with histology. *J Am Acad Dermatol.* October 2004;51(4):547–555.

Thai KE, Fergin P, Freeman M, et al. A prospective study of the use of cryosurgery for the treatment of actinic keratoses. *Int J Dermatol.* September 2004;43(9):687–692.

CHAPTER 8 Dermatochalasis

Dermatochalasis is a condition characterized by upper eyelid skin and muscle redundancy and laxity and is attributable to chronological aging and chronic sun exposure.

EPIDEMIOLOGY

Incidence: very common

Age: most frequently observed in persons over 50 years

Sex: no predilection

Race: most common in fair-skinned individuals (skin phototypes I and II); less common in darker skinned individuals (skin phototypes IV–VI)

Precipitating factors: chronological aging; chronic sun exposure

PATHOGENESIS

Upper eyelid skin and muscle hypertrophy and prolapse.

PHYSICAL EXAMINATION

Early findings include a double lid crease with only modest hooding. Severe findings include prominent eyelid hooding with upper and lateral visual field obstruction. Coexisting brow ptosis may further compromise the peripheral vision.

DIFFERENTIAL DIAGNOSIS

Blepharochalasis (recurrent idiopathic eyelid inflammation with resultant relaxation of the upper lid skin); upper eyelid hooding secondary to eyebrow ptosis.

DERMATOPATHOLOGY

Epidermal acanthosis with flattening of the dermal–epidermal junction. Dermal collagen breakdown with formation of amorphous masses and increase in glycosaminoglycans.

COURSE

Chronic progressive course; visual eye fields may be affected.

KEY CONSULTATIVE QUESTIONS

• Any associated symptoms including visual obstruction, dry eyes

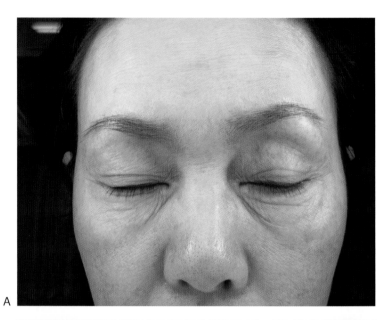

A

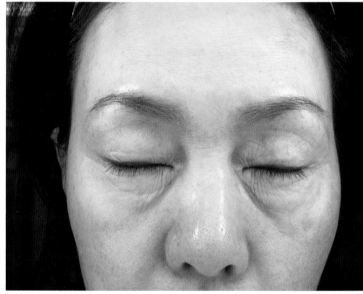

B

Figure 8.1 (A) *A 59-year-old female concerned about her sunken eyes and forehead wrinkles.* **(B)** *Improvement of the blephaloptosis, sunken eyes, and forehead wrinkles 9 months following upper lid blepharoplasty and lavator aponeurotica advancement (photographs courtesy of Harue Suzuki, MD, Kyoto, Japan)*

- Underlying medical conditions
- Prior treatment and response

MANAGEMENT

Prevention: strict sun avoidance.

TREATMENT

- Topical therapy: daily sunscreen application with UVB/UVA coverage
- Surgical therapy
  - Coronal browlift—upper face rejuvenation
  - Trichophytic browlift—upper face rejuvenation
  - Blepharoplasty—upper and lower eyelid rejuvenation (Fig. 8.1)
  - Carbon dioxide laser—upper and lower eyelid rejuvenation
  - Nd:YAG 1064 laser—upper and lower eyelid rejuvenation

PITFALLS TO AVOID

- A conservative approach to surgical removal of this skin is vital to prevent a "startled" appearance.
- Retention of all or portions of any herniated fat pads helps minimize the skeletonized appearance often noted to develop with age and loss of facial volume.

BIBLIOGRAPHY

Carter S, Seiff S, Choo P. Lower eyelid CO_2 laser rejuvenation: a randomized prospective clinical study. *Ophthalmology.* 2001;108:437–441.

Lemke BN, Stasior OG. The anatomy of eyelid ptosis. *Arch Ophthalmol.* 1932;100:981–986.

Mayer TG, Fleming RW. *Aesthetic and Reconstructive Surgery of the Scalp.* St. Louis: Mosby Year Book; 1992.

Shorr N, Enzer Y. Considerations in aesthetic eyelid surgery. *J Dermatol Surg Oncol.* 1992;1:1081–1095.

CHAPTER 9 Poikiloderma of Civatte

Poikiloderma of Civatte (POC) is a condition that is attributable to chronic sun exposure of the neck and the chest. The severity of findings is dependent on the duration and intensity of sun exposure, constitutive skin color (Fitzpatrick skin type), and the capacity to tan.

EPIDEMIOLOGY

Incidence: common

Age: most frequently observed in persons over 40 years

Sex: slight female predominance

Race: most common in fair-skinned individuals (skin phototypes I and II); rarely seen in darker skinned individuals (skin phototypes IV–VI)

Precipitating factors: chronic sun exposure including intentional sun exposure since youth and occupational exposure; trauma; chronological aging

PATHOGENESIS

UVB is the most damaging ultraviolet radiation; with high dose UVA contributing to the noted changes. In addition, visible and infrared radiations have been shown to augment the action of UVB.

PHYSICAL EXAMINATION

Telangiectases, mild atrophy, reticulated hyperpigmentation, and hypopigmentation affecting the lateral and posterior aspect of the neck, anterior chest, and jawline. Submental neck is spared. Perifollicular sparing noted (Figs. 9.1 and 9.2).

DERMATOPATHOLOGY

Epidermal acanthosis with flattening of the dermal–epidermal junction. Focal increase in epidermal basilar melanocytes; irregular basilar hyperpigmentation. Dermal collagen breakdown with formation of amorphous masses and increase in glycosaminoglycans. Telangiectasia noted.

DIFFERENTIAL DIAGNOSIS

Rothmund–Thomson syndrome; radiation dermatitis.

COURSE

Chronic progressive course.

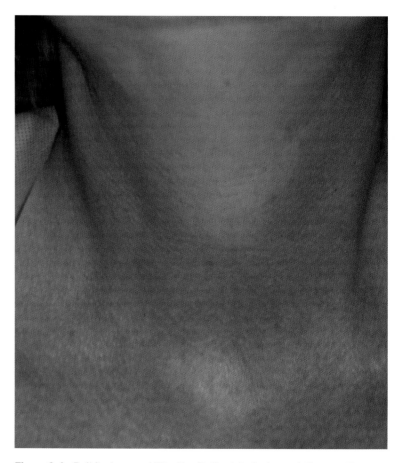

Figure 9.1 *Poikiloderma of Civatte. Reticulated pigmentation, erythema, and atrophy can be seen with characteristic sparing of the submental area. The erythematous component is more prominent in this patient*

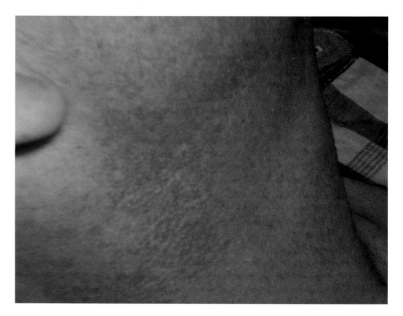

Figure 9.2 *Poikiloderma of Civatte—the pigmented component is more prominent in this patient*

KEY CONSULTATIVE QUESTIONS

- Past and current sun exposure history
- Occupation
- Hobbies/sporting activities
- Past treatments and response

MANAGEMENT

Prevention: strict sun avoidance.

TREATMENT

- Topical therapy: daily sunscreen application with UVB/UVA coverage
- Surgical therapy: great caution must be followed with any surgical treatment administered to minimize the risk of scar formation, hypopigmentation with "fingerprinting," and textural changes. The neck is particularly prone to scarring. A test site is recommended. Multiple sessions are generally required

  - Pulsed dye laser—low fluences utilized (Scleroplus 595 nm, 3–4.5 J/cm^2, 7-mm spot, DCD 30/20 with 10% overlapping passes). Improvement in telangiectasia and atrophy seen. Limited benefit for dyspigmentation

  - Intense pulsed light (Starlux, 20–30 ms, 28–34 J/dm^2, 10% pass overlap)—improvement of all components possible

  - Versapulse 532-nm laser—low fluences necessary (Fig 9.3)

  - Fraxel laser (250 ms, 6–7 J/cm^2, eight passes)—all components targeted. Can be safely utilized in all treatment sites. Postoperative sunburn-like erythema lasting up to 1 week and bronzing lasting 1 day expected

PITFALLS TO AVOID

- A conservative approach must be followed with any treatment used for POC given the significant risk of uneven removal of the pigmentation and erythema resulting in a "footprint" like appearance. (Figure 9.4) This mottled appearance can occur normally during the course of treatment. The patient must be aware of this possibility. Continued treatment to the residual lesions generally results in a resolution of this side effect.

- Patients must be aware of the difficulty in improving this condition. Multiple treatments are expected for endpoint of lightening.

- POC with a primary erythematous component typically responds better than POC with a primarily hyperpigmented component.

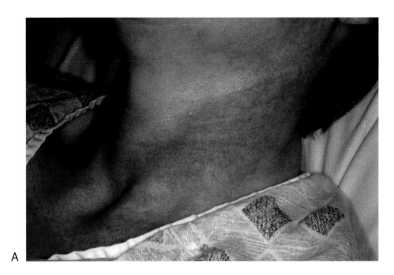

A

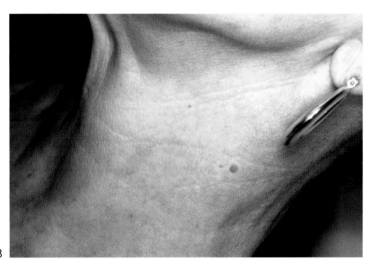

B

Figure 9.3 (A) *Poikiloderma of Civatte pretreatment.* **(B)** *Poikiloderma of Civatte following three Versapulse 532-nm laser treatments. Marked reduction in erythematous component is observed*

BIBLIOGRAPHY

Batta K, Hindson C, Cotterill JA, Foulds IS. Treatment of poikiloderma of Civatte with the potassium titanyl phosphate (KTP) laser. *Br J Dermatol.* June 1999; 140(6):1191–1192.

Geronemus R. Poikiloderma of Civatte. *Arch Dermatol.* April 1990;126(4):547–548.

Goldman MP, Weiss RA. Treatment of poikiloderma of Civatte with an intense pulsed light source. *Plast Reconstr Surg.* May 2001;107(6):1376–1381.

Langeland J. Treatment of poikiloderma of Civatte with the pulsed dye laser: a series of seven cases. *J Cutan Laser Ther.* April 1999;1(2):127.

Lautenschlager S, Itin PH. Reticulate, patchy and mottled pigmentation of the neck. Acquired forms. *Dermatology.* 1998;197(3):291–296.

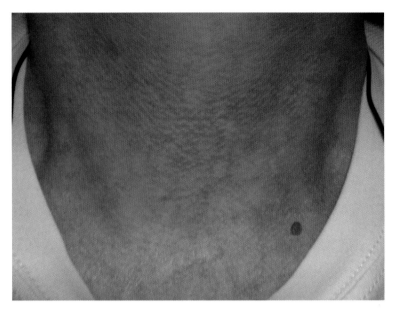

Figure 9.4 *"Footprinting" of the anterior neck after a single intense pulsed light (IPL) source treatment for Poikiloderma of Civatte. This subsequently resolved with continued IPL treatments*

SECTION
TWO

Disorders of Sebaceous Glands

CHAPTER 10 Acne Vulgaris

Acne vulgaris is a chronic inflammatory disease of the pilosebaceous unit. Acne lesions favor the face, neck, upper back, chest, and upper arms. Multiple clinical variants exist and they include comedonal acne, papulopustular acne, nodulocystic acne, acne conglobata, and acne fulminans.

EPIDEMIOLOGY

Incidence and age: predominantly a disorder of adolescence. Affects 85% of individuals between 12 and 24 years of age. May affect all age groups

Race: lower incidence in African-Americans and Asians

Sex: more severe forms in males

Precipitating factors: genetic predisposition, endocrine disorders, stress, mechanical factors (friction, pressure, occlusion), contact with acnegenic materials (oils, chlorinated hydrocarbons, cosmetics), drugs (steroids, lithium, androgens, hydantoin)

PATHOGENESIS

Many patients with nodulocystic acne have a first-degree relative with a history of severe acne. The primary pathophysiology involves altered follicular keratinization resulting in obstruction of sebaceous follicles, increased sebum production, hyperproliferation of *Propionibacterium acnes*, and increased production of chemotactic factors which result in inflammation.

PHYSICAL EXAMINATION

Comedones (closed and open), erythematous papules, pustules, nodules, and cysts. May resolve with residual hyperpigmentation or scarring.

DIFFERENTIAL DIAGNOSIS

Acne rosacea, steroid acne, acne mechanica, pityrosporum folliculitis, and bacterial folliculitis.

LABORATORY DATA

■ Endocrine Studies

Screen for free and total testosterone, dehydroepiandrosterone, and FSH/LH ratios to exclude polycystic ovary syndrome or other hormonal abnormalities especially in women with moderate to severe acne, hirsutism, irregular menses, and weight gain.

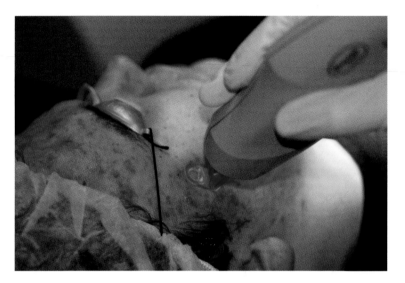

Figure 10.1 *An 18-year-old male with cystic acne being treated with 1450-nm diode laser*

■ Dermatopathology

Pathology of early lesion (comedone) reveals obstruction of the follicular infundibulum by cornified cells leading to dilatation. Later lesions reveal follicular rupture with lymphocytes, neutrophils, and macrophages. Scarring may be seen.

COURSE

This disease demonstrates a chronic course and remits spontaneously in the early to mid third decade in the majority of patients. However, acne may persist much longer in some patients.

MANAGEMENT

Early treatment of acne is essential for the prevention of lasting cosmetic disfigurement associated with scarring (see scar treatment chapters). Many acne patients benefit from combination therapies. A thorough history and physical examination are paramount to administering a maximally effective plan. This should include current cosmetics and sunscreens, skin type, lifestyle, occupation, medications, past treatments and response, menstrual and oral contraceptive history.

■ Topical Treatment

Topical treatment may be required for the duration of this condition. Topical formulations should be applied to the lesions as well as to the adjacent acne-prone clinically normal skin.

- Retinoids: tretinoin, adapalene, tazarotene.
- Antibacterial agents: benzoyl peroxide, clindamycin, erythromycin.
- Keratolytic agents: salicylic acid, α-hydroxy acid, azelaic acid, sodium sulfacetamide, and sulfur.

■ Systemic Treatment

- Antibiotics: tetracycline, doxycycline, minocycline are most commonly used. Alternatives include erythromycin, azithromycin, and amoxicillin.
- Hormones: oral contraceptives and spironolactone for women with persistent acne on lower face, chin, and neck.
- Isotretinoin: for severe nodulocystic acne that has failed other topical and systemic therapies.

■ Surgical Treatment

- Comedone extraction: expression of keratinous contents of open comedones by applying the comedone extractor to the comedones and applying pressure. A

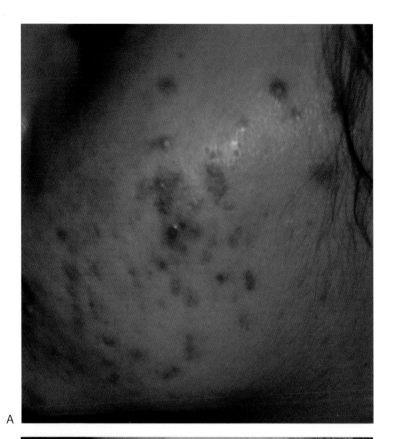

A

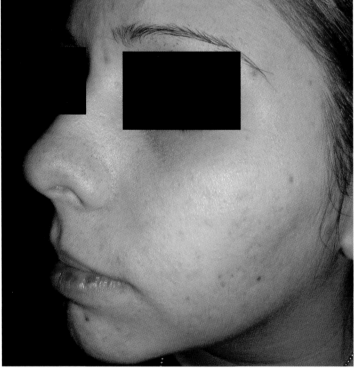

B

Figure 10.2 (A) *Facial inflammatory acne vulgaris unresponsive to multiple topical and oral treatment regimens.* **(B)** *Marked improvement of acne 6 months following five 1450 nm diode laser treatments (Smoothbeam, Candela Corp., Wayland, MA), 6 mm spot, 14 J/cm², DCD 30 ms*

nick may be made to the overlying skin with an #11-blade or 18-gauge needle to ease in the extraction. The Schamberg, Unna, and Saalfield comedone expressors are most commonly utilized. Comedone extraction is contraindicated for inflamed comedones or pustules due to increased scar risk.

- Intralesional steroid injection: Triamcinolone acetonide (2–5 mg/mL) is injected into inflamed cystic lesions using a 30-gauge needle. Maximum dose injected should not exceed 0.1 mL per lesion to avoid atrophy.

- Chemical peels: serial salicylic acid peels, glycolic acid peels (20–70%), and TCA peels (10–20%) have been utilized to reduce the number of comedones and improve post-inflammatory hyperpigmentation and persistent erythema. Peels may be performed every 2–3 weeks, with increasing strengths applied as tolerated. Mild irritation may be observed. Adjunctive therapy is generally necessary. Chemical peels are not effective for cystic acne.

- Microdermabrasion: this is primarily effective for comedonal acne. It is usually performed every 2–3 weeks.

■ Light Treatment

- Lasers: lasers and light treatments are not the first-line therapy for acne but can be useful as an alternative or adjuvant to medical therapy when required.

  - 1450-nm diode laser (Smoothbeam laser, Candela Corp., Wayland, MA): treatment fluences from 10 to 14 J/cm^2, 6-mm spot size and dynamic cooling device setting of 30–40 ms can result in mild to moderate improvement of inflammatory back and facial acne with a significant reduction in lesion count after an average of three to five treatments, separated by 2–6 week intervals (Fig. 10.1, 10.2). It is important to deliver non-overlapping pulses to prevent scarring. Topical lidocaine cream applied prior to treatment is needed to minimize the treatment-associated pain.

  - Pulsed dye laser (PDL): studies examining the efficacy of PDL for inflammatory acne have produced conflicting data. A single low fluence (1.5–3 J/cm^2) 585-nm PDL treatment has been shown in one study to improve mild to moderate facial inflammatory acne. A subsequent study published by Orringer et al. showed no significant improvement in inflammatory facial acne utilizing PDL. However, PDL can improve post-acne erythema. Fluences of 5.5–7 J/cm^2 with pulse durations of 3–6 ms are most commonly employed. Serial treatments are needed to achieve the greatest benefit.

- Phototherapy: multiple light sources have been reported to significantly improve acne with minimal side effects. These sources include high-intensity narrow-band blue light, high-intensity metal halide lamp, high-energy broad-spectrum blue-light as well as mixed blue and red light.

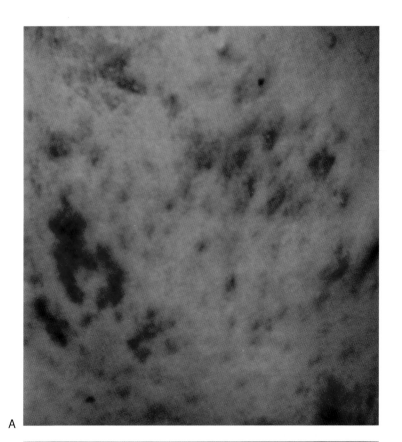
A

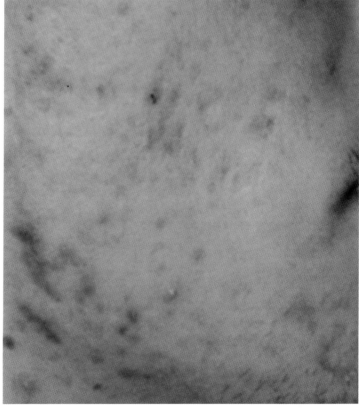
B

Figure 10.3 (A) *Severe acne before treatment.* **(B)** *After three treatments of photodynamic therapy with topical 5-aminolevulinic acid and pulsed dye laser, 7 mm spot, 6 J/cm^2, 6-ms pulse duration (courtesy of Mark Nestor, MD, PhD)*

- Photodynamic therapy (PDT): PDT utilizing the topical administration of 5-aminolevulinic acid (ALA, Levulan Kerastick, DUSA Pharmaceuticals, Inc., Wilmington, MA) activated by light exposure is another potentially effective modality to treat acne (Figs. 10.3-10.4). Short contact ALA-PDT (15–60 min drug incubation) was capable of improving acne significantly in a variety of clinical studies. Different light sources have been utilized including blue light (405–420 nm), red light (635 nm), and intense pulsed light (430–1200 nm).

BIBLIOGRAPHY

Elman M, Lebzelter J. Light therapy in the treatment of acne vulgaris. *Dermatol Surg.* February 2004;30(2, pt 1): 139–146.

Friedman PM, Jih MH, Kimyai-Asadi A, Goldberg LH. Treatment of inflammatory facial acne vulgaris with the 1450-nm diode laser: a pilot study. *Dermatol Surg.* February 2004;30(2, pt 1):147–151.

Orringer JS, Kang S, Hamilton T, et al. Treatment of acne vulgaris with a pulsed dye laser: a randomized controlled trial. *JAMA.* 2004;291:2834-2839.

Paithankar DY, Ross EV, Saleh BA, Blair MA, Graham BS. Acne treatment with a 1,450 nm wavelength laser and cryogen spray cooling. *Lasers Surg Med.* 2002;31(2): 106–114.

Pollock B, Turner D, Stringer MR, Bojar RA, Goulden V, Stables GI, Cunliffe WJ. Topical aminolaevulinic acid-photodynamic therapy for the treatment of acne vulgaris: a study of clinical efficacy and mechanism of action. *Br J Dermatol.* September 2004;151(3):616–622.

Seaton ED, Charakida A, Mouser PE, et al. Pulsed-dye laser treatment for inflammatory acne vulgaris: a randomised controlled trial. *Lancet.* 2003;362:1347–1352.

Taub AF. Photodynamic therapy for the treatment of acne: a pilot study. *J Drugs Dermatol.* November–December 2004;3(suppl 6):S10–S14.

White GM. Recent findings in the epidemiologic evidence, classification, and subtypes of acne vulgaris. *J Am Acad Dermatol.* August 1998;39(2, pt 3):S34–S37.

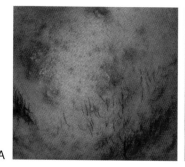
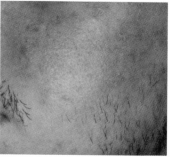

Figure 10.4 (A) *Facial inflammatory acne prior to photodynamic therapy.* **(B)** *Marked reduction of the inflammatory acne after three sessions of photodynamic therapy (courtesy of Mark Nestor, MD, PhD)*

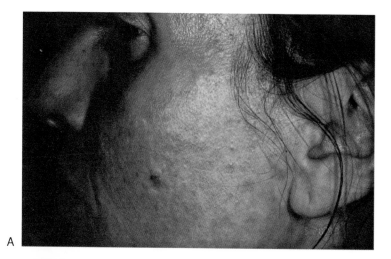

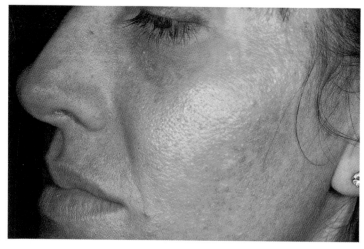

Figure 10.5 (A) *Mild acne scarring and dyschromia prior to Er:YAG laser resurfacing.* **(B)** *Four months after Er:YAG laser resurfacing utilizing a 5 mm spot at 1 J with four passes results in significant improvement (Jeffrey D, Kenneth A, Roy G, Beatrice AM, eds. Illustrated Cutaneous & Aesthetic Laser Surgery. McGraw-Hill, Inc.; 2000)*

CHAPTER 11 | Rosacea

Acne rosacea is a chronic vascular and acneiform disorder of the pilosebaceous unit that affects predominantly the central face including the central cheeks, nose, and chin. The eyes and the eyelids can occasionally be involved. Typically, there is an increased reactivity of capillaries to heat, leading to flushing and ultimately telangiectasia. Subtypes of rosacea include (a) vascular rosacea (erythematotelangiectatic), (b) papulopustular rosacea, (c) sebaceous hyperplasia (phymatous rosacea) including rhinophyma (nasal sebaceous hyperplasia), and (d) ocular rosacea. Granulomatous rosacea is a variant of rosacea.

EPIDEMIOLOGY

Incidence: common

Age: 30–50 years; peak incidence between 40 and 50 years

Sex: female predilection; male predominance for rhinophyma

Race: most common in fair-skinned individuals (skin phototypes I and II); rarely seen in darker skinned individuals (skin phototypes IV–VI)

Precipitating factors: excessive sun exposure, caffeine, spicy foods, hot foods and beverages, heat, alcohol, seborrhea, topical corticosteroid use, and underlying Parkinson's disease

PATHOGENESIS

Multiple factors are involved in the pathogenesis of rosacea including vascular hyperactivity, *Demodex folliculorum* mites, *Helicobacter pylori*, and hypersensitivity to *Propionibacterium acnes*.

PHYSICAL EXAMINATION

Variable clinical features can be present depending on the severity and the subtype of rosacea. Early features include transient and nontransient flushing, erythematous papules, and pustules. No comedones are noted. Late features include telangiectasias, sebaceous hyperplasia, nasal thickening and enlargement (rhinophyma), and lymphedema. Ocular involvement is frequently seen.

DIFFERENTIAL DIAGNOSIS

Acne vulgaris, seborrheic dermatitis, perioral dermatitis, steroid rosacea, systemic lupus erythematosus, and lupus miliaris disseminatus faciei.

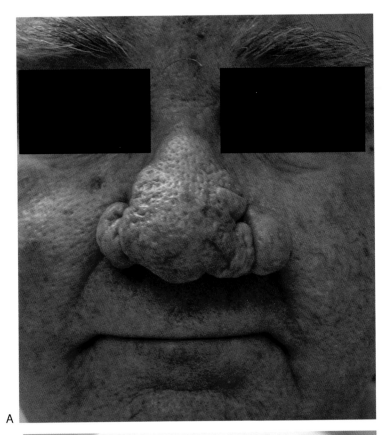

A

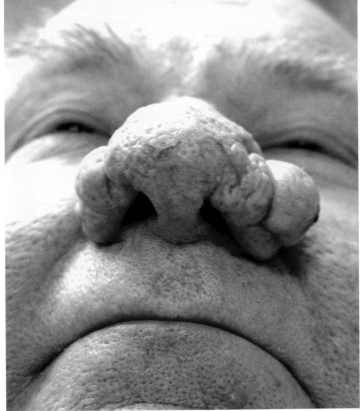

B

Figure 11.1 (A, B) *Severe rhinophyma prior to electrosurgery.*

DERMATOPATHOLOGY

Vascular ectasia as well as perifollicular and perivascular lymphohistiocytic infiltrates are the most common findings. *Demodex folliculorum* is usually detected in the follicles. Noncaseating epithelioid granulomas are seen in the granulomatous variant. Sebaceous hyperplasia and fibrosis are seen in rhinophyma.

COURSE

Chronic with frequent recurrences. May spontaneously resolve after several years.

MANAGEMENT

▨ Prevention

Reduction or elimination of exacerbants; sun avoidance.

▨ Topical Therapy

Metronidazole (0.75–1%) once or twice daily, 10% sodium sulfacetamide with 5% sulfur once daily, azelaic acid once daily, alone or in combination are helpful in suppressing the papulopustular component of rosacea.

▨ Systemic Therapy

- Tetracycline, 1000–1500 mg daily in divided doses, until clear; then taper to a maintenance dose of 250–500 mg daily.

- Minocycline and doxycycline, 50–100 mg twice daily, with a tapering to once daily use.

- Oral isotretinoin is reserved for severe cases not responding to oral antibiotics and requires close follow-up. A low-dose regimen may be effective.

▨ Surgical Therapy

Rhinophyma
Multiple surgical modalities have been used to correct the hypertrophic changes of rhinophyma. It is important to examine a photograph of the patient prior to the onset of the rhinophymatous change in order to help guide the surgeon in the remodeling of the nose. A regional nerve block with additional local anesthesia is sufficient in the majority of cases for perioperative pain management. Direct injection of anesthesia requires multiple infiltrations and is less effective and far more painful.

- Electrosurgery: electrosection (cutting) is very effective in debulking and recontouring the rhinophymatous nose with the added advantage of a relatively bloodless field. It is similar in efficacy to CO_2 laser treatment and less expensive (Fig. 11.1).

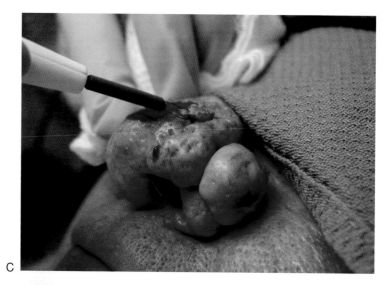

C

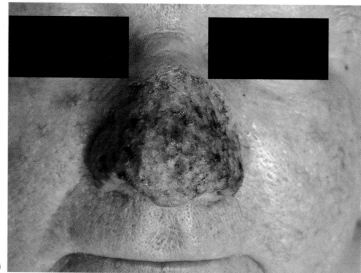

D

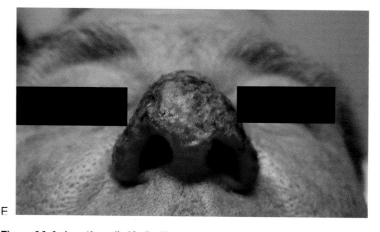

E

Figure 11.1 (*continued*) (C, D, E) *Debulking and recontouring of the rhinophymatous nose in a relatively bloodless field utilizing large wire loop electrosurgery. Impressive flattening of the rhinophymatous nose after electrosurgery. The wound is left to heal by secondary intention (courtesy of Suzanne Olbricht, MD)*

– The hypertrophied tissue is removed with care to preserve the pilosebaceous units.

○ Overcorrection will produce scarring and contractures. Wound contracture with healing may pull the nasal tip upward.

○ Permanent depigmentation may result from overvigorous treatment.

– The Ellman Surgitron can be used with a large wire loop in blended waveform "fully rectified" mode which provides cutting with hemostasis, at a power control between 4 and 5.

– A vacuum evacuator should be utilized for eliminating plumes of smoke.

– Any remaining bleeding points can be coagulated at the end of the procedure by switching to the coagulation "partially rectified" mode.

– The wound is allowed to heal by secondary intention.

– The patients are instructed to keep the wound moist by multiple applications of petroleum jelly daily until reepithelialization is complete approximately 2 weeks post-op.

• Excision by the far-infrared lasers (i.e., CO_2 or Er:YAG) followed by vaporization is also very effective with a relatively bloodless surgical field. A scanned CO_2 laser is the optimal device given the need to debulk large, thick areas of skin. The pulsed CO_2 laser can also be used in the continuous wave mode to remove the bulk of the rhinophyma and in the pulsed mode to sculpt and resurface the remainder of the nose.

• Dermabrasion has been successfully employed. The aerosolized particles produced during the procedure, the amount of procedural blood produced, and the existence of effective alternative treatments have reduced the use of this technique.

Telangiectasias

Laser and flashlamp treatments based on selective light absorption by hemoglobin are usually very effective for removing telangiectasias and partially effective in inhibiting flushing. Patients must be aware that over time they are likely to develop more telangiectasias.

• Laser treatment: multiple effective options are available.

– Pulsed dye lasers (PDL) are the treatment of choice for facial telangiectasias.

○ The traditional PDL with a short pulse duration of 0.45 or 1.5 ms provides the most effective treatment for facial telangectasias. However, posttreatment purpura occurs which generally lasts 10–14 days.

○ A variable-pulse PDL (595 nm, Candela V-beam, Wayland, MA) with stuttered pulse durations (i.e., 0.45, 1.5, 3, 6, 10, 20, 30, 40 ms) can provide a reduced purpura treatment of facial telangiectasias,

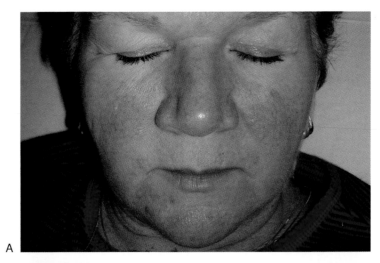

A

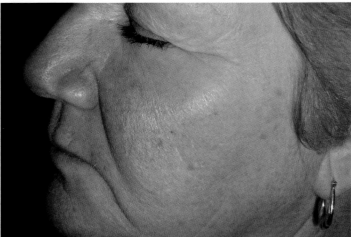

B

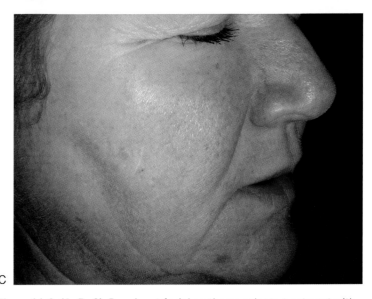

C

Figure 11.2 (A, B, C) *Prominent facial erythema prior to treatment with intense pulse light.*

but is somewhat less effective and usually requires multiple treatments.

- ⌐ Commonly, subpurpuric fluences of less than 10 J/cm² at pulse duration of 10 ms, with a 7 mm spot size are utilized.

- ⌐ Better efficacy of the variable-pulse PDL in treating facial telangiectasias can be achieved by utilizing purpuric fluences or with a pulse stacking of subpurpuric pulses (stacked 2–4 subpupuric pulses at a 1.5 Hz repetition rate, 7.5 J/cm², 10 ms pulse duration, 10 mm spot size, DCD of 30/20).

- ○ Facial edema, erythema, and discomfort can occur after extensive treatment with the purpura-free variable-pulse PDL. However, these undesired effects are generally better tolerated when compared to a purpura-inducing laser treatment.

- The variable pulse width 1064 nm Neodymium:YAG (Nd:YAG) laser has proven to be effective in the treatment of facial telangiectasias. Shorter pulse widths with higher fluences might be necessary for effective treatment of smaller vessels but have an increased risk of blister and scar formation.

- Frequency-doubled 532 nm Nd:YAG laser also called, potassium-titanyl-phosphate (KTP) laser, provides effective absorption of hemoglobin with a pulse duration of 1–50 ms making it ideally suited to treat superficial vessels without purpura formation. Tracing of individual vessels is a useful technique for patients with a countable number of discrete, visible vessels.

- Flashlamp (pulsed light) treatment: intense pulse light (IPL) provides another effective, purpura-free method for reducing facial telangiectasias and erythema (Figs. 11.2-11.3). For example, fluences of 30–40 J/cm² with a 20 ms pulse duration are effective with the Starlux Lux G handpiece (Palomar Medical Technologies, Burlington, MA). The treatment endpoint is immediate vessel clearance or selective vessel darkening. Multiple treatments may be required for the greatest treatment benefit.

- Other treatment options include electrosurgery, cryotherapy, and infiltration of sclerosing agents. These are less selective, often less effective, and more likely to result in scarring than PDL or IPL treatment.

BIBLIOGRAPHY

Aferzon M, Millman B. Excision of rhinophyma with high-frequency electrosurgery. *Dermatol Surg.* August 2002; 28(8):735–738.

Alam M, Dover JS, Arndt KA. Treatment of facial telangiectasia with variable-pulse high-fluence pulsed-dye laser: comparison of efficacy with fluences immediately above and below the purpura threshold. *Dermatol Surg.* July 2003;29(7):681–684. Discussion 685.

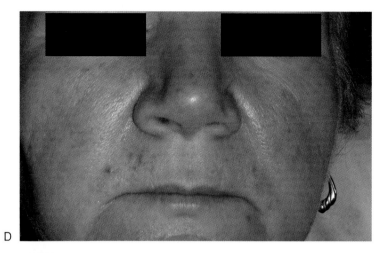

D

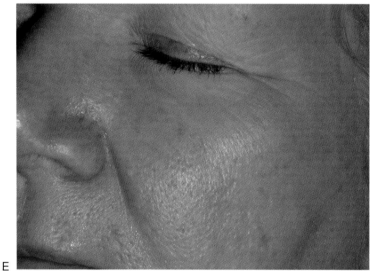

E

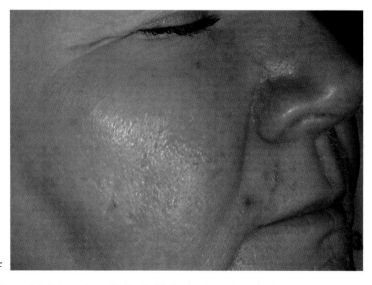

F

Figure 11.2 (*continued*) (**D, E, F**) *Reduction of the facial erythema after two treatments with intense pulse light, Starlux Lux G handpiece*

Alam M, Omura NE, Dover JS, Arndt KA. Clinically significant facial edema after extensive treatment with purpura-free pulsed-dye laser. *Dermatol Surg.* September 2003;29(9):920–924.

Fincher EF, Gladstone HB. Use of a dual-mode erbium:YAG laser for the surgical correction of rhinophyma. *Arch Facial Plast Surg.* July–August 2004;6(4):267–271.

Jasim ZF, Woo WK, Handley JM. Long-pulsed (6-ms) pulsed dye laser treatment of rosacea-associated telangiectasia using subpurpuric clinical threshold. *Dermatol Surg.* January 2004;30(1):37–40.

Mark KA, Sparacio RM, Voigt A, Marenus K, Sarnoff DS. Objective and quantitative improvement of rosacea-associated erythema after intense pulsed light treatment. *Dermatol Surg.* 2003;29(6):600–604.

Rohrer TE, Chatrath V, Iyengar V. Does pulse stacking improve the results of treatment with variable-pulse pulsed-dye lasers? *Dermatol Surg.* February 2004;30(2, pt 1):163–167. Discussion 167.

Sarradet DM, Hussain M, Goldberg DJ. Millisecond 1064-nm neodymium:YAG laser treatment of facial telangiectases. *Dermatol Surg.* 2003;29(1):56–58.

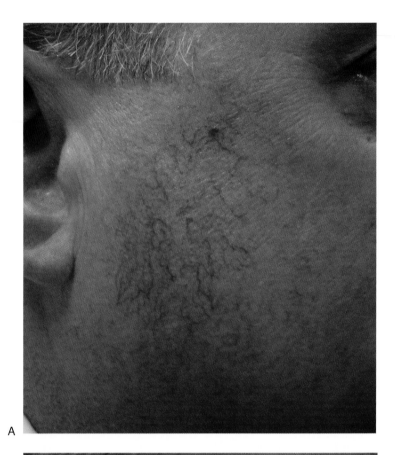

A

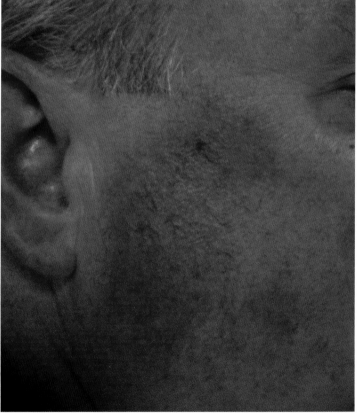

B

Figure 11.3 (A) *Prominent facial telangiectasias prior to treatment with intense pulse light.* **(B)** *Post-treatment erythema immediately after intense pulsed light treatment*

CHAPTER 12 Sebaceous Hyperplasia

Sebaceous hyperplasia appears as 1–3 mm yellow umbilicated papules with overlying telangiectasias on the face of middle-aged individuals. They represent a benign proliferation of sebaceous glands. The lesions are sometimes mistaken for basal cell carcinoma.

EPIDEMIOLOGY

Incidence: very common

Age: most commonly middle age and elderly but can appear in young individuals as well

Race: more common in Caucasians

Sex: equal

Precipitating factors: organ transplantation is a rare precipitant

PATHOGENESIS

Unknown.

PATHOLOGY

Increased numbers of large, mature sebaceous lobules are clustered around a central duct in the upper dermis. The lobules lie closer than normal to the epidermis.

PHYSICAL LESIONS

There are single or multiple 1–3 mm yellow umbilicated papules with overlying telangiectasias that appear on the face. The forehead, cheeks, and nose are the most common locations. It can rarely present on the areola.

DIFFERENTIAL DIAGNOSIS

Most commonly mistaken for basal cell carcinoma.

LABORATORY EXAMINATION

None is indicated. Biopsy if considering basal cell carcinoma.

COURSE

Benign, but do not regress or resolve without therapy.

KEY CONSULTATIVE QUESTIONS

Any history of the lesion bleeding.

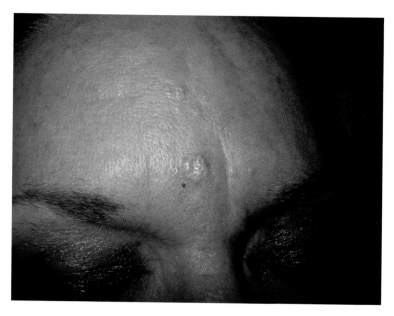

Figure 12.1 *Large sebaceous hyperplasia on the forehead*

MANAGEMENT

There is no medical indication to treat sebaceous hyperplasia. Still, some individuals are significantly bothered by its appearance and request removal, particularly in the circumstance of multiple lesions. Treatments include oral, destructive, laser, and photodynamic therapies. Each has its side effects and risk of recurrence.

TREATMENTS

■ Destructive Modalities

- "Light" cryotherapy and electrosurgery are quick, inexpensive means of treating sebaceous hyperplasia.
- Local excision is another means of removal that produces a scar as a side effect.

■ Oral Medications

- Isotretinoin (1 mg/kg/day) showed improvement after 6 weeks of therapy in a small study of three patients.
- Continued improvement was seen with subsequent use of topical tretinoin or lower dose isotretinoin.
- Should be seen as an alternative treatment.

■ Laser Therapy

- Pulsed dye laser (PDL) (585 nm) has been shown to improve sebaceous hyperplasia.
  - Successful treatment has been shown with 3-stacked 5-mm pulses at fluences of 7 and 7.5 J/cm^2.
  - Most lesions respond after one treatment with flattening, shrinking, or resolution.
  - Seven percent of lesions recurred completely.
  - One study showed clearance in two patients treated with the PDL at 585 nm, 6.5–8 J/cm^2, and a pulse width of 300–450 μs. Two to three treatments were performed.
- The 1450-nm diode laser has been studied in 10 patients for the treatment of sebaceous hyperplasia (Figs. 12.2–12.3).
  - Each patient was treated 1–5 times.
  - Fluences of 16–17 J/cm^2 were employed, with cooling durations of 40–50 ms.
  - After two to three treatments with the diode laser, 84% of lesions decreased in size greater than 50%, and 70% decreased greater than 75%. Patient and physician satisfaction was high.
  - Side effects included one case of an atrophic scar and one case of hyperpigmentation.
- Erbium:YAG laser ablation can also improve sebaceous hyperplasia.
- Laser-assisted photodynamic therapy with topical 20% 5-aminolevulinic acid and PDL irradiation (595 nm)

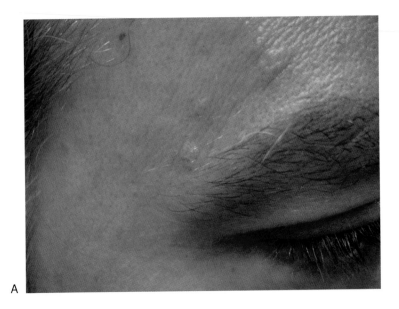

A

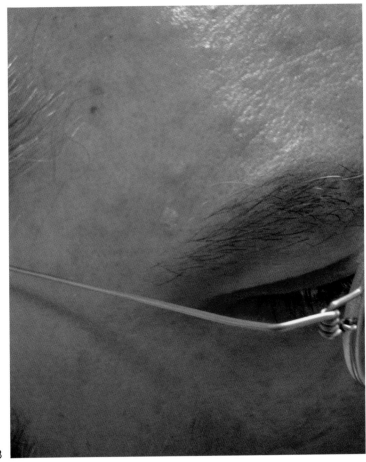

B

Figure 12.2 (A) *Patient with sebaceous hyperplasia on the right temple and forehead.* **(B)** *Improvement 1 month after treatment with 1450 nm diode laser (Smoothbeam, Candela Corp., Wayland, MA) utilizing a 6 mm spot with a fluence of 14 J/cm^2 and a pulse duration of 35 ms*

achieved more effective improvement of sebaceous hyperplasia than PDL alone.

– Treatments were performed at 1–6 week intervals.

– Both therapies showed greater improvement than no therapy at all. There were no long-term results.

– Side effects were limited to mild temporary redness, edema, and crusting.

PITFALLS TO AVOID/ OUTCOME EXPECTATIONS/ COMPLICATIONS/ MANAGEMENT

• Patients should be informed that complete resolution is difficult and not always permanent.

• Destructive modalities such as cryotherapy and electrodessication can produce pigmentary changes and even scarring if done too aggressively. Recurrences are common.

• Local excision leaves a scar.

• Oral therapy with isotretinoin is clearly an alternative treatment and is not as efficacious as other modalities and carries with it the risk of significant side effects such as teratogenicity, dry skin and mucous membranes, high triglycerides and cholesterol, diffuse skeletal hyperostosis, liver function abnormalities, reduced night vision, pseudotumor cerebri, leukopenia, possible depression, and suicidal ideation. Topical tretinoin can produce skin irritation.

• Laser therapy must be used with caution, especially in dark skin phototypes, given the risk of hyperpigmentation. There can be scarring, redness, edema, and crusting as noted above as well. Recurrence is not uncommon.

BIBLIOGRAPHY

Aghassi D, Gonzalez E, Anderson RR, Rajadhyaksha M, Gonzalez S. Elucidating the pulsed-dye laser treatment of sebaceous hyperplasia in vivo with real-time confocal scanning laser microscopy. *J Am Acad Dermatol.* 2000;43(1, pt 1):49–53.

Alster TS, Tanzi EL. Photodynamic therapy with topical aminolevulinic acid and pulsed dye laser irradiation for sebaceous hyperplasia. *J Drugs Dermatol.* 2003;2(5): 501–504.

Grimalt R, Ferrando J, Mascaro JM. Premature familial sebaceous hyperplasia: successful response to oral isotretinoin in three patients. *J Am Acad Dermatol.* 1997;37(6):996–998.

No D, McClaren M, Chotzen V, Kilmer SL. Sebaceous hyperplasia treated with a 1450-nm diode laser. *Dermatol Surg.* 2004;30(3):382–384.

Schonermark MP, Schmidt C, Raulin C. Treatment of sebaceous gland hyperplasia with the pulsed dye laser. *Lasers Surg Med.* 1997;21(4):313–316.

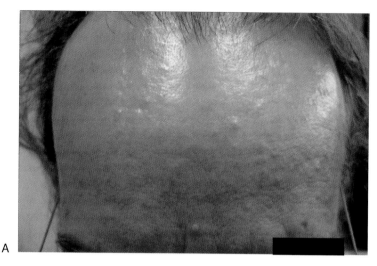

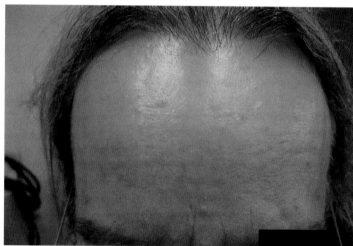

Figure 12.3 (A) *Sebaceous hyperplasia—before.* **(B)** *10 days later after one treatment—1450 nm diode laser, 14.5 J/cm², 35 ms cooling, single pulse per lesion*

SECTION THREE

Disorders of Eccrine Glands

CHAPTER 13 Hyperhidrosis

Hyperhidrosis is the secretion of excessive amounts of sweat from the eccrine sweat glands at rest and at normal room temperature. It produces both physical and social discomfort. The most commonly affected areas are the axillae, palms, and plantar feet. It can present in a bilateral or symmetric fashion. The most common cause of hyperhidrosis is idiopathic.

EPIDEMIOLOGY

Incidence: no good epidemiologic studies of prevalence

Age: palmoplantar: birth; axillary: puberty

Race: no racial predilection

Sex: equal

Precipitating factors: idiopathic, emotional, central nervous system injury/disease, drug, surgical injury are the most common causes. In most cases, there is a family history.

PATHOGENESIS

Eccrine glands are primarily innervated by sympathetic fibers that are cholinergic rather than adrenergic in neural response.

PHYSICAL FINDINGS

- Palmoplantar: excessive sweat and sweat droplets producing a moist appearance and clammy feel.
- Axillary: staining of shirts in the underarm area.

DIFFERENTIAL DIAGNOSIS

Clinical appearance does not suggest other disorders.

LABORATORY EXAMINATION

Starch-iodine or ninhydrin test are useful in defining areas of sweating (Fig. 13.1).

DERMATOPATHOLOGY

No characteristic findings. Biopsy plays no role in management.

COURSE

Does not remit spontaneously; may improve slightly with age.

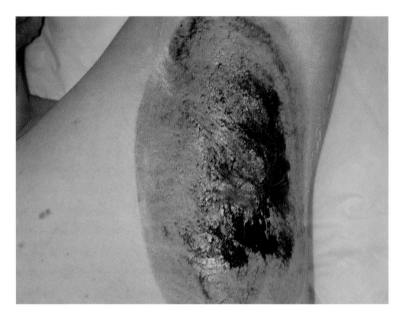

Figure 13.1 *An example of the starch-iodine test in the left axilla. Note the prominent dark blue-black discoloration at sites of hyperhidrosis*

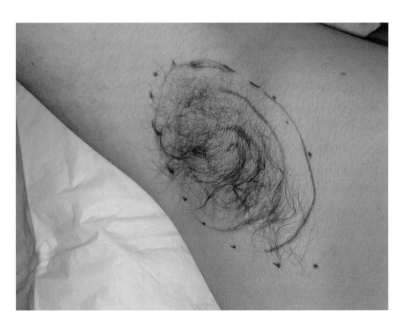

Figure 13.2 *Injection sites marked on right axilla of a male prior to botulinum toxin A injection*

KEY CONSULTATIVE QUESTIONS

- Medication history
- Past treatments and response
- Assess for systemic abnormality
- Recent surgery

MANAGEMENT

The goal of the treatment is to substantially decrease sweat production to improve physical and social discomfort; not complete elimination. There are multiple treatments for hyperhidrosis (Fig. 13.4). Botulinum toxin A is a very effective treatment providing temporary reduction in sweating. Topical medications are only modestly effective. Surgical therapy is more effective than topical therapy. Compensatory hyperhidrosis secondary to sympathectomy limits its use at present except as a final therapeutic modality.

TOPICAL MEDICATIONS

- Aluminum chloride hexahydrate

  - Application of 10–30% aluminum chloride hexahydrate with or without occlusion for 6–8 h nightly for 3–4 days can be beneficial but is complicated by local irritation. Retreatment once or twice weekly for maintenance is recommended. Treated skin should be washed the following morning.

  - In the axillae, it is applied at night to unshaven skin and washed off in the morning.

  - Frequency of application diminishes with improvement.

- Tap water iontophoresis can be effective

  - The procedure requires continual application for 15–20 min 2–3 times per week.

  - Blistering and burning have been reported as side effects.

  - Contraindications include pregnancy, cardiac pacemakers, and metal implants.

ORAL MEDICATIONS

Oral anticholinergics including bornaprin, glycopyrronium bromide, propantheline, and methanthelium bromide are of limited efficacy. They produce dose-related anticholinergic side effects.

SURGERY

Surgical procedures include

- Endoscopic or classic sympathectomy is usually reserved as a final therapeutic option for palmar hyperhidrosis. Surgery provides long-lasting control. General anesthesia is required. Side effects include bleeding,

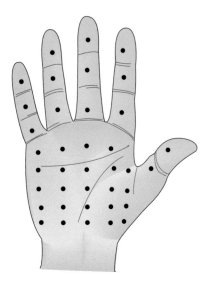

Figure 13.3 *Appropriate injection sites of botulinum toxin A for treatment of palmar hyperhidrosis. Each injection should be approximately 1-2 cm apart*

scar formation, infection, reaction to anesthesia, compensatory hyperhidrosis, gustatory sweating, pneumothorax, and Horner's syndrome.

- Selective gland removal is reserved for axillary hyperhidrosis.

- Liposuction for axillary hyperhidrosis involves subdermal liposuction. The liposuction cannula is held with the bevel side up at the subdermal level for suctioning of this region.

BOTULINUM TOXIN A

Botulinum toxin A provides temporary effective treatment for this condition. It is a bacterial toxin that decreases sweating by irreversibly blocking acetylcholine release from cholinergic presynaptic vesicles (Fig. 13.6).

■ Anesthesia

- Topical anesthetic cream and/or ice generally can provide sufficient anesthetic effect.

- Still, nerve blocks should be considered prior to plantar and palmar treatments to minimize the associated pain.
  - Plantar: sural and posterior tibial nerves.
  - Palmar: ulnar and median nerves.

■ Treatment

- A starch-iodine test performed prior to treatment can help delineate the areas to be injected. Iodine is placed on the affected area, followed by the application of cornstarch producing a prominent dark blue-black discoloration. The starch-iodine poste should be washed off prior to Botox injections.

- Effective Botox dilutions vary. A Botox A (100 U/vial) dilution of 2.0 U/0.1 cc is effective.

- Injections are performed at 1–2 cm intervals throughout the affected area (Figs. 13.2-13.3). Two units should be injected per site.

- A total dose ranging from 50–100 U/axilla, palm, or sole can be injected, for a total dose of 100–200 U for both treatment sites. A decreased dose can be used for localized hyperhidrosis.

- Temporary hand and finger muscle weakness may be a complication of palmar botulinum toxin A injections, especially with increasing dosages. Patients should use caution when holding cups and other objects supported by the thenar muscle while the weakness is present. This weakness generally dissipates within 3–4 weeks.

- Decreased sweating is observed within 1–2 weeks. Benefits generally are noted between 3 and 9 months.

- Side effects may include local muscle weakness for palmar injections, bruising, antibody resistance, and rarely an anaphylactic reaction.

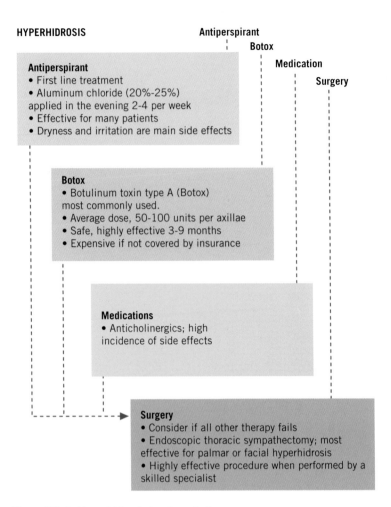

HYPERHIDROSIS

Antiperspirant
- First line treatment
- Aluminum chloride (20%-25%) applied in the evening 2-4 per week
- Effective for many patients
- Dryness and irritation are main side effects

Botox
- Botulinum toxin type A (Botox) most commonly used.
- Average dose, 50-100 units per axillae
- Safe, highly effective 3-9 months
- Expensive if not covered by insurance

Medications
- Anticholinergics; high incidence of side effects

Surgery
- Consider if all other therapy fails
- Endoscopic thoracic sympathectomy; most effective for palmar or facial hyperhidrosis
- Highly effective procedure when performed by a skilled specialist

Figure 13.4 *Hyperhidrosis treatment diagram*

PITFALLS TO AVOID

- Temporary hand and finger muscle weakness may be a complication of palmar injections of botulinum toxin A, especially with increasing dosages.
- Botox injections are contraindicated in patients with underlying neuromuscular conditions as well as in pregnant and lactating patients.
- Decreased doses should be considered for patients on ACE inhibitors, which can potentiate Botox effects.
- It is important to counsel that the benefits of Botox are temporary and require repeat treatments.
- None of the therapies is universally efficacious. The patient must be aware that the treatment endpoint is a reduction in sweating and not complete elimination.
- Treatment side effects may be considerable depending on the treatment chosen and must be reviewed at depth with the patient prior to any treatment initiation.

BIBLIOGRAPHY

Campanati A, Lagalla G, Penna L, Gesuita R, Offidani A. Local neural block at the wrist for treatment of palmar hyperhidrosis with botulinum toxin: technical improvements. *J Am Acad Dermatol.* 2004;51(3):345–348.

Glaser DA. Treatment of axillary hyperhidrosis by chemodenervation of sweat glands using botulinum toxin type A. *J Drugs Dermatol.* 2004;3(6):627–631.

Goh CL. Aluminum chloride hexahydrate versus palmar hyperhidrosis. *Int J Dermatol.* 1990;29:368–370.

Hamm H. The place of botulinum toxin type A in the treatment of focal hyperhidrosis. *Br J Dermatol.* 2004;151(6): 1115–1122.

Heckmann M, Ceballos-Bauman AO, Plewig G. Botulinum toxin A for axillary hyperhidrosis (excessive sweating). *N Engl J Med.* 2001;344:488–493.

Herbst F, Plas EG, Fuggo R, Fritsch A. Endoscopic thoracic sympathectomy for primary hyperhidrosis of the upper limbs: a critical analysis and long-term results in 480 operations. *Ann Surg.* 1994;220:86–90.

Lowe N, Campanati A, Bodokh I, Cliff S, Jaen P, Kreyden O, Naumann M, Offidani A, Vadoud J, Seukeran DC, Highet AS. The use of topical glycopyrrolate in the treatment of hyperhidrosis. *Clin Exp Dermatol.* 1998;23:204–205.

Reinauer S, Nuesser A, Schauf G, Holzle E. Iontophoresis with alternating current and direct current offset (A/C iontophoresis): a new approach for treatment of hyperhidrosis. *Br J Dermatol.* 1993;129:166–169.

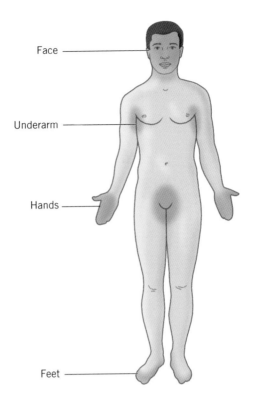

Figure 13.5 *The sites of hyperhidrosis*

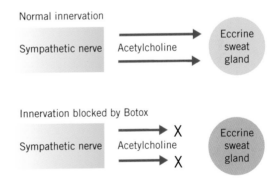

Figure 13.6 *Mechanism of action of Botox in hyerhidrosis. Blocking acetelycholine release from cholinergic presynaptic vesicles.*

SECTION FOUR

Disorders of Hair Follicles

CHAPTER 14 | Male Pattern Hair Loss

Male pattern hair loss, also known as androgenetic alopecia, presents after puberty with bitemporal hair loss that progresses to the loss of hair on the vertex, frontal, and temporal scalp. Parietal and occipital hair is usually unaffected. It is a nonscarring form of alopecia that occurs in genetically susceptible males. It represents a normal physiological process and is the most common form of alopecia. Nonetheless, many men seek treatment for androgenic alopecia because of unhappiness with its cosmetic appearance and association with aging.

EPIDEMIOLOGY

Incidence: 30% of males over 30, more than half of males over 50

Age: begins after puberty

Precipitating factors: polygenetic inherited predisposition. No diagnostic tests exist to determine the etiology and natural progression

PATHOGENESIS

There is a diminution in the size of affected terminal follicles that regress to become vellus follicles that eventually disappear. There is an increase in telogen hairs and a decrease in anagen hairs. This process is believed to result from both a polygenetic inherited susceptibility as well as androgenic stimulation. The most important androgen in this process is dihydrotestosterone.

PHYSICAL EXAMINATION AND NATURAL PROGRESSION

Typically, frontal and temporal hair loss/thinning is present first. Begins in puberty and progresses over decades. The rate and extent of hair loss varies from individual to individual. Some progress to complete baldness in early twenties and others gradually thin over decades.

DIFFERENTIAL DIAGNOSIS

In males, the pattern of hair loss is characteristic suggesting no other diagnoses.

LABORATORY EXAMINATION

In males, no laboratory workup is typically required.

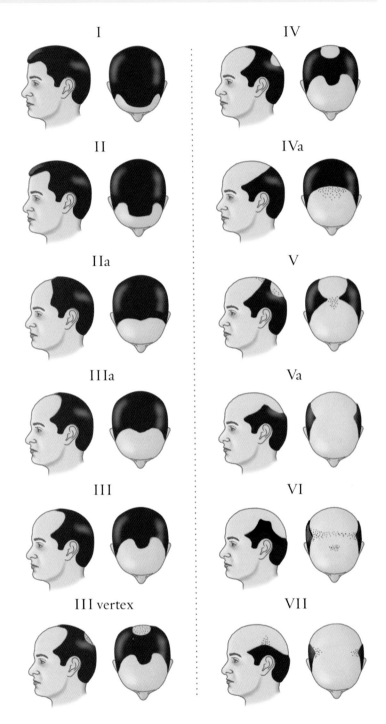

Figure 14.1 *Norwood classification of the natural progression of male pattern hair loss*

TABLE 14.1 ■ Minoxidil and Finasteride—The Only Two FDA Approved Medications for Male Pattern Hair Loss

	Finasteride	Minoxidil
Mechanism of action	5-α reductase type II inhibitor blocking the conversion of testosterone to dihydrotestosterone	Unknown
Key to success	Emphasize maintenance over regrowth of hair and compliance for at least 6–8 months to see benefit	Emphasize maintenance over regrowth of hair and compliance 6–8 months to see benefit
Side effects	2% of men experience sexual dysfunction. Reversible within days if discontinued	Dryness and pruritus of the scalp. Rare allergic reaction
	No allergic reactions, blood monitoring or drug interactions. Pre menopause of females should never handle or take medication. Women may have some benefit	
Clinical onset of action	6–8 months	6–8 months
Dose	1 mg qd with or without food	Two to four drops 1–2 times daily to frontal and vertex of scalp
Candidate selection		
Norwood II–IV	Highly effective	Highly effective
Norwood IV–VII	Somewhat effective	Somewhat effective

MEDICAL THERAPY

■ Key Consultative Questions

- Age of onset
- Rate of hair loss
- Past medical history
- Medications used to date and success of therapy
- Patient expectation of any medical or surgical therapy

■ FDA Approved Medical Therapy (Table 14.1)

Minoxidil and finasteride are the only two FDA approved medications for male pattern hair loss.

HAIR TRANSPLANTATION

■ Definition

Based on the theory of donor dominance, hair follicles maintain their genetic destiny wherever they grow on our scalp. Hair transplanted from the posterior scalp will grow for as long as it was genetically programmed to grow. For the vast majority of men, transplanted hair will grow for decades.

The era of 10–25 hair grafts harvested by 3–4 mm punches is over. Hair naturally grows in 1–4 hair follicular bundles. Contemporary hair transplantation utilizes a large number of 1–4 hair grafts. The result is consistently natural appearing transplanted hair for men and women.

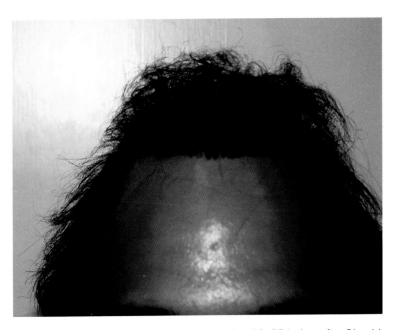

Figure 14.2 *Unnatural "pluggy" hairline using 10–25 hair grafts. Should never happen in 21st century*

THE CONSULT

■ Key Questions

- How long have you noticed hair loss?
- Rate of hair loss?
- Which medications whether prescription or alternative have been tried and for how long?
- Expectations?

■ Physical Examination

- Norwood stage (Fig. 14.1)
- Donor density
- Caliber of hair follicles

Ideal candidate: high donor density, thick caliber hair follicle, realistic expectation (Figs. 14.3-14.4)

Poor candidate: poor donor density, below average hair caliber, unrealistic expectations

■ Key Points to Emphasize *Before* Hair Transplantation

- Ongoing rate of hair loss affects the perceived density of a hair transplant
- Fine hair follicles will create thin natural coverage and thick caliber follicles will create more perceived density
- Ongoing hair loss will affect the cosmetic appearance of a transplant
- Visible donor scar or scars if hair is shaved in posterior scalp
- Limited donor supply!

  Key to success: physician and patient have similar expectations of what the procedure will and will not achieve over the short (1–3 years) and long-term (10–20 years).

■ Medication and Transplantation

Medication to maintain existing hair will maximize the density from a transplant but medications should always remain elective. Hairline design and distribution of recipient sites should always assume ongoing hair loss.

SURGICAL PROCEDURE

■ Pre-op Instructions

- No specific blood tests
- Medical clearance if appropriate

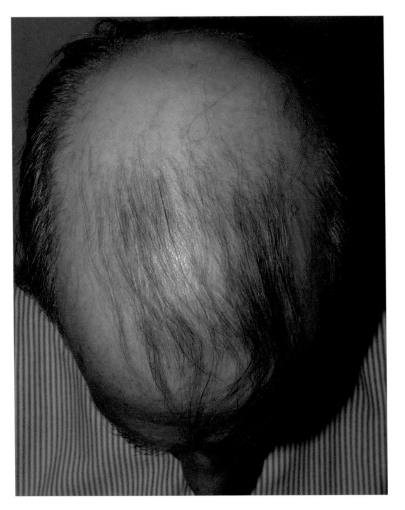

Figure 14.3 *Realistic expectations using 1–4 hair grafts. Before Norwood V*

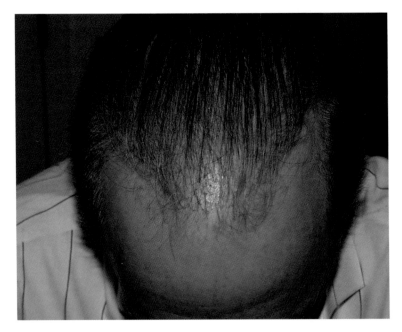

Figure 14.4 *Realistic expectations using 1–4 hair grafts. After 1100 1–4 hair grafts*

- Photographs
- Informed written consent
- Optional prophylactic antibiotic

■ Day of Procedure

- Written consent with post-op instructions reviewed
- Introduce hair transplant team
- Review procedure and goals with patient

■ Donor Region—Only Limiting Factor in Hair Transplantation (Figs. 14.5-14.10)

Anesthesia in donor region

- 1% lidocaine with 1:200,000 epinephrine
- 0.25% marcaine with 1:200,000 epinephrine
- 30–60 cc saline
  Saline in donor region provides
  - anesthesia
  - hemostasis
  - less transection of hair follicles
  - less likely to transect the occipital arteries

TABLE 14.2 ■ Advantages and Disadvantages of Follicular Unit Extraction (FUE)

Advantage	Disadvantage
–No linear donor scar	–More time consuming
–Often minimally visible scarring in trimmed donor region; advantage for patients with short hairstyle	–More FUE sessions to equal density from ellipse
–Can be used for patients with extensive scarring in posterior scalp from multiple previous surgeries	–Greater transection of hair follicles with potential decreased yield

Donor harvesting techniques (Tables 14.2–14.3)

- elliptical strip harvesting: >95% of patients
- follicular unit extraction: <5% of patients (Figs. 14.11)

Elliptical strip harvesting

- Undermining donor region rarely necessary
- Double layer of sutures rarely necessary
- Sutures or staples to close in single layer
- Sutures or staples out in 7–10 days
  Key to success in donor harvesting of ellipse

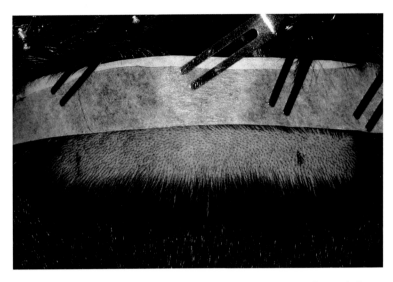

Figure 14.5 *Trim donor region with moustache trimmer, and tape hair up so donor suture will not be visible in the post-op period*

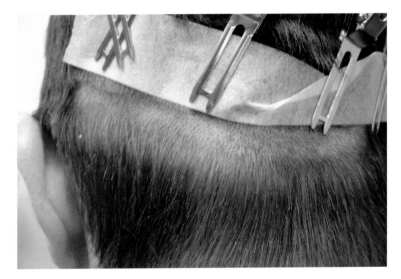

Figure 14.6 *Patient in prone position*

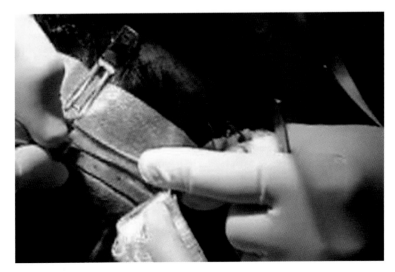

Figure 14.7 *Donor strip should not be more than 1 cm wide. Strips >1 cm have an increased risk of creating a hypertrophic scar*

TABLE 14.3 ■ Donor Harvesting Techniques. Elliptical Strip Harvesting Versus Follicular Unit Extraction

	Ellipse	Follicular unit extraction
Minimal transection of donor hair	Yes	No
Number of 1–4 grafts safely harvested per procedure	1500–2000	200–500
Time to harvest donor hair	15–20 min	1–2 h
Visible donor scar with hair length >1 cm	No	No
Visible donor scar with hair length <0.5 cm	Yes	Likely not
Overall percentage of cases used	>95%	<5%

- Donor strip width <1 cm
- After lidocaine/marcaine, add saline to donor region to provide hemostasis, anesthesia and reduce transection of hair follicles
- Do not rush!

■ Follicular Unit Extraction

Definition: Removal of follicular groupings from the posterior scalp using 1-mm punches.

■ Graft Creation

All grafts should mimic the natural 1–4 follicular bundles that naturally occur on the scalp.

Keys to success in creating 1–4 hair grafts
- Good ergonomics and instruments
- Do not allow grafts to dry. They must always be in saline
- Well-trained staff of three to four surgical assistants

Staff training
- Enthusiasm/interest in procedure
- Patience; 6–12 months for an assistant to learn to create 200–300 grafts per hour

■ Anesthesia in Recipient Region

- Field block and local infiltration with 1% lidocaine with 1:200,000 epinephrine and 0.25% marcaine with 1:200,000 epinephrine
- Supraorbital and supratrochlear block is optional
- Superficial infiltration in dermis not subcutaneous tissue will grant good hemostasis

■ Hairline Design

Definition: A hairline is an irregular ill-defined transition zone from skin to increasing density of terminal pigmented hair follicles.

- Frontal, temporal, and posterior hairlines should all be *irregular*

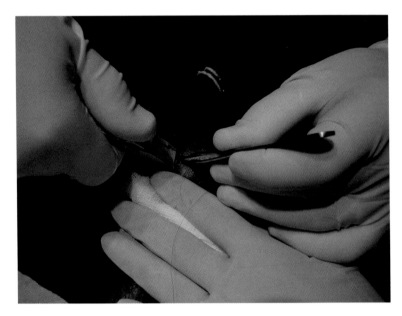

Figure 14.8 *Closing donor region with staples*

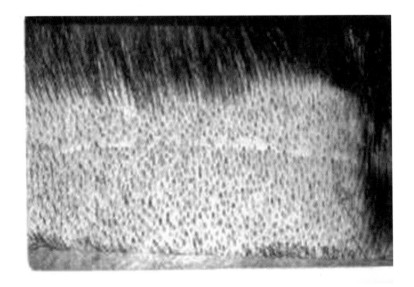

Figure 14.9 *A 2 mm linear scar 1 year after surgery from donor strip <1 cm wide*

- When designing a frontal temporal hairline always assume progression of hair loss to Norwood stage V
- Frontal hairline at least 9 cm above glabella
- Be conservative

◾ Recipient Site Creation (Fig. 14.17)

Commonly used needles to create recipient sites

- #18, #19, or #20 gauge needle
- SP 88–90 gauge needle
- 0.5–1.0 mm cag needle

Key points

- Distribute recipient sites randomly and closely together and in a distribution that will appear natural if all hair is lost in the frontal two-thirds of the scalp
- Avoid trauma to existing hair follicles
  - Magnification in recipient sites
  - Follow the natural 15–30° angle of hair follicles in the frontal two-thirds of the scalp
- Excellent hemostasis using 1:100,000 epinephrine
- 10–30 sites per cm² depending on the amount of existing hair and area (cm²) to distribute grafts

◾ Graft Placement (Fig. 14.18)

Two or three surgical assistants place the grafts into recipient sites using microvascular forceps.

Keys to success

- Handle grafts in perifollicular tissue—never crush hair follicles
- Keep all grafts in chilled saline—never allow a graft to desiccate
- Staff training
- Excellent hemostasis using 1:100,000 epinephrine
- Patience

◾ Postoperative Period

- Overnight dressing to protect grafts
- Oral steroids 40 mg qd for 3–4 days to reduce frontal edema
- Tylenol #3, one tablet q 4–6 h for 1 day PRN. There should be no discomfort morning after surgery
- Shower in morning after surgery. Avoid trauma to transplanted zone
- Normal activities. No heavy exercise for 5–7 days
- Topical antibiotic to donor wound for 7–10 days
- Sutures or staples removed 7–10 days after surgery

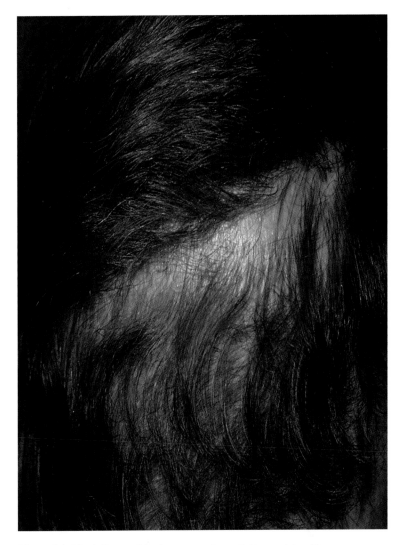

Figure 14.10 *A 2 cm wide donor scar from 1.5 cm wide ellipse*

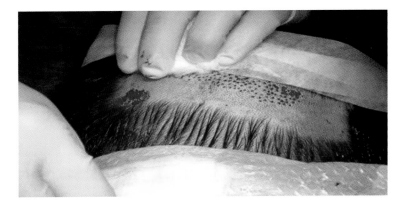

Figure 14.11 *Follicular unit extraction using 1 mm sites*

■ Common Post Hair Transplant Side Effects

- Frontal edema lasting 3–5 days post-op
- Pruritus in donor and/or recipient zone
- Transitory folliculitis
- Telogen effluvium in patients with diffuse thinning

■ Rare Side Effects

- Hypertrophic scarring in donor region in ellipses less than 1 cm
- Persistent numbness or discomfort in donor or recipient zone
- Cystic nodules
- Poor quality growth of transplanted hair
- Infection

■ Postsurgical Period After Sutures/Staples Removed

- Resume full sports 1 week after surgery
- Dye hair 2 weeks after surgery
- Initial follow up 6 months after surgery
- Subsequent follow-ups every 3 months up to 15 months
- Full cosmetic result 9–15 months after surgery

■ Corrective Hair Transplant Surgery (Table 14.4)

For the majority of men, corrective hair transplant surgery is cosmetically and emotionally mandatory not elective.

Consult

Key question: what is your chief concern and goal for possible corrective surgery?

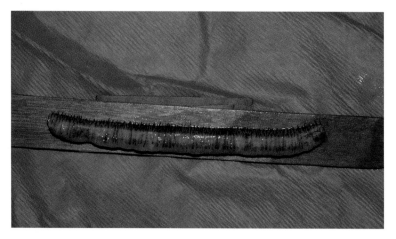

Figure 14.12 *Donor ellipse with natural follicular bundles*

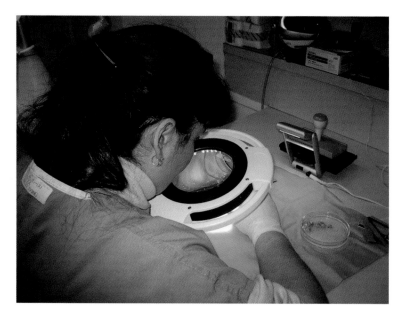

Figure 14.13 *Magnification helps visualize 1–4 hair bundles and minimize transection when separating with surgical prep blades*

TABLE 14.4 ■ **Treatment Options for Corrective Hair Transplant Surgery**

Treatment option	Advantage	Disadvantage
Adding 1–3 hair grafts between existing large 10–25 hair "plugs"	Dramatically soften hairline and add further density to existing "plugs"	Donor region may be depleted
		Patient not psychologically able to go through another hair transplant procedure
Excision of grafts	Patient requesting "I would rather just be bald" Status quo ante	Potential visible erythematous scar for weeks to months Permanent scar and/or dyschromia
Laser hair removal	Noninvasive	40–80% improvement after—five to seven does not work on bland hair
Combination	Reduce "pluggy" grafts Majority of patients utilize a combination of the above for optimal results	As above

BIBLIOGRAPHY

Avram MR. Polarized light-emitting diode magnification for optimal recipient site creation during hair transplant. *Dermatol Surg.* September 2005;31(9, pt 1):1124–1127. Discussion 1127.

Epstein JS. The treatment of female pattern hair loss and other applications of surgical hair restoration in women. *Facial Plast Surg Clin North Am.* May 2004;12(2):241–247.

Harris JA. Follicular unit transplantation: dissecting and planting techniques. *Facial Plast Surg Clin North Am.* May 2004;12(2):225–232.

Leavitt M, Perez-Meza D, Rao NA, Barusco M, Kaufman KD, Ziering C. Effects of finasteride (1 mg) on hair transplant. *Dermatol Surg.* October 2005;31(10):1268–1276. Discussion 1276.

Limmer BL. Elliptical donor stereoscopically assisted micrografting as an approach to further refinement in hair transplantation. *J Dermatol Surg Oncol.* December 1994; 20(12):789–793.

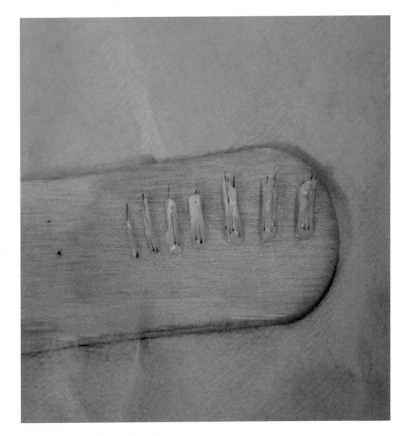

Figure 14.14 *1–4 hair grafts*

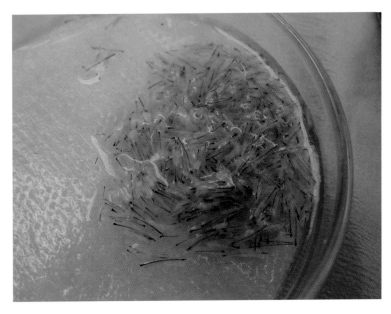

Figure 14.15 *1–4 hair grafts in chilled saline*

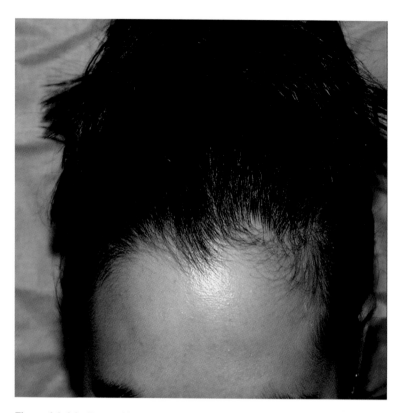

Figure 14.16 *Natural irregular frontal hairline*

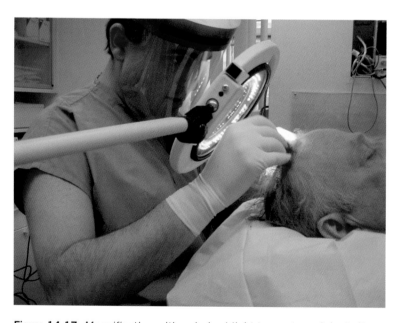

Figure 14.17 *Magnification with polarized light to create recipient sites*

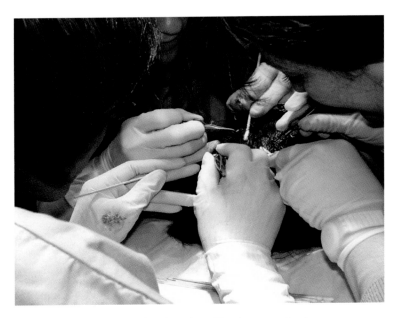

Figure 14.18 *Placing 1–4 hair grafts with microvascular forceps*

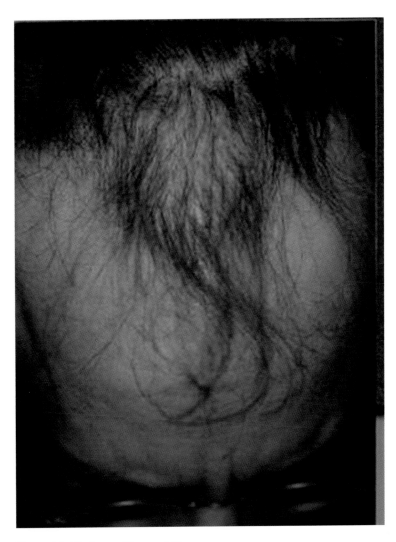

Figure 14.19 *Pre-op Norwood III*

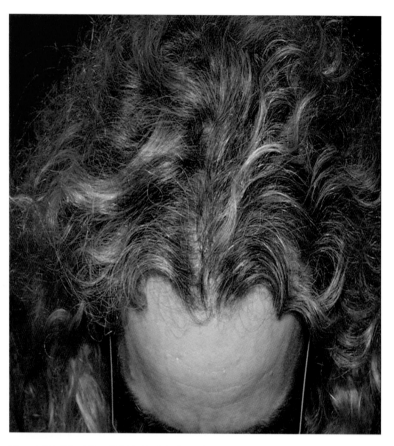

Figure 14.20 *After 2400 1–4 hair grafts*

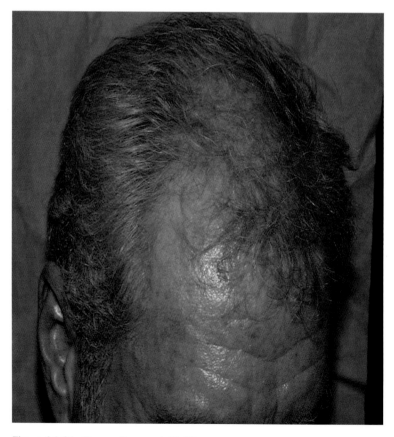

Figure 14.21 *Pre-op Norwood III–IV*

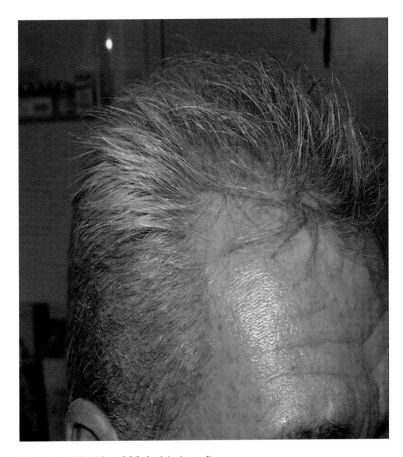

Figure 14.22 *After 900 1–4 hair grafts*

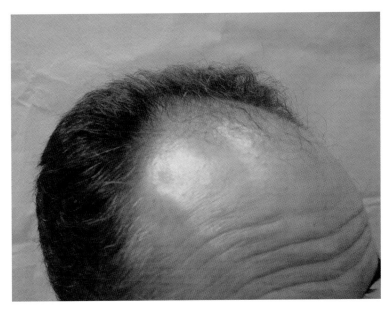

Figure 14.23 *Pre-op Norwood IV–V*

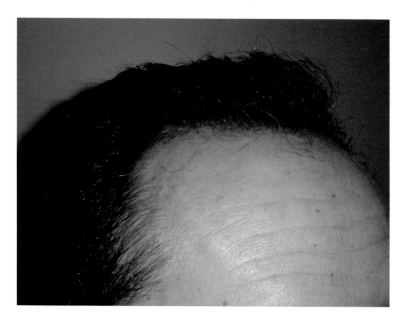

Figure 14.24 *After 1430 1–4 hair grafts*

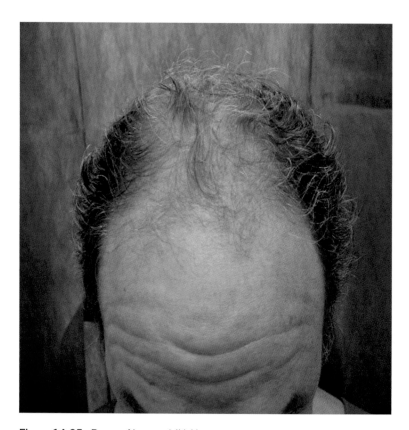

Figure 14.25 *Pre-op Norwood IV–V*

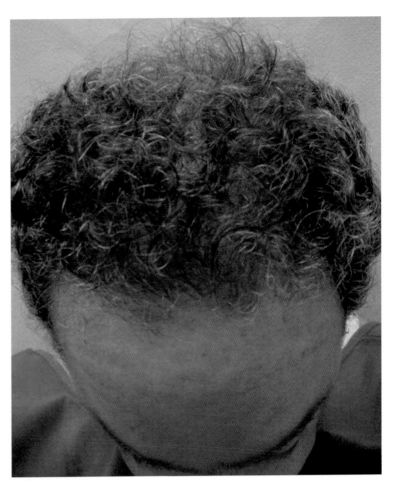

Figure 14.26 *After 1000 1–4 grafts*

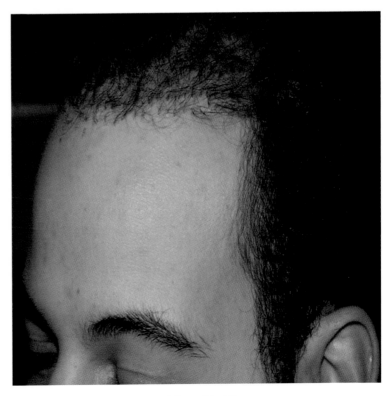

Figure 14.27 *Straight "pluggy" frontal hairline*

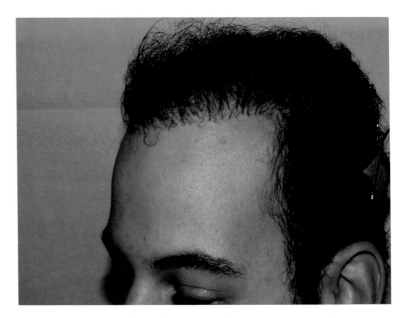

Figure 14.28 *After 650 1–3 hair grafts. Note improvement. Not completely natural hairline*

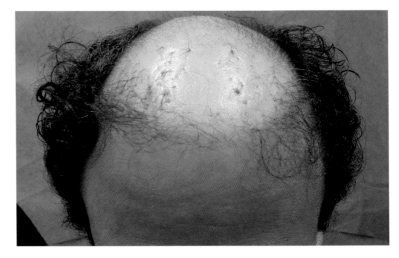

Figure 14.29 *Straight "pluggy" hairline. Depressed scars*

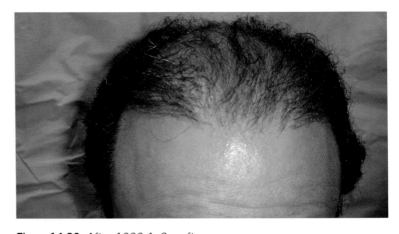

Figure 14.30 *After 1000 1–3 grafts*

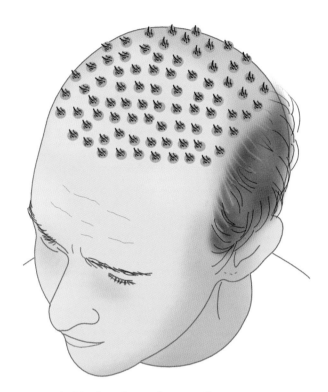

Illustration 14.1 *Obsolete 4 mm pluggy grafts*

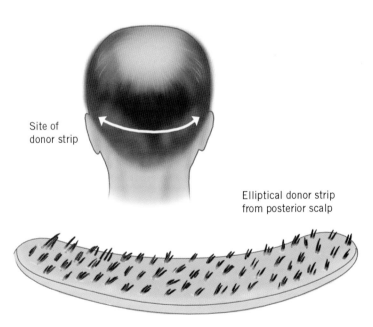

Site of
donor strip

Elliptical donor strip
from posterior scalp

Illustration 14.2 *Elliptical donor strip from posterior scalp*

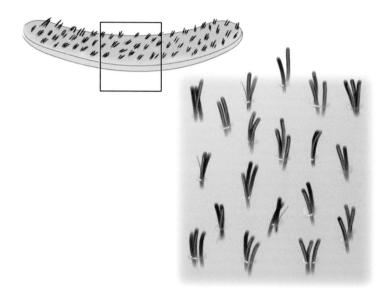

Illustration 14.3 *1–3 hair follicular groupings within donor strip*

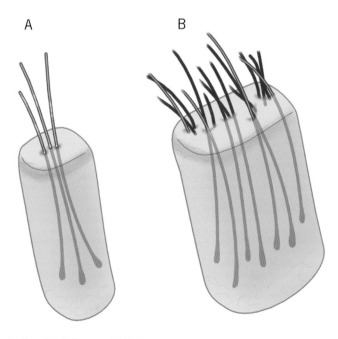

Illustration 14.4 *Versus 10–20 hair "pluggy" graft. Natural 1–3 follicular groupings*

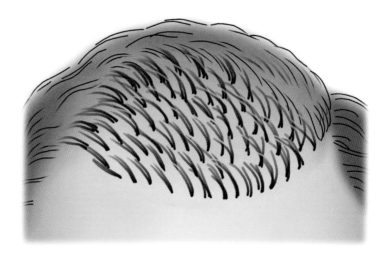

Illustration 14.5 *Straight artificial pluggy hairline using 10–20 hair grafts.*

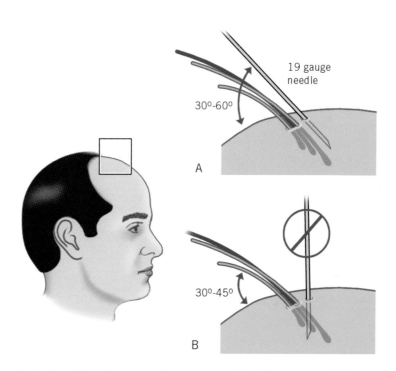

Illustration 14.6 *Recipient sites created at 15–45° angles not 90°*

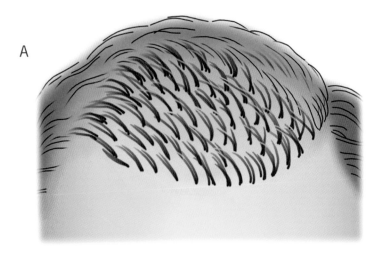

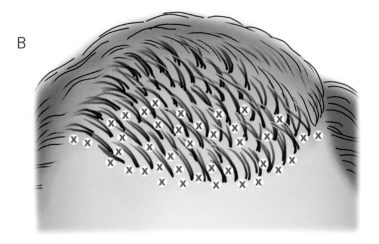

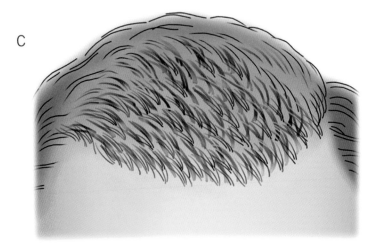

Illustration 14.7 *Corrective hair transplant adding 1–3 hair grafts between and in front of "pluggy" grafts*

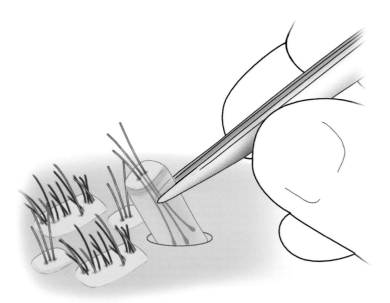

Illustration 14.8 *Adding 1–3 hair grafts between large "pluggy" grafts to improve cosmatic appearance*

CHAPTER 15 Female Pattern Hair Loss

Female pattern hair loss, also known as androgenetic alopecia, presents with a diffuse thinning of the mid-scalp with a characteristic maintenance of the frontal hairline. It may also present with the typical bitemporal hair recession seen in male pattern alopecia. Parietal and occipital hair is usually unaffected. As with males, it is a nonscarring form of alopecia. Female pattern hair loss is particularly problematic for women for whom hair loss produces greater social and self-esteem difficulties than for men with male pattern hair loss.

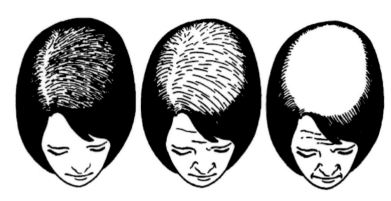

Figure 15.1 *Ludwig scale of female pattern hair loss*

EPIDEMIOLOGY

Incidence: nearly 30% of females over 30

Age: begins in twentier and in third decade

Race: none reported in females

Precipitating factors: polygenetic inherited predisposition is present. It is not one parent's fault!

PATHOGENESIS

There is a diminution in the size of affected terminal follicles that regress to become vellus follicles that eventually disappear. There is an increase in telogen hairs and a decrease in anagen hairs. Hormones play a role but the exact pathophysiology is uncertain.

COURSE

Begins in twenties and progresses over decades. The rate and extent of hair loss varies.

TABLE 15.1 ■ **Male Versus Female Pattern Hair Loss**

	Male	Female
Differential diagnosis	None	Telogen effluvium, medications, hormonal disorder, diet, hair styling, trauma
Natural progression	Unstable, receding hairlines, balding	Stable hairlines, gradual diffuse thinning, no balding
Caliber of hair	Variable between individuals	Variable between individuals
Emotional impact	Emotionally upsetting and an actual change in physical appearance but societal acceptance	Emotionally upsetting and an actual change in physical appearance but **no** societal acceptance
Hair care	Regular shampooing and cutting of hair. Ok to wear a hat!	Regular shampooing and cutting of hair, semi-permanent dye. Avoid tight braids, straightening, hot combs, bleach

KEY CONSULTATIVE QUESTIONS

- Duration of hair loss
- Menstrual history
- Medication history
- Nutrition, dieting, weight loss
- Hair care—bleaching, braiding
- Family history of hair loss
- History of major unexpected emotional or physical stress
- Medical history i.e. thyroid disease, iron deficiency

PHYSICAL EXAMINATION

Nonscarring alopecia—no erythema, scale, atrophy in skin with female pattern hair loss

DIFFERENTIAL DIAGNOSIS OF FEMALE PATTERN HAIR LOSS

- Telogen effluvium
- Poor hair styling—chemicals, excessive dying
- Iron deficiency, thyroid disease, chronic medical disease, polycystic or other endocrine imbalance
- Medication-related hair loss
- Poor nutrition, weight loss
- Trichotillomania
- Diffuse alopecia areata—rare

KEY QUESTIONS TO DISTINGUISH DIFFERENTIAL DIAGNOSIS

- How long has your hair loss persisted?
- Changes in diet or weight loss over past 6–12 months?
- Any new prescription, OTC medications or supplements?
- Any major surgery or unusual emotional stress?
- Any change in hair care? Chemicals to hair?

KEY POINTS

- Patients may have a combination of etiologies
- If there is any questioning after history and physical examination, scalp biopsy is indicated.
- Thyroid function tests, iron studies, ANA, RPR
- Referral to gynecologist and/or endocrinologist if appropriate on history and/or examination

MEDICAL THERAPY

Topical minoxidil (2 and 5% solution) are the only FDA approved medications for female pattern hair loss

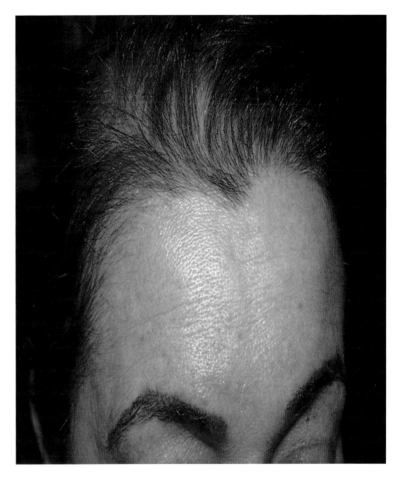

Figure 15.2 *"See through" frontal hairline*

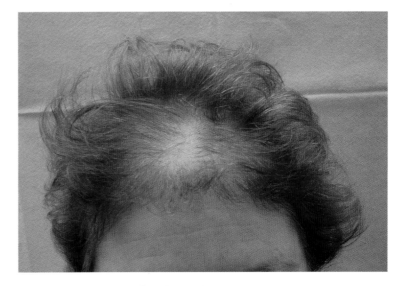

Figure 15.3 *Lugwig II "See through"*

(Table 15.2). The mechanism of action is unknown. It is safe for long-term application.

TABLE 15.2 ■ Minoxidil

Mechanism of action	Unknown
Onset of action	6–8 months
Side effects	Dryness, pruritus, "greasy hair"
Use with pregnancy or breast-feeding	No
5% versus 2%	5% slightly more effective but more "greasy" slight increased risk of hirsutism

KEYS TO SUCCESS

- Compliance: must use for 6–8 months to produce the desired effect.
- Emphasize maintenance over regrowth of hair. Minoxidil stops hair loss in the majority of patients and grows back pigmented terminal hair in a minority of patients.

NON-FDA APPROVED MEDICATIONS

- Finasteride, a type II 5-α reductase inhibitor, is contraindicated in women of childbearing age. Studies demonstrate some efficacy in postmenopausal females.
- Oral androgen receptor antagonists such as spironolactone and cyproterone acetate are other alternatives with limited proof of efficacy in both premenopausal and postmenopausal females. They are contraindicated in pregnant patients, given the risk of producing sexual defects in a male fetus. They should, therefore, be discontinued months prior to a planned pregnancy.

SURGICAL

■ Consultation

Chief complaint: "see through" frontal hairline, "limited styling options," "fear of windy days."

■ Key Questions

- How long has hair loss persisted on?
- Medical workup to date
- Medication used to treat hair loss and for how long
- Patient's chief cosmetic concern
- Patient's goal for hair transplantation

PHYSICAL EXAMINATION

- Donor density
- Caliber of hair loss
- Extent of hair loss

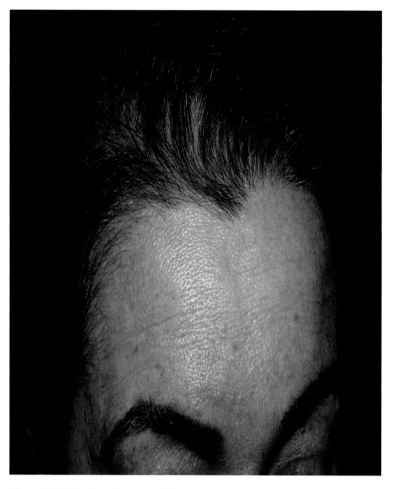

Figure 15.4 *Ludwig I–II: note intact hairline*

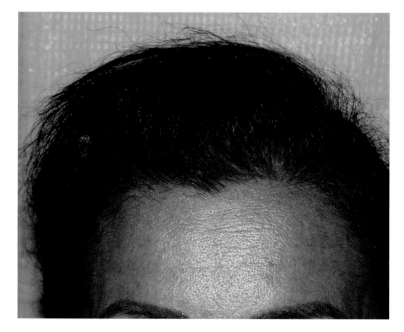

Figure 15.5 *After 700 1–4 hair grafts: frontal one-third of scalp*

KEY POINTS

- Emphasize unpredictable donor density. The transplanted hair will grow for as long as it was genetically programed to grow
- Increased risk of postsurgical telogen effluvium
- Ongoing hair loss will affect perceived density of hair transplant

SURGICAL APPROACH: FEMALE VERSUS MALE HAIR TRANSPLANTATION (Table 15.3)

Hair transplantation for men and women utilize the same donor harvesting techniques, graft creation, instruments, anesthesia, pre and postsurgery course.

FEMALE SURGICAL PLANNING

Transplant frontal one-third of scalp only! This will address chief complaint and reduce the risk of telogen effluvium.

- Chief complaint: "see through" frontal hairline
- Stable hair line
- Diffuse thinning—no bald spots
- Risk of telogen effluvium

◼ Pre-operative

- B-HCG in appropriate patient
- Consent
- Photos
- Medical clearance if appropriate
- Ok to dye hair up until day before procedure
- Oral antibiotic 1 h before surgery

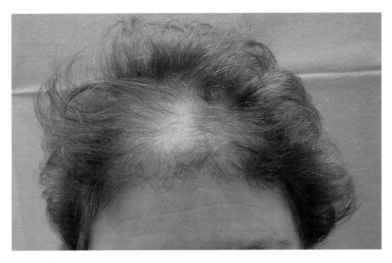

Figure 15.6 *Ludwig I–II pre-op*

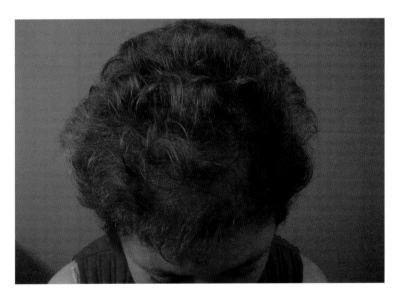

Figure 15.7 *After 900 1–4 hair grafts frontal one-third scalp*

TABLE 15.3 ◼ Surgical Approach: Female Versus Male Hair Transplantation

	Male	Female
Donor density	More predictable	Less predictable long-term
Hairline design	Unstable and receding frontal temporal and posterior hairline Need to design hair transplant for long-term natural cosmetic appearance (>10 years)	Stable hairlines. Major cosmetic advantage over men for surgical planning
Caliber of hair	Variable between individuals	Variable between individuals
Medication use with hair transplantation	If existing hair remains, medication will add density by limiting further hair loss Medication always remains elective Need to design hair transplant assuming ongoing hair loss and receding hairlines	All women should use minoxidil to help maintain existing hair and decrease risk of postsurgery telogen effluvium Density = number of hair follicles transplanted – ongoing hair loss
Expectations	Key to success	Key to success

▓ Procedure

- Introduce staff
- Review surgical plan
- Review postsurgical care anesthesia, instruments, donor harvesting, graft creation, grafts placement are the same as for men.

▓ Postoperative Instructions

- Overnight dressing to protect grafts as they heal.
- Resume regular activities. Light exercise 2–3 days after surgery. Full exercise when staples/sutures removed 7–10 days post-op.
- If any discomfort or pain, take Tylenol #3 with food q 4–6 h. Fifty-percent of patients take no pain medication and the other 50% take one or two tablets. If a patient has any discomfort or pain after the day of surgery, they should contact their physician.
- Complete course of antibiotic.
- Prednisone 40 mg QD for 3–4 days to prevent frontal edema. If a patient cannot or will not take prednisone, ice to forehead for 10 min every 30 min over the dressing for the first afternoon/evening of surgery to reduce but not eliminate edema. Edema begins 24 h after surgery, peaks 72 h postsurgery and disappears 5–6 days postsurgery. Rare periorbital ecchymoses.
- The morning after surgery the dressing is removed. All patients are encouraged to shower to help reduce post-surgery hemorrhagic crusting. Patients should NOT pick or rub scabs; this may permanently damage transplanted hair.
- After shower, blow dry with warm not hot air on low power.
- Apply topical antibiotic or aquaphor to donor region twice daily for 10 days.
- Resume minoxidil 48–72 h postsurgery.

▓ Postoperative Period

- Continue minoxidil 1–2 times daily.
- Telogen effluvium may begin 2–3 weeks after surgery and continue for 2–3 months.
- If telogen effluvium occurs, hair density will decrease but will rarely be cosmetically noticeable.
- Can dye hair 2 weeks after surgery.
- Initial follow-up 6 months after surgery and then every 3 months until 15 months when final density from the procedure will appear.

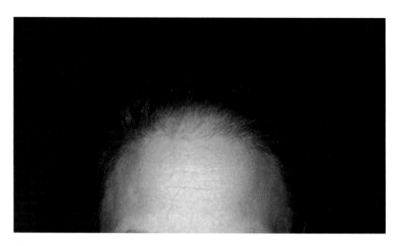

Figure 15.8 *Ludwig III pre-op. Note thin but intact*

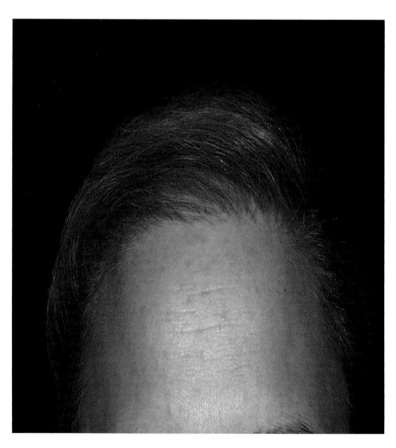

Figure 15.9 *After 650 1–4 hair grafts frontal one-third scalp grafts.*

KEYS TO SUCCESS WITH FEMALE HAIR TRANSPLANTATION

- Emphasize ongoing hair loss will affect long-term density of hair transplant
- Discuss the risk of postsurgical telogen effluvium
- Minoxidil will help reduce not eliminate the risk of telogen effluvium and help slow or stop ongoing hair loss for the majority of patients
- Unpredictable future loss of donor hair. Transplanted hair will grow for as long as it was genetically programed
- Limit the majority of transplanted grafts to frontal one-third of scalp for maximum cosmetic impact
- Well-trained staff

HAIR TRANSPLANTATION TO CORRECT ALTERED TEMPORAL HAIRLINE FROM LIFTING PROCEDURE

After female pattern hair loss, transplanting to correct scars left from lifting procedures such as facelifts and browlifts are the most common reasons for hair transplantation in women.

CHIEF COMPLAINT (Figs. 15.12-15.13)

"I cannot wear my hair up or back."

CONSULT

▓ Key Points

- After hair loss following a lift, wait at least 12 months before considering surgery.
- The loss may be a telogen effluvium and the hair may grow back on its own.
- Hair growth in scar tissue is unpredictable. The majority of patients have excellent growth but a small minority do not.
- Emphasize greater risk of frontal and potentially periorbital edema. It is not medically concerning, but may impact postoperative cosmetic appearance of the patient.

▓ Procedure

Preoperative, intraoperative and postoperative medication, technique, and wound care are the same for male and female hair transplantation. When creating recipient sites, follow the natural direction of hair growth in the temporal region.

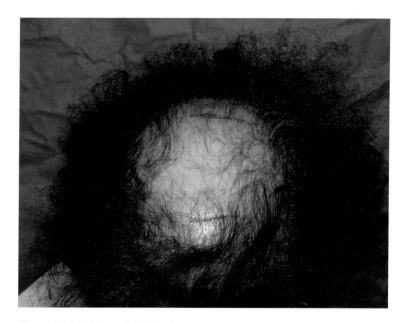

Figure 15.10 *Pre op Ludwig III*

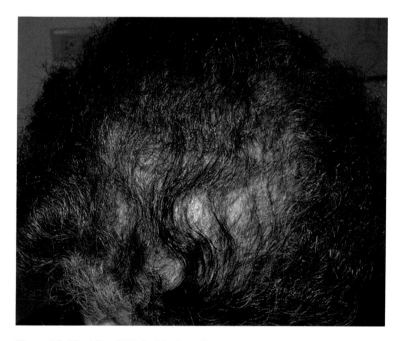

Figure 15.11 *After 900 1–4 hair grafts*

■ Keys to Success

- Wait at least 12 months after loss before considering surgery
- Follow the natural angle of hair in the temporal region, i.e., 15° angle pointing down toward the neck
- With appropriate patient selection, there is high patient satisfaction

BIBLIOGRAPHY

Avram MR. Accurately communicating the extent of a hair transplant procedure. A proposal of a follicular-based classification scheme. *Dermatol Surg.* September 1997;23(9):817–818.

Avram MR. Polarized light-emitting diode magnification for optimal recipient site creation during hair transplant. *Dermatol Surg.* September 2005;31(9, pt 1):1124–1127. Discussion 1127.

Avram MR, et al. The potential role of minoxidil in the hair transplantation setting. *Dermatol Surg.* October 2002; 28(10):894–900. Discussion 900.

Epstein JS. The treatment of female pattern hair loss and other applications of surgical hair restoration in women. *Facial Plast Surg Clin North Am.* May 2004;12(2):241–247.

Harris JA. Follicular unit transplantation: dissecting and planting techniques. *Facial Plast Surg Clin North Am.* May 2004;12(2):225–232.

Leavitt M, Perez-Meza D, Rao NA, Barusco M, Kaufman KD, Ziering C. Effects of finasteride (1 mg) on hair transplant. *Dermatol Surg.* October 2005;31(10):1268–1276. Discussion 1276.

Limmer BL. Elliptical donor stereoscopically assisted micrografting as an approach to further refinement in hair transplantation. *J Dermatol Surg Oncol.* December 1994; 20(12):789–793.

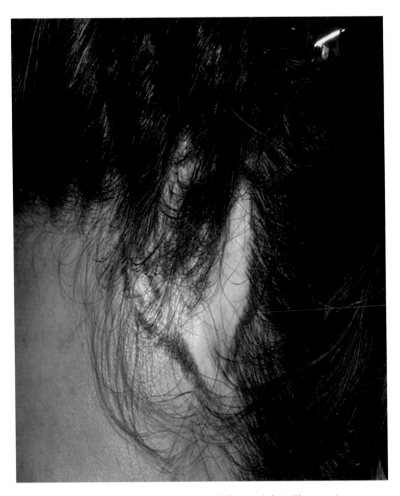

Figure 15.12 *Pre-op temporal scar—chief complaint: "I cannot wear my hair back"*

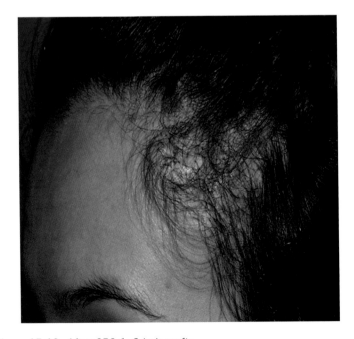

Figure 15.13 *After 650 1–3 hair grafts*

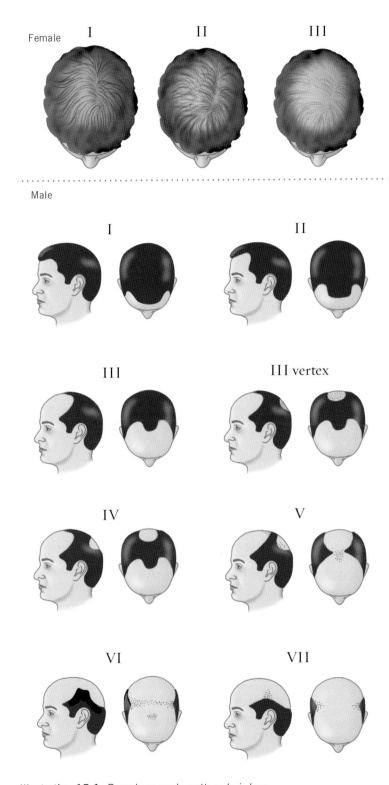

Illustration 15.1 *Female vs male pattern hair loss*

CHAPTER 16 Hirsutism

Hirsutism represents a male pattern overgrowth of terminal and vellus hairs in women. Far from being solely a cosmetic concern, hirsutism can be an important manifestation of an underlying endocrine disorder arising from increased androgenic activity. Often, it results from an overproduction of adrenal and ovarian hormones and may accompany other signs of virilization. Its appearance produces social anxiety, distress, and ostracism in affected patients. It also merits an appropriate medical workup. By contrast, hypertrichosis features fine hairs in androgen-sensitive as well as androgen-insensitive areas. Normal racial and ethnic variations may cause confusion with these disorders.

EPIDEMIOLOGY

Incidence: common

Age: usually postpubertal but age of onset can vary in the setting of medication, tumor, or endocrine abnormality.

Race: racial and cultural factors affect the perception of what constitutes abnormal hair growth. Skin type affects treatment options as well.

Sex: female

Precipitating Factors: hirsutism is caused by a host of endocrine abnormalities. Adrenal causes include Cushing's disease, ectopic ACTH production, primary androgen-producing neoplasms, and congenital adrenal hyperplasia. Ovarian causes can be related to polycystic ovarian syndrome and primary tumors among other causes. Finally, medications such as oral contraceptive pills, anabolic steroids, and androgens may cause hirsutism.

PHYSICAL EXAMINATION

There is an overgrowth of hair in androgen-sensitive hair follicles. Common sites include the beard area of the face, chin, preauricular face, linea alba, periareolar area, and chest. Depending on the severity of the condition, other signs of virilization such as increased muscle mass, deep voice, male pattern hair loss, and clitoral enlargement may be present.

DIFFERENTIAL DIAGNOSIS

While both hirsutism and hypertrichosis feature hair overgrowth, these conditions can be differentiated by the location and quality of the hair growth. Hirsutism is characterized by terminal hair overgrowth in androgen-dependent areas,

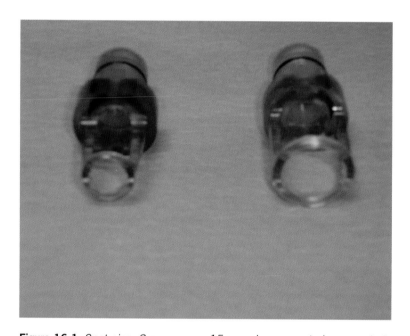

Figure 16.1 *Spot size, 8 mm versus 15 mm. Larger spot sizes penetrate deeper and allow quicker treatments*

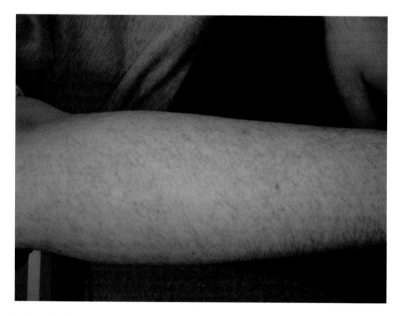

Figure 16.2 *Hair trimmed prior to treatment*

while hypertrichosis features fine hairs in androgen-sensitive as well as androgen-insensitive areas. Normal racial and ethnic variations may cause confusion with these disorders.

LABORATORY TESTS

The laboratory workup should be guided by the patient's clinical findings as well as by a detailed patient history. Testing can help establish if there is an adrenal or ovarian source of the hair growth. Ovarian, adrenal, and pituitary tumors should be ruled out in cases of rapid onset by an endocrinologist and/or a gynecologist. Total testosterone levels, dehydroepiandrosterone sulfate levels, urinary free cortisol levels, dexamethasone suppression test, prolactin levels, ACTH stimulation, LH/FSH ratio, 17-hydroxy progesterone levels, and pelvic ultrasound may all represent important components of a thorough endocrinologic workup.

COURSE

Course is dependent on the etiology of the hirsutism.

KEY CONSULTATIVE QUESTIONS

- Menstrual history—regular or irregular
- Medication history
- Onset and progression of symptoms
- Family history
- History of endocrine abnormalities

MANAGEMENT

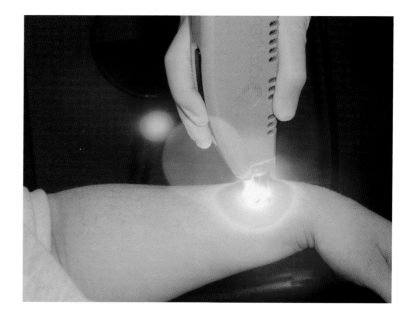

Figure 16.3 *Laser light firing*

The primary goal of the treatment is to determine the underlying cause of the hirsutism and treat. After determining the cause and insuring appropriate medical therapy, the goal can transition to reversing the abnormal hair growth. There are multiple means by which temporary and permanent hair removal can be achieved.

■ Consultation with Endocrinology

In cases of hirsutism, the first priority is to uncover the source of the aberrant hair growth. Numerous laboratory investigations as detailed above may be required. Consultation and referral to an endocrinologist is strongly recommended as part of such a workup.

■ Nonlaser Therapies

There are several temporary means to conceal hair overgrowth. They include makeup, bleaches, and hydrogen peroxide. Shaving also can temporarily hide hair growth.

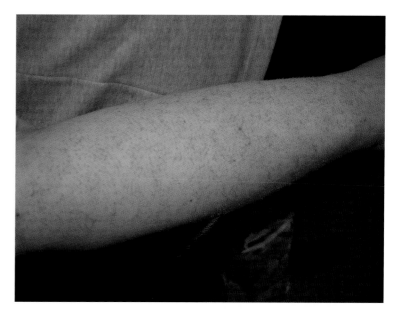

Figure 16.4 *Characteristic post treatment perifollicular erythema*

Hair removal can be achieved with depilation, epilation, laser therapy, electrolysis, and topical eflornithine.

Depilation

Depilation is the process of removing part of the hair shaft. Its effects are temporary. There are chemical and mechanical methods of depilation. Chemical depilatories, such as thioglycolate salts and sulfides of alkali metals, dissolve hair shafts. They can produce localized irritation at the site of treatment. Mechanical depilation can be quite crude including shaving of hair as well as rubbing hair with a pumice stone.

Epilation

Epilation is the process of removing the entire hair shaft. It provides more longevity than depilation but is not permanent. It includes waxing, plucking, threading, and electrical devices that remove the hair shaft. Each of these options is relatively inexpensive but can produce pain and irritation as side effects. Plucking can result in localized infection, ingrown hairs, and even scarring. Each of these treatments can be used in combination with topical eflornithine on the face of women.

Topical eflornithine

Topical eflornithine twice daily has been approved by the FDA for temporary hair removal on the face of women. It should only be used on the face and not on other parts of the body. It decreases the rate of hair growth by inhibiting ornithine decarboxylase. It should be used in conjunction with other hair removal methods, such as shaving, waxing, or plucking. Discontinuation of treatment results in a resumption of hair growth. Side effects include local irritation. It should not be used during pregnancy.

▣ Electrolysis

• Removal can be permanent

• Electrolysis uses direct electrical current to destroy the dermal papilla of the hair follicle. A fine needle placed directly into the hair follicle delivers the electrical current to the follicle's base without producing scarring. The site of treatment is shaved several days prior to therapy and topical anesthetic cream can be used 1 h prior to the procedure to reduce pain. Side effects include scar, hypo/hyperpigmentation, and infection. It is most appropriate for small areas of treatment

• Need for multiple treatments for limited treatment zone

• Greater risk of side effects, painful

• Not practical for large areas of the body

▣ Laser Hair Removal

Lasers are the treatment of choice for permanent reduction of unwanted, pigmented terminal hair follicles. Laser hair removal is quick, relatively nonpainful, especially compared to electrolysis. Furthermore, it can cover a far more extensive area of affected skin with less pain in less

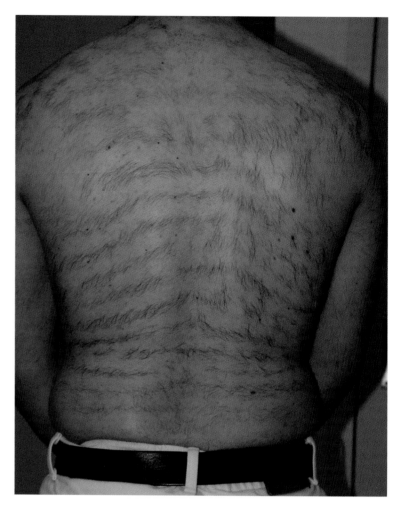

Figure 16.5 *Bizarre growth of back hair on a male due to poor technique (i.e. improper spacing and overlap)*

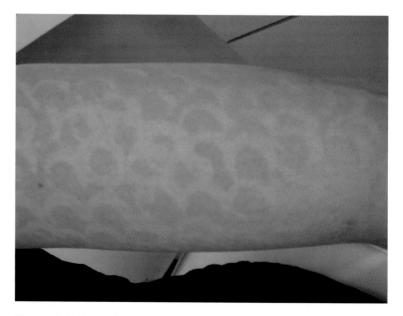

Figure 16.6 *Extensive dyschromia secondary to inappropriate fluence and pulse duration*

time. An average of five to seven treatments are needed for greater than 50% reduction.

Mechanism of action

Lasers are based on the selective photothermolysis. The light is absorbed by the pigment in hair follicles. Therefore if hair follicles have no pigment (i.e., blond or gray hair), lasers do not work.

■ Patient Consultation

- Hair color
- Skin type—all skin types can benefit from laser hair removal
- Past medical history
- Medications
- Past treatments
- Emphasize the need for five to seven treatments on an average to remove the majority of unwanted hair
- Improvement is variable
- Low risk of no improvement or *increased* hair (especially in females of meditervanean heritage)
- Risk of hyper or hypopigmentation that may last months; rarely permanent
- Scarring is rare
- Likelihood of at least some pain; the amount of pain associated with the procedure is a reflection of the caliber and density of hair in the treated region
- Ideal candidate has dark course hair and light skin phototype
- Average candidate—fine/light brown hair with increased hair on lateral cheeks
- Poor candidate—blond/gray hair should not be treated with current lasers. Additionally, patients with unrealistic expectations or medical contraindications should not be treated

■ Patient Consultation Prior to Treatment

- Sun avoidance is crucial. If a patient is tanned, the procedure should be postponed until the tan completely fades. If the procedure is performed on tanned skin, the risk of dyschromia is markedly increased
- Shave hair prior to arriving in the office. Alternatively, the hair can be trimmed in the office with a moustache trimmer. This will focus the majority of energy to the pigmented hair follicles in the skin
- A topical anesthetic cream can be applied 1 h prior to therapy to decrease the pain during the procedure. It is important to advise the patient to apply topical anesthetic over a limited surface of the skin to avoid any risk of lidocaine toxicity
- Hair waxing should not be performed 2–3 weeks before treatment.

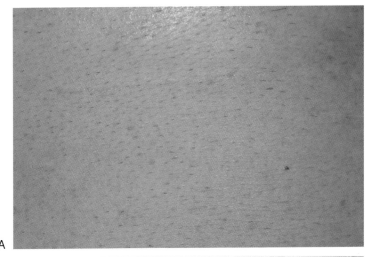

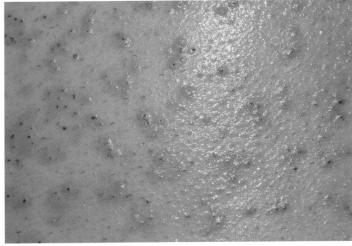

Figure 16.7 (A) *Appearance of skin prior to laser hair removal.* **(B)** *Appropriate clinical endpoint shows perifollicular erythema after treatment with a 810 nm diode laser*

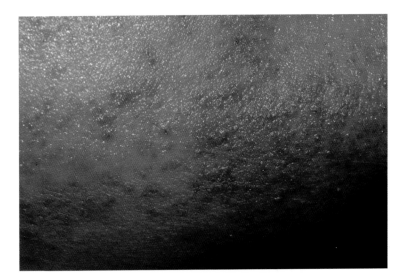

Figure 16.8 *Appropriate clinical endpoint of perifollicular erythema in this 24-year-old female with type VI skin and polycystic ovarian syndrome treated with the long-pulsed 1064 nm Nd:YAG laser*

- If there is a history of recurrent herpes simplex virus, prophylaxis should be provided before laser hair removal on face
- Pregnancy: there are no clear studies demonstrating safety or risk. It is important to educate pregnant patients desiring hair removal as to this uncertainty. Most physicians will not treat patients while pregnant. If treatment is pursued, it is recommended to treat only limited areas during third trimester after medical clearance from an obstetrician

◼ Just Prior to Treatment

- Written consent
- Photography
- Trim hair

◼ Laser Hair Removal Technique (Figs. 16.1-16.8) (Table 16.1)

Key concepts for optimal results

- For skin types I–III, use relatively high energy with a shorter pulse duration for optimal results
- Skin types IV–VI *must* use longer pulse duration with higher energies
- If uncertain as to treatment parameters, perform test sites with variable fluencies and pulse durations
- All machines utilize cooling of epidermal skin via cryogen, contact cooling, or gel
- Optimal cooling settings must be utilized to lower the risk of dyschromia
- Use larger spot sizes for deeper penetration and more rapid treatment of larger areas
- Safety goggles for patient and medical team
- Use the largest spot size possible for target region
- Overlap laser pulses 10% over the entire treatment region

TABLE 16.1 ◼ **Laser Hair Removal Technique**

Laser type	Safest skin type	Wavelength (nm)	Pulse duration	Energy (J/cm^2)	Comments
Ruby	I–III	694	1–20 ms	10–40 J/cm^2	First laser used for hair removal; slower to use
Alexandrite	I–III	755	Skin types I–III 3 ms; skin types III and IV 10–20 ms	Skin types I–III 20–25 J/cm^2; skin type IV 15–20 J/cm^2	3 ms and 10–20 ms pulse duration demonstrate equal efficacy
Diode	I–V	810	3–100 ms	30–40 J/cm^2	Longer pulse duration for treatment of skin types IV and V
Nd:YAG	I–VI	1064	Skin types I–III 10-20 ms; skin types IV–VI 25–100 ms	Skin types I–III 30–50 J/cm^2; skin types III–VI 25–35 J/cm^2	Safest device for removing hair in skin types IV–VI
Intense pulsed light—noncoherent light	I–IV	550–1200	1.5–3.5 ms	25–50 J/cm^2	Most variable results

LASER SAFETY

Hazard: ocular

Dangers
Cornea, retina, or lens can be damaged

Damage can occur from direct exposure or reflected beams, i.e. patient jewelry, watches

Q-switched lasers are most hazardous, can cause blindness

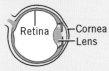

Enhance Safety
Baseline eye exam

Laser goggle optical density (OD) should be equal to or greater than 7 (check goggles)

Inspect goggles for visible damage or degradation of the filter media

Always check that appropriate goggles for wavelength are used

Remove, ebonize or cover any reflective surfaces in laser room, i.e. mirrors, metallic garbage cans

Remove patient jewelry, watches

Hazard: fire

Dangers
All lasers can potentially cause fire hazards

Most commonly seen with CO_2 lasers

Damage can occur from direct exposure or reflected beams

Enhance Safety
Remove, ebonize, or cover any relfective surfaces in laser room, i.e. mirrors, metallic garbage cans

Avoid alcohol or ensure that it is fully vaporized prior to start of treatment

Drape treatment site with wet gauze or towels

Remove all flammable items, i.e. dry gauze, towels, drapes

Coat exposed hair with water-based jelly

Decrease FiO_2 to 40% when treating near endotracheal tubes

Hazard: plume, splatter, infection

Dangers
Intact virions and viral DNA such as HPV may be present in the plume of CO_2 lasers

Tissue particles can splatter and aerosolize with Q-switched lasers

Enhance Safety
Use mask

Smoke evacuator

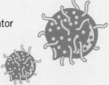

Hazard: electrocution

Dangers
Even with power off, can cause shock/electrocution

Enhance Safety
Only qualified laser technicians should open lasers

Check for water spills, hose ruptures or condensations

Hazard: general

Dangers
Anticipate dangers

Enhance Safety
Always immediately put laser on standby mode when not treating patient

Ensure proper sign is on the door of laser room

Educate staff members as to laser safety

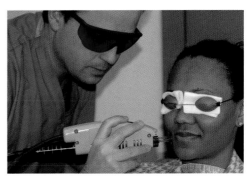

A

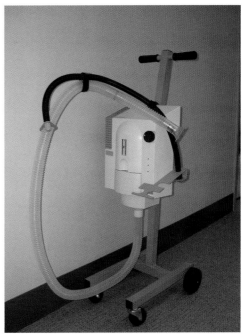

B

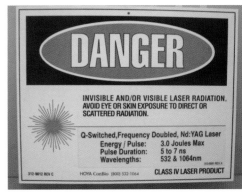

C

Figure 16.9 *Laser safety. It is important to emphasize that lasers present special safety concerns for physicians, staff, and patients. Among the risks are ocular injury, fire, electrocution, and dissemination of infectious disease. No lasers should be operated in the absence of a detailed knowledge of laser safety issues between the physician and the staff. Educating staff members is an essential component of safe laser practices. Periodic laser safety training is required by many hospitals and remains good practice for private physician offices as well. (A) Patient and all personnel are wearing protective eyewear. Note gauze is moist to reduce the risk of fire. (B) Smoke evacuator. (C) Safety sign placed outside appropriate laser room to ensure proper warning of laser use*

■ Post-treatment Instructions to Patient

- Expect redness for up to several hours after treatment

- If redness or pain persists for more than 12 h, call the office

- Once redness fades, patient may continue to wear makeup

- Avoid sun for 48 h; no tanning

- Hair removal is not entirely immediate. Some hair will fall out 1–3 days after treatment

- Do not worry if some hair persists after treatment

- Call the office if discoloration develops in the treated sites

- Call the office with questions or concerns

PITFALLS TO AVOID/ COMPLICATIONS/ MANAGEMENT (Figs. 16.5-16.6)

- There is no effective mechanism for laser removal of light or blond hair

- Excessive fluencies or incorrect pulse duration may produce epidermal damage and dyschromia. These effects are typically temporary but can be permanent. If there is any doubt regarding laser parameters, perform a test site

- Skin types IV–VI require longer pulse durations and lower fluencies

- Coincident tattoos and lentigines may experience lightening. Patients should be informed of this possibility

- Always keep contact cooling against the skin to avoid burning

- Overlap (10%) in the treated zone. Do not leave "gaps" that can create bizarre hair growth patterns as hair regrows

- For Nd:YAG lasers, patients may experience pain even after topical anesthesia

BIBLIOGRAPHY

Azziz R. The evaluation and management of hirsutism. *Obstet Gynecol.* 2003;101(5, pt 1):995–1007.

Battle EF, et al. Laser-assisted hair removal for darker skin types. *Dermatol Ther.* 2004;17(2):177–183.

Bouzari N, et al. Laser hair removal: comparison of long-pulsed Nd:YAG, long-pulsed alexandrite, and long-pulsed diode lasers. *Dermatol Surg.* 2004;30(4, pt 1):498–502.

Goldberg DJ. Laser hair removal. *Dermatol Clin.* 2002;20(3):561–567.

Tanzi EL, Alster TS. Long-pulsed 1064-nm Nd:YAG laser-assisted hair removal in all skin types. *Dermatol Surg.* 2004;30(1):13–17.

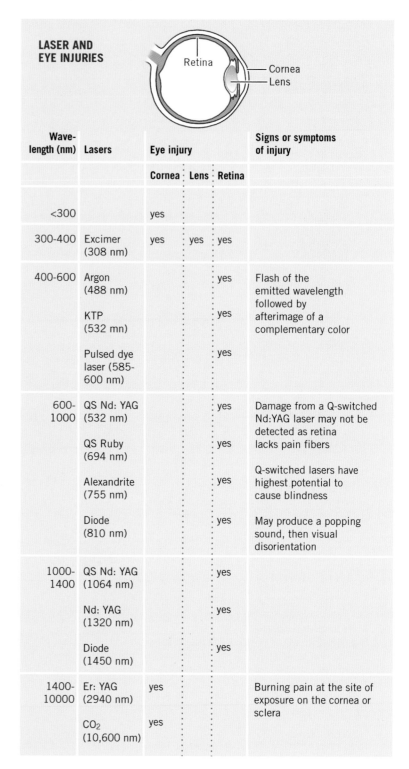

Wavelength (nm)	Lasers	Eye injury			Signs or symptoms of injury
		Cornea	Lens	Retina	
<300		yes			
300-400	Excimer (308 nm)	yes	yes	yes	
400-600	Argon (488 nm)			yes	Flash of the emitted wavelength followed by afterimage of a complementary color
	KTP (532 mn)			yes	
	Pulsed dye laser (585-600 nm)			yes	
600-1000	QS Nd: YAG (532 nm)			yes	Damage from a Q-switched Nd:YAG laser may not be detected as retina lacks pain fibers
	QS Ruby (694 nm)			yes	
	Alexandrite (755 nm)			yes	Q-switched lasers have highest potential to cause blindness
	Diode (810 nm)			yes	May produce a popping sound, then visual disorientation
1000-1400	QS Nd: YAG (1064 nm)			yes	
	Nd: YAG (1320 nm)			yes	
	Diode (1450 nm)			yes	
1400-10000	Er: YAG (2940 nm)	yes			Burning pain at the site of exposure on the cornea or sclera
	CO₂ (10,600 nm)	yes			

Figure 16.10 *Lasers and eye injuries (http://www.eyesafety.4ursafety.com/laser-eye-safety.html)*

CHAPTER 17 Pseudofolliculitis

Pseudofolliculitis is a common, chronic inflammatory disorder that presents with inflammatory papules and pustules in the beard distribution of males, particularly those with darker skin phototypes and tightly coiled hair. Nonetheless, pseudofolliculitis can present in any skin that is regularly shaved and in all skin phototypes. In females it is most commonly seen in the axillary and pubic areas. It tends to present in a more mild form in lighter skin phototypes.

EPIDEMIOLOGY

Incidence: over 50% of African-American males

Age: begins with shaving

Race: more common in beard distribution of males with darker skin phototypes

Sex: male > females

Precipitating factors: shaving in any region of the body

PATHOGENESIS

This disorder is induced by shaving. Shaving sharpens curled hair. Sharpened, tightly curled hairs pierce into the skin adjacent to the hair follicle and invade into the dermis producing an inflammatory reaction.

DERMATOPATHOLOGY

Hair penetration results in epidermal invagination with associated microabscess, mixed inflammatory infiltrate, and foreign body giant reaction at the tip of the invading hair. Dermal fibrosis may be observed.

PHYSICAL LESIONS

Most commonly, it presents with follicular papules, pustules, and post-inflammatory hyperpigmentation in the beard and anterolateral neck of males and underarms and bikini areas of females. Papules can develop into cysts. Scar formation may be observed. The upper cutaneous lip is typically spared.

DIFFERENTIAL DIAGNOSIS

Acne vulgaris, folliculitis.

LABORATORY EXAMINATION

None.

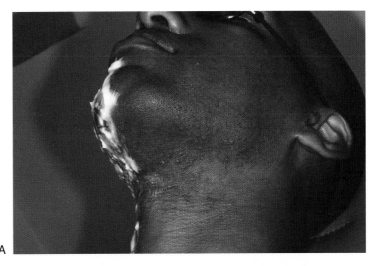

A

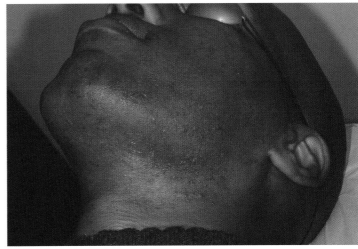

B

Figure 17.1 (A) *A young male with type VI skin phototype and pseudofolliculitis barbae prior to treatment.* **(B)** *Same patient 3 months later after several treatments with long-pulsed 1064 nm Nd:YAG laser (photographs courtesy of E. Victor Ross, MD)*

COURSE

Begins with shaving and continues until cessation or modification in the shaving technique.

MANAGEMENT

The goal of the treatment is to prevent the formation of the papules, pustules, scarring, and post-inflammatory hyperpigmentation associated with this disorder. There are multiple treatment options available to accomplish this goal. Cessation of shaving is the most successful treatment but it is impractical and undesirable for many patients. Laser therapy is highly effective with high patient satisfaction.

TREATMENT

■ Shaving Cessation

The most simple, inexpensive, and effective treatment for pseudofolliculitis is the cessation of shaving. Many patients will find this option undesirable or not practical.

■ Modification of Shaving Technique

A proper shaving technique may prevent or significantly decrease the risk of pseudofolliculitis. Among these practices are lifting—not plucking ingrown hairs, thoroughly wetting the area prior to applying shaving cream, using a sharp razor, shaving in the direction of the hair growth, and avoiding shaving in more than one direction in the same area. The Bump Fighter Razor prevents the shaved hair from being cut too short. Additionally, cutting the hair twice daily with hair clippers prevents hairs from piercing into the skin.

■ Topical Treatment

Topical antibiotics are effective in treating the inflammation and occasional impetiginization associated with this condition. Topical tretinoin, benzoyl peroxide, and glycolic acids can be helpful adjuncts.

■ Laser Hair Removal (Figs. 17.1-17.2)

• Skin types I–III

  – The long-pulsed alexandrite laser (755 nm), diode laser (810 nm), intense pulse light (590–100 nm), and long-pulsed Nd:YAG (1064 nm) have the appropriate wavelengths to selectively target the chromophore melanin found in the hair bulb.

  – Multiple treatments (average of 5–10) every 4–8 weeks achieve an average of 50–75% permanent reduction of follicular papules/pustules.

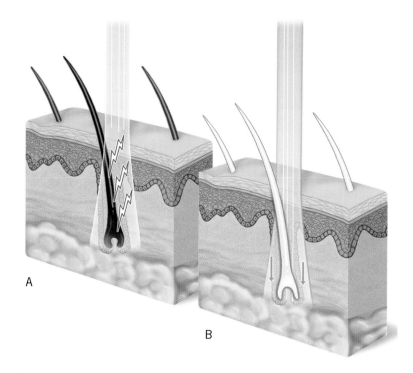

A

B

Figure 17.2 *Pseudofolliculitis—laser therapy: pigmented versus unpigmented hair follicle*

- Skin types IV–VI
  - The long-pulsed 1064 nm Nd:YAG laser is the treatment of choice in skin phototypes IV–VI. It is safe and effective. Long pulse durations are necessary for epidermal protection. Pulse durations of 30–100 ms are generally recommended. Optimal fluences range from 30 to 40 J/cm^2. Treatment is performed with nonoverlapping pulses utilizing cooling to the epidermis via cryogen, contact cooling, or gel.
  - Typically, 5–10 treatments spaced every 4–8 weeks are needed for 50–75% permanent reduction.

PITFALLS TO AVOID/ OUTCOME EXPECTATIONS/ COMPLICATIONS/MANAGEMENT

- Suntanned patients should not be treated with laser hair removal. Once the tan/inflammation subsides, hair removal can begin.
- Do not pluck or wax hair prior to or during the course of laser hair removal.
- Patients with unpigmented hair (blond, grey, red) will not benefit from laser hair removal and should not be treated.
- There is the risk of transient and long-term hyperpigmentation and hypopigmentation. Transient erythema, scabbing, and risk of scar formation also exist.
- A minority of patients will see <75% improvement. A small minority will see little or no improvement.
- Future maintenance treatments may be needed.
- A small minority of patients will experience a paradoxical increase in hair growth, particularly females of Mediterranean descent.
- Treatment may not benefit preexisting hyperpigmentation and will not improve scars.
- It is important to inform patients that side effects are often delayed in skin phototypes IV–VI and may not be observed for 1–2 weeks after treatment. Test spot is advised for these patients (Figs. 17.3-17.4).

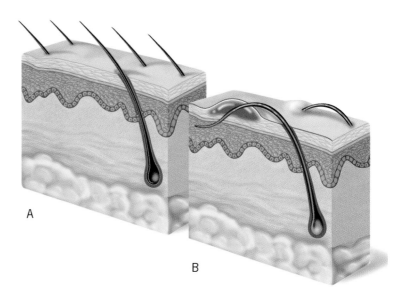

Figure 17.3 *Etrology and Pseudofolliculitis*

BIBLIOGRAPHY

Battle EF Jr, Hobbs LM. Laser-assisted hair removal for darker skin types. *Dermatol Ther.* 2004;17(2):177–183.

Bridgeman-Shah S. The medical and surgical therapy of pseudofolliculitis barbae. *Dermatol Ther.* 2004;17(2): 158–163.

Haedersdal M, Wulf HC. Evidence-based review of hair removal using lasers and light sources. *J Eur Acad Dermatol Venereol.* January 2006;20(1):9–20.

Kontoes P, et al. Hair induction after laser-assisted hair removal and its treatment. *J Am Acad Dermatol.* January 2006;54(1):64–67.

Ross EV, Cooke LM, Timko AL, Overstreet KA, Graham BS, Barnette DJ. Treatment of pseudofolliculitis barbae in skin types IV, V, and VI with a long-pulsed neodymium: yttrium aluminum garnet laser. *J Am Acad Dermatol.* 2002;47(2): 888–893.

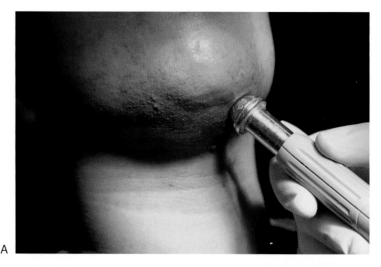

A

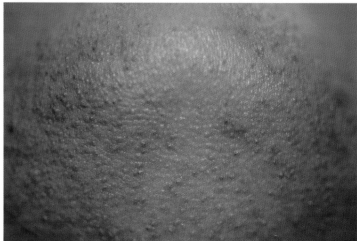

B

Figure 17.4 **(A)** *Test spot treatment under chin and on cheek is advised for darker skin phototypes before treating pseudofolliculitis.* **(B)** *Two weeks after test spot treatment, some hair removal is achieved with no pigmentary changes*

SECTION
FIVE

Disorders of Pigmentation

CHAPTER 18 Café Au Lait Macule

Café au lait macules (CALMs) are benign well-demarcated, light brown macules that typically present in early childhood. The pigmentation is typically uniform. Lesions may be multiple or isolated. They grow in proportion to the growth of the child. They are present in as many as 20% of the population and, rarely, can be associated with a host of genodermatoses.

EPIDEMIOLOGY

Incidence: 10–20% of the population

Age: birth and early childhood

Race: more common in African-Americans than Caucasians

Sex: none

Precipitating factors: most commonly these are benign, isolated findings in healthy children. Multiple CALMs can be associated with genodermatoses such as neurofibromatosis, tuberous sclerosis, Bloom's syndrome, McCune–Albright syndrome, Russell–Silver syndrome, Watson's syndrome, and Westerhof's syndrome

PATHOGENESIS

Unknown.

PATHOLOGY

Increased melanin in basal keratinocytes. Clinically darker lesions contain more melanocytes than lighter ones.

PHYSICAL LESIONS

Lesions are well-demarcated, uniformly pigmented macules that vary in color from hues of tan to light brown to brown. They can present anywhere on the body but spare mucous membranes. Their size can range from a few millimeters to over 20 cm.

DIFFERENTIAL DIAGNOSIS

Post-inflammatory hyperpigmentation, Becker's nevus, melasma, lentigines, ephelides, berloque dermatitis, and congenital nevus.

LABORATORY EXAMINATION

Biopsy is not indicated. Additional laboratory workup may be appropriate in the event of suspicion of an underlying systemic disorder.

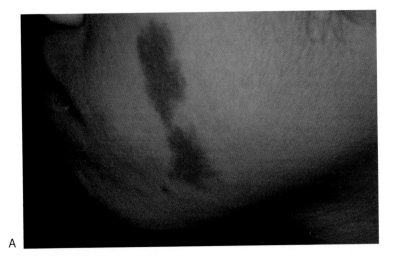

A

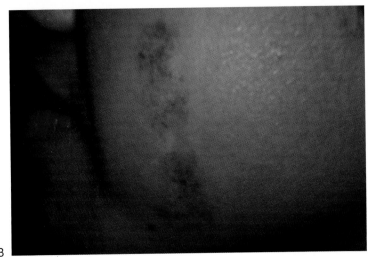

B

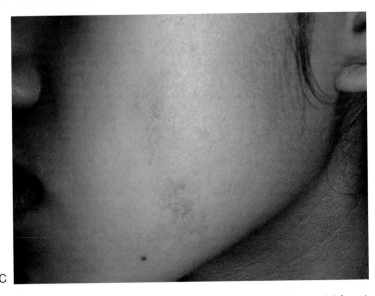

C

Figure 18.1 (A) *Café au lait macule on left cheek of a 17-year-old female prior to treatment.* **(B)** *Erythema and lightening of café au lait macule after one treatment with 694 nm Q-switched ruby laser.* **(C)** *Significant clearing after four treatments with Q-switched ruby laser*

COURSE

They grow in proportion to the growth of the child. Once a child has fully grown, CALMs do not change in size or color. There is no increased risk of malignant transformation.

KEY CONSULTATIVE QUESTIONS

- Time of onset
- Failure to meet milestones
- Photosensitivity
- Intellectual impairment
- History of multiple fractures
- CNS disorders or tumors
- Poor growth
- Scoliosis
- Ophthalmologic impairment

MANAGEMENT

CALMs do not require treatment unless their appearance is disfiguring or distressing to the patient or parents. Multiple lesions may suggest an underlying systemic disorder. If there is any indication of underlying systemic abnormalities in the setting of multiple CALMs, referral to appropriate pediatric specialists is indicated. Laser therapy is often employed as a treatment. Cryotherapy and surgical excision are alternatives to laser therapy but carry the risk of pigmentary alterations, poor cosmesis, pain, and scarring.

LASER TREATMENT (Figs. 18.1-18.3)

Prior to treatment, a test site should be performed to assess for efficacy and hyperpigmentation. CALMs respond variably to multiple modalities of laser therapy.

- Q-switched lasers including the frequency-doubled Q-switched Nd:YAG (532 nm, 3 mm spot, 1.0–1.5 J/cm^2), Q-switched ruby (694 nm, 6.5 mm, 3.0–4.5 J/cm^2), and the Q-switched alexandrite (755 nm, 3-mm spot, 2.5–3.5 J/cm^2), have been most commonly employed for selective pigment removal.

    - In one study, Q-switched ruby and frequency-doubled Q-switched Nd:YAG treatments, each at 6 J/cm^2, produced variable responses including

        ○ Significant lightening, which was most frequently observed

        ○ Clearance with recurrence

        ○ Darkening

    - Q-switched lasers have a decreased risk of textural change versus other laser therapies, but still carry the risk of hyperpigmentation.

    - Results are variable with about 50% of lesions showing a response.

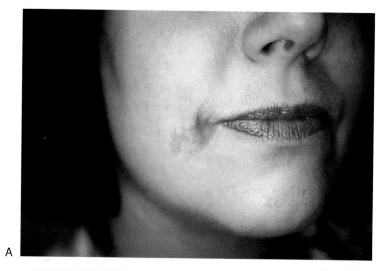

A

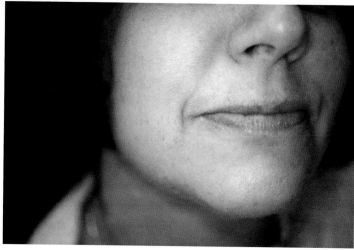

B

Figure 18.2 (A) *Café au lait macule adjoining right lateral commissure of lips.* **(B)** *Near clearance after three treatments with a 755 nm Q-switched alexandrite laser*

– While full resolution can be obtained with the Q-switched lasers, there are frequent recurrences. Frustratingly, recurrences may occur 6 months to 1 year after treatment. Sometimes lightening, rather than full resolution, is the best obtainable result. All of these lasers produce equivalent results in the treatment of CALMs.

TOPICAL TREATMENT

CALMs are not responsive to topical bleaching creams.

PITFALLS TO AVOID/ OUTCOME EXPECTATIONS/ COMPLICATIONS/MANAGEMENT

* Unfortunately, despite their superficial nature, CALMs can be difficult to treat completely.

* Lightening, rather than full clearance, is often the best result; even after multiple treatments.

* There is a high risk of recurrence of CALMs up to 1 year after treatment.

* Studies indicate a risk for hyper and hypopigmentation associated with the Q-switched lasers, especially in darker skin phototypes.

* Treating above the therapeutic threshold may result in prolonged healing and increased risk of pigmentary changes.

* Patients with darker skin types should be treated cautiously and conservatively given the lower therapeutic threshold.

* Laser treatment of tanned patients should be avoided.

BIBLIOGRAPHY

Alora MB, Arndt KA. Treatment of a cafe-au-lait macule with the erbium:YAG laser. *J Am Acad Dermatol.* 2001; 45(4):566–568.

Grossman MC, Anderson RR, Farinelli W, Flotte TJ, Grevelink JM. Treatment of café au lait macules with lasers: a clinicopathologic correlation. *Arch Dermatol.* 1995;131: 1416–1420.

Levy JL, Mordon S, Pizzi-Anselme M. Treatment of individual cafe au lait macules with the Q-switched Nd:YAG: a clinicopathologic correlation. *Cutan Laser Ther.* 1999;1(4): 217–223.

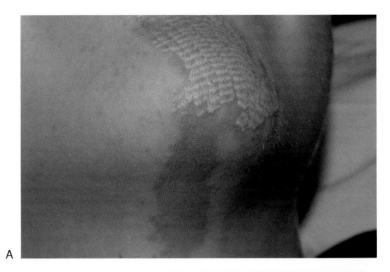

A

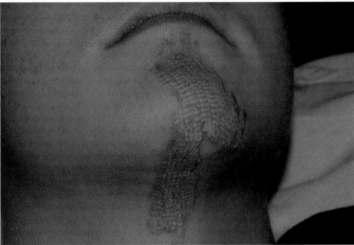

B

Figure 18.3 (A) *Treatment of café au lait macule on the chin of a young man with a 532 nm frequency doubled Q-switched Nd:YAG laser.* **(B)** *Completion of treatment of café au lait macule with the appropriate clinical endpoint of tissue whitening and erythema*

CHAPTER 19 Ephelides

Ephelides, more commonly known as freckles, are benign, small, well-demarcated, brown macules found on the sun-exposed skin of blond, light brown, and red-haired individuals. They present in early childhood and decrease in older age. They can be distinguished from lentigines in that they darken in times of high sun exposure and fade during periods of limited sun exposure.

EPIDEMIOLOGY

Incidence: very common, particularly in fair-skinned patients

Age: early childhood

Race: more common in Caucasians, but also seen in Asians

Sex: equal

Precipitating factors: individuals with light hair and complexion such as blonds and redheads

PATHOGENESIS

The brown pigmentation associated with ephelides results from increased production of melanin in sun-exposed areas of the skin.

PATHOLOGY

Keratinocytes display an increase in melanin especially in the basal layer, but there is no substantial increase in the number of melanocytes in ephelides.

PHYSICAL LESIONS

Ephelides are well-demarcated light brown to dark brown macules of several millimeters diameter that present in sun-exposed areas of the skin.

DIFFERENTIAL DIAGNOSIS

The differential diagnosis includes other benign lesions such as lentigines and junctional nevi.

LABORATORY EXAMINATION

None.

COURSE

They present in early childhood. They darken in periods of high sun exposure and lighten during periods of limited sun exposure.

KEY CONSULTATIVE QUESTIONS

Sun exposure

MANAGEMENT

There is no medical indication to treat ephelides. The cosmetic appearance, however, may displease some individuals. Sun avoidance and sunscreens protect against darkening of ephelides. Bleaching creams, such as hydroquinone, and topical retinoids can produce lightening. Cryotherapy and laser treatment are also effective. Recurrence is frequent, particularly with sun exposure.

TREATMENTS

■ Topical Treatment

Topical bleaching creams may provide some lightening. Multiple formulations are available differing in their product contents and strengths.

- Hydroquinone (2–4%) creams have traditionally been employed.
  - Twice daily application of the cream to the ephelides over 3–6 months is generally necessary to achieve noted benefits.
  - Side effects include irritation, pruritus, peeling, and dryness of the treated areas.
  - If erythema and irritation occur, exercise caution to avoid hyperpigmentation.
  - Patients must discontinue the treatment if any lightening of nonlesional skin is observed.
  - Bleaching creams are contraindicated in pregnant and lactating women.
- Retinoids
  - Retinoids have been added in products such as Solage (2% mequinol and 0.01% tretinoin) and Triluma (0.01% fluocinolone acetonide, 4% hydroquinone, and 0.05% tretinoin) to provide an exfoliative benefit.
  - Triluma application must be limited in duration due to the possibility of side effects with repeated corticosteroid usage.
- Azelaic acid (20%) cream is slightly effective for ephelides and lentigines.
- Kojic acid (1–2.5%) cream.

Chemical Peels

Chemical peels can be helpful in reducing the appearance of ephelides.

- Over-the-counter α-hydroxy acid peels are a beneficial adjunct to physician-strength chemical peels. The

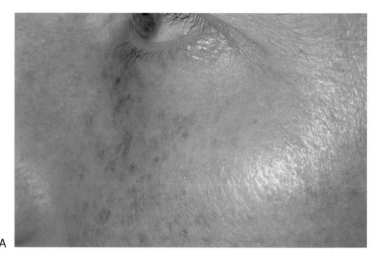

A

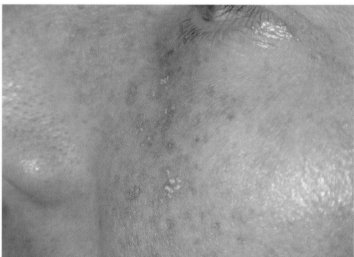

B

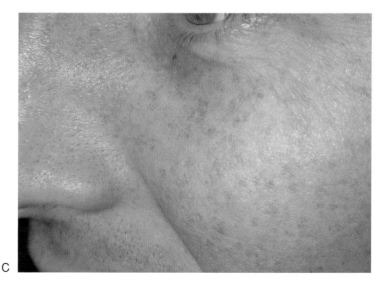

C

Figure 19.1 (A) *A 38-year-old male from Southern California with extensive ephelides.* **(B)** *Same patient with post-treatment whitening immediately after frequency-doubled Q-switched Nd:YAG (532 nm) laser therapy.* **(C)** *Significant improvement 2 weeks after single treatment with frequency-doubled Q-switched Nd:YAG (532 nm) laser utilizing a fluence of 1.5 J/cm² and a 2.0 mm spot size*

continual exfoliation achieved from consistent use of the peels will result in mild lightening.

- Glycolic acid peels (35–70%) are administered every 2–3 weeks utilizing increasing strengths as tolerated. Lightening of ephelides may be observed after four to six peels. Strict photoprotection is stressed.

- Jessner peels (resorcinol, lactic acid, and salicylic acid) are administered every 6–8 weeks.
  - Strict photoprotection for 2–3 months is advised.
  - Multiple treatments are recommended.
  - Contraindicated in pregnant and lactating women.

- Combination Jessner/10% trichloroacetic (TCA) peels may also be employed in a similar fashion as the Jessner peel.
  - The Jessner peel results in exfoliation allowing for greater penetration of the TCA peel.
  - Multiple peels are generally needed. Contraindicated in pregnant and lactating women.

- Caution to avoid pigmentary changes; care must be utilized in treating skin phototypes III–V, in particular with medium-depth peels.

- A test site should be considered.

Cryotherapy

Cryotherapy can produce lightening of freckling.

- Has a risk of hypo or hyperpigmentation at treated sites.
- Recurrence is common.

▇ Laser Therapy (Figs. 19.1-19.2)

Laser therapy can be effective in treating ephelides.

- The frequency-doubled Q-switched Nd:YAG (532 nm), Q-switched alexandrite (755 nm), and Q-switched ruby lasers (694 nm) are all effective.

- One study used the frequency-doubled Nd:YAG (532 nm) to treat ephelides in 20 patients with type IV skin. Eighty percent of patients showed better than 50% improvement. Recurrence was common. Hypopigmentation, textural changes, and hyperpigmentation all resolved within 2–6 months after final treatment.

- In another study, 197 Asians were treated with the Q-switched alexandrite (755 nm) at 7.0 J/cm^2, with a pulse width of 100 ns at 8-week intervals. Clinical follow-up after an average of 1.5 treatment sessions showed a 76% decrease in the number of ephelides. No scarring, textural changes, or pigmentary changes were noted.

- Lasers are most effective for darker lesions.

- Caution should be employed when treating patients with darker skin types to avoid hyperpigmentation that may persist for months.

- Recurrence of freckling after treatment, however, is common.

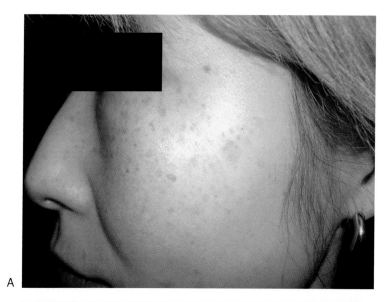
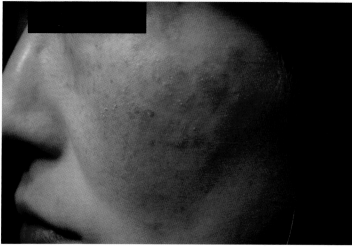

Figure 19.2 (A) *A 40-year-old Japanese female with ephelides and lentigines prior to 694-nm Q-switched ruby laser treatment.* **(B)** *Immediate tissue whitening and erythema after treatment*

- Sunscreen and sun avoidance are mandatory adjuncts to laser therapy.

PITFALLS TO AVOID/ COMPLICATIONS/ MANAGEMENT

- Laser treatment of ephelides is frequently successful but often transient.
- Patients should be informed that recurrence is highly likely, especially with sun exposure.
- Daily strict photoprotection with a sunscreen with UVA/UVB protection and/or a physical block such as titanium dioxide or zinc oxide are stressed as well as sun avoidance.
- If bleaching creams produce erythema, caution is advised as irritation and erythema can produce hyper-pigmentation.
- Patients should be counseled regarding the possibility of post-inflammatory pigmentation changes after treat-ment. Laser removal of ephelides may also produce an unattractive, spotty hypopigmentation.

BIBLIOGRAPHY

Jang KA, Chung EC, Choi JH, Sung KJ, Moon KC, Koh JK. Successful removal of freckles in Asian skin with a Q-switched alexandrite laser. *Dermatol Surg.* 2000;26(3): 231–234.

Mishima Y, Ohyama Y, Shibata T, et al. Inhibitory action of kojic acid on melanogenesis and its therapeutic effect for various human hyperigmentation disorders. *Skin Res.* 1994;36(2):134–150.

Nakagawa M, Kawai K. Contact allergy to kojic acid in skin care products. *Contact Dermatitis.* 1995;31(1): 9–13.

Ngujen QH, Bui TP. Azelaic acid: pharmacokinetic and pharmacodynamic properties and its therapeutic role in hyperpigmentary disorders and acne. *Int J Dermatol.* 1995;34(2):75–84.

Rashid T, Hussain I, Haider M, Haroon TS. Laser therapy of freckles and lentigines with quasi-continuous, fre-quency-doubled, Nd:YAG (532 nm) laser in Fitzpatrick skin type IV: a 24-month follow-up. *J Cosmet Laser Ther.* 2002;4(3–4):81–85.

CHAPTER 20 Lentigines

There are two major types of lentigines: lentigo simplex and solar lentigos. They are benign lesions. Although both are clinically identical, they appear in entirely different clinical settings. Lentigo simplex typically first present in childhood as multiple well-demarcated, brown or black macules that can appear on any part of the skin or mucous membranes. They are clinically indistinguishable from a junctional nevus. There is no association with sun exposure in this type of lentigo. In contrast, solar lentigos, more commonly known as "liver spots," are well-defined, brown macules that appear on sun-exposed skin of adults. They increase in number with age. They most often appear on the dorsal hands, shoulders, and face of lightly pigmented and red-haired patients.

EPIDEMIOLOGY

Incidence: very common, particularly in fair-skinned patients

Age: bimodal distribution in childhood and in sun-damaged skin of adults

Race: more common in Caucasians

Sex: equal

Precipitating factors: sun exposure is closely related to solar lentigines. Multiple lentigines are associated with a few genodermatoses including LEOPARD syndrome, LAMB syndrome, and Peutz–Jeghers syndrome

PATHOGENESIS

Unknown.

PATHOLOGY

There is a uniform elongation of the rete ridges of the epidermis along with increased melanin in melanocytes and basal keratinocytes. Additionally, there is an increased number of melanocytes in the basal layer. Melanophages are present in the papillary dermis.

PHYSICAL LESIONS

Well-defined brown macules. Lentigo simplex macules tend to be evenly distributed and small, measuring only a few millimeters. Solar lentigos have a predilection for the sun-exposed areas of the dorsal hands and face. They can be larger than lentigo simplex.

DIFFERENTIAL DIAGNOSIS

Seborrheic keratosis, junctional nevi, ephelides, lentigo maligna, melanoma may all mimic lentigines (Table 20.1).

TABLE 20.1 ■ **Lentigo Versus Ephelid**

	Solar Lentigo	Ephelid
Presents in childhood	No	Yes
Permanent	Yes	No
Decreases with age	No	Yes
High recurrence after treatment	Yes	Yes
Increase in melanin	Yes	Yes
Increase in melanocytes	Yes	No

LABORATORY EXAMINATION

Biopsy is indicated if there is suspicion of a lentigo maligna or melanoma. Medical workup is appropriate if suspicion for a genodermatosis.

COURSE

There is a bimodal distribution for lentigines. They appear in childhood and in sun-exposed adults.

KEY CONSULTATIVE QUESTIONS

- Has there been any change in the color or size of the lesion?
- Does the lesion bleed?
- Sun exposure
- Sunscreen use

MANAGEMENT

There is no medical indication to treat lentigines. The cosmetic appearance, however, displeases many due to the perception that lentigines are associated with aging. Cryotherapy and laser treatment are the mainstays of treatment. Laser therapy is more effective than one-time application of cryotherapy. Cryotherapy, however, is an effective and less expensive option for the patient. Chemical peels, topical tretinoin, local dermabrasion, and topical bleaching agents represent other treatment options.

TOPICAL MEDICATIONS

- Bleaching creams such as 4% hydroquinone can lighten lesions over a period of several months.

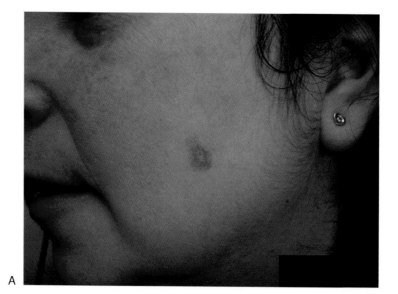

A

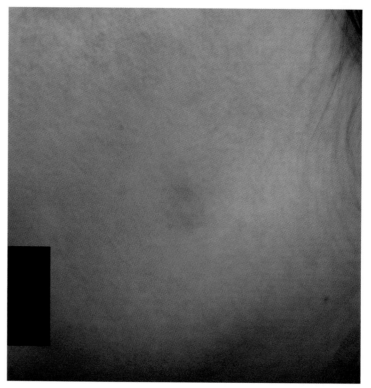

B

Figure 20.1 (A) *Lentigo on left cheek of a female.* **(B)** *Signficant improvement after one treatment with a 532 nm Q-switched Nd:YAG laser at a fluence of 1.0 J/cm² and a 2 mm spot size*

- Topical tretinoin can produce lightening.
- Combination of hydroquinone and retinoid, i.e., Triluma (4% hydroquinone, 0.05% tretinoin, 0.01% fluocinolone acetinonide) can be effective.
- Retreatment is often necessary.
- If any of these topical medications produce significant inflammation or irritation, it is important to discontinue their use to avoid producing post-inflammatory hyperpigmentation.

CRYOTHERAPY

- This is a cheap, swift, and effective means for treating lentigines.
- Application of cryotherapy can be accomplished with a small cotton-tip applicator for approximately 5 s.
- It is often less effective than one-time treatment with a Q-switched laser.
- Cryotherapy has been found superior to argon and CO_2 laser for lentigines.

CHEMICAL PEELS

Thirty-five percent TCA (trichloroacetic acid) peels can be effective.

LASER LIGHT SOURCE TREATMENT

Multiple different therapies are effective for treating lentigines.

- Intense pulsed light, frequency-doubled Q-switched Nd:YAG (532 nm) (Fig. 20.1), Q-switched alexandrite (755 nm), Q-switched ruby (694 nm), Q-switched Nd:YAG (1064 nm), pulsed dye (595 nm), fractional resurfacing, and KTP lasers (532 nm) are all effective.
- With Q-switched lasers:
  - Perform a test spot on darker skin types.
  - Treatment endpoint for Q-switched lasers is tissue whitening. For the Q-switched Nd: YAG (1064 nm), small pinpoint bleeding may be seen.
  - A 1-week healing time can be expected.
  - Legs respond more slowly than the face and hands.
- The frequency-doubled Q-switched Nd:YAG (532 nm) laser has been shown to improve lentigines safely and effectively.
  - In one study, 37 patients were treated once with a fluence of 2–5 J/cm^2, a 2.0 mm spot size, and a 10 ns pulse width.
  - Higher fluences provided best results with 60% of patients showing 75% or better clearances.
  - Minor, transient hypopigmentation, hyperpigmentation, and erythema were noted in a few patients.

– Has been shown to produce better clearing than 35% TCA peel.

– Has been shown to treat lentigines more effectively than cryotherapy.

• The Q-switched ruby (694 nm) laser has also been shown to be effective.

– In one treatment, substantial clearing occurred at fluences of 4.5 and/or 7.5 J/cm^2 and a pulse width of 40 ns.

• Fractional resurfacing (Fraxel Laser; Reliant technologies, San Diego, CA) is also effective.

– Treatment is generally performed at energies between 6 and 8 mJ/cm^2, and a density setting of 250 MTZ/cm^2.

– Eight passes are delivered with appropriate overlap to a total density of 2000 MTZ/cm^2.

– Mild to moderate erythema, resembling a sunburn reaction, is often observed. Postprocedure swelling is also not uncommon, especially at higher fluences.

– The erythema resolves in 3–7 days and can be covered with makeup.

– Long-term data are currently lacking.

• Intense pulse light is also effective.

– Seventy-four percent clearance of lentigines in 18 patients with one treatment.

PITFALLS TO AVOID/COMPLICATIONS/ MANAGEMENT/OUTCOME EXPECTATIONS

• Laser and light source treatment for lentigines is frequently successful.

• Patients should be counseled regarding the possibility of post-inflammatory pigmentation changes after treatment especially on the lower legs.

• Recurrence after treatment is not uncommon.

• Biopsy any lesion that demonstrates any clinical atypia prior to treating with laser or cryotherapy. Laser therapy of a malignant lesion such as a lentigo maligna may mask its clinical appearance and thus cause a delay in diagnosis.

BIBLIOGRAPHY

Bjerring P, Christiansen K. Intense pulsed light source for treatment of small melanocytic nevi and solar lentigines. *J Cutan Laser Ther*. 2000;2:177–181.

Kilmer SL. Laser eradication of pigmented lesions and tattoos. *Dermatol Clin*. 2002;20(1):37–53.

Kilmer SL, Wheeland RG, Goldberg DJ, Anderson RR. Treatment of epidermal pigmented lesions with the frequency-doubled Q-switched Nd:YAG laser. A controlled, single-impact, dose-response, multicenter trial. *Arch Dermatol*. 1994;130(12):1515–1519.

Li YT, Yang KC. Comparison of the frequency-doubled Q-switched Nd:YAG laser and 35% trichloroacetic acid for the treatment of face lentigines. *Dermatol Surg.* 1999; 25(3):202–204.

Stern RS, Dover JS, Levin JA, Arndt KA. Laser therapy versus cryotherapy of lentigines: a comparative trial. *J Am Acad Dermatol.* 1994;30(6):985–987.

Todd MM, Rallis TM, Gerwels JW, Hata TR. A comparison of 3 lasers and liquid nitrogen in the treatment of solar lentigines: a randomized, controlled, comparative trial. *Arch Dermatol.* 2000;136(7):841–846.

Taylor CR, Anderson RR. Treatment of benign pigmented epidermal lesions by Q-switched ruby laser. *Int J Dermatol.* 1993;32(12):908–912.

CHAPTER 21 Melasma

Melasma is an acquired brown macular hyperpigmentation usually of the face. It is far more common in females than in males. It usually presents bilaterally and symmetrically on the face, but extensor forearms may also be involved. There are three histologic variants of melasma: epidermal, dermal, and mixed dermal and epidermal. Epidermal melasma responds best to therapy. Sun exposure, pregnancy, and oral contraceptive pills are all associated with its presentation (Fig. 21.1).

EPIDEMIOLOGY

Incidence: common

Age: young females

Race: Central and South American, Middle Eastern, Indian, East Asian females are most frequently affected

Sex: females > males (9:1)

Precipitating factors: pregnancy, oral contraceptive pills, sun exposure, hormone replacement therapy

PATHOGENESIS

Unknown.

DERMATOPATHOLOGY

In epidermal melasma, there is increased melanin deposition in the epidermis, particularly in the basal and

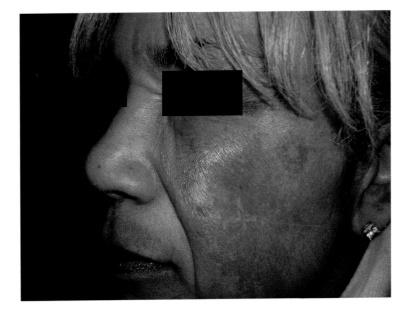

Figure 21.1 *Female with extensive melasma recalcitrant to multiple topical regimens for several years*

suprabasal layers. In dermal melasma, there are perivascular melanin-containing macrophages in the superficial and mid-dermis. Mixed-type melasma exhibits features of each of the above findings.

PHYSICAL LESIONS

Patients present with well-demarcated light brown to dark brown symmetric macular hyperpigmentation. In about two-thirds of patients it appears on the central face including the forehead, nose, upper cutaneous lip, and chin. It presents less frequently on the malar areas and jawline. More rarely, it appears on the dorsal forearms. Dermal melasma has more of a blue-gray hue. Mixed-type melasma has a brown-gray coloration.

DIFFERENTIAL DIAGNOSIS

Post-inflammatory hyperpigmentation, exogenous ochronosis, drug-induced/photo-hyperpigmentation, nevus of Ota, erythema dyschromicum perstans.

LABORATORY EXAMINATION

Wood's lamp examination accentuates the increased epidermal pigmentation in melasma but does not highlight its dermal component.

COURSE

The pigmentation presents over a period of weeks. It occurs most commonly in summertime, with high estrogen states, during pregnancy, and prior to menstruation. It may fade completely months after delivery or after discontinuation of oral contraceptive pills. It may reappear in subsequent pregnancies.

KEY CONSULTATIVE QUESTIONS

- Medication history
- Pregnancy
- Sun exposure
- Time of onset
- Previous treatments

MANAGEMENT

There is no medical indication to treat melasma. Nevertheless, many patients understandably are distressed by its appearance and desire treatment. The goal of the treatment is to lighten or remove the pigmentation. Prior to initiating therapy, it is essential to determine which form of melasma is being treated, i.e., epidermal

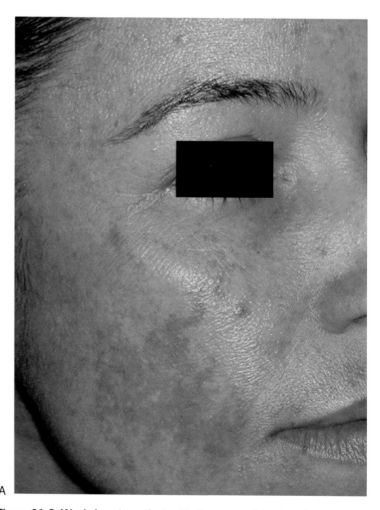

A

Figure 21.2 (A) *A female patient with therapy-resistant melasma on the right face*

TABLE 21.1 ■ **Treatment of Pigmented Lesions on the Face**

	Retinoid/ hydroquinone	Glycolic acid peels	Q-switched laser	Ablative resurfacing	Fractional resurfacing
Melasma	Variable improvement	Multiple light peels in conjunction with sunscreen and topical retinoid/ hydroquinone	No	Yes; but careful patient selection and long post-laser recovery	Yes
Post-inflammatory hyperpigmentation	Yes; weeks to months to see clinical improvement	Unpredictable benefit	No	No	No
Lentigo	Minimal/moderate improvement after months of use	Minimal/moderate change with three to four peels	Yes; one to two treatments are highly successful	Yes; post-inflamma-tory erythema chief obstacle	Yes
Nevus of Ota	None	None	Yes; multiple treat-ments result in improvement	No	No

versus mixed-type versus dermal melasma (Fig. 21.4). There are multiple topical and laser therapies available (Fig. 21.3). Treatment is frustrating and often ineffective. Dermal and mixed-type melasma are least responsive to therapy. In all melasma patients, sunscreen and sun avoidance are essential components of therapy.

TOPICAL TREATMENT (Table 21.1)

There are a host of topical treatments for melasma.

- Numerous formulations containing bleaching agents such as 4% hydroquinone are effective treatments to lighten or resolve pigmentation. They are most effective over a long period of treatment. If the skin becomes significantly irritated from treatment, discontinue its use to avoid post-inflammatory hyperpigmentation.
- Retinoids such as topical 0.1% tretinoin applied once daily for 40 weeks has been shown to be effective.
- Combination therapy of 0.05% tretinoin, 4% hydroquinone, and 0.01% fluocinolone acetonide, i.e., Triluma, produce favorable clinical results with decreased irritation. Treatment duration is limited by side effects of prolonged topical steroid use including skin atrophy and acne.
- Azelaic acid has also been shown to produce improvement.

CHEMICAL PEELS

Chemical peels are effective for melasma.

- In one study, there was no difference in results when comparing Jessner's solution versus 70% glycolic acid peels after performing three peels 1 month apart on each side of the face.

- Glycolic acid peels performed every 3 weeks in combination with daily sunscreen and a combination glycolic acid/hydroquinone cream has been shown to be effective.

- Serial superficial chemical peels such as salicylic acid and glycolic acid peels are the safest peels in darker skin phototypes.

LASERS

▪ Q-switched Lasers

Q-switched laser treatment for melasma is not recommended given its high incidence of post-inflammatory hyperpigmentation. Additionally, it is not dramatically effective except in some cases of superficial melasma.

▪ Ablative Laser

In cases refractory to topical creams and chemical peels, erbium:YAG laser produced significant, temporary improvement in 10 patients in one study but was complicated by subsequent post-inflammatory hyperpigmentation in all 10 patients.

▪ Fractional Resurfacing (Fig. 21.2)

Fractional resurfacing (Fraxel Laser; Reliant technologies, San Diego, CA) can be successful for some cases of melasma, especially epidermal types.

- Long-term data are lacking.

- Treatment is generally performed at energies between 6 and 8 mJ/cm^2 with a density setting of 250 MTZ/cm^2.

- Eight passes are delivered with appropriate overlap for a total density of 2000–3000 MTZ/cm^2.

- Pre and post-treatment use of hydroquinone and longer intervals between treatments may reduce post-inflammatory hyperpigmentation in darker skin phototypes.

PITFALLS TO AVOID/COMPLICATIONS/ MANAGEMENT/OUTCOME EXPECTATIONS

- All forms of melasma are difficult and frustrating to treat.

- Dermal melasma is particularly difficult.

- Patients should be apprised of the recalcitrant nature of this condition.

- Postpartum state and discontinuance of oral contraceptive pills are frequently successful therapies.

- Some treatments worsen its appearance.

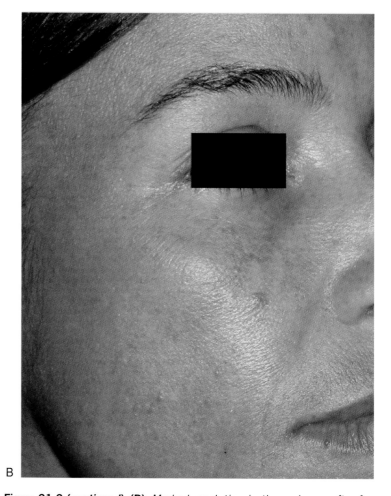

B

Figure 21.2 (*continued*) (B) *Marked resolution in the melasma after four treatment sessions with Fraxel laser (7 mJ/MTZ, total density of 2000 MTZ/cm^2) (courtesy of Howard Conn, MD)*

* Strict sun avoidance is crucial with a sunscreen with UVA/UVB protection and/or a physical block such as titanium dioxide or zinc oxide during and after any treatment regimen.

BIBLIOGRAPHY

Finkel LJ, Ditre CM, Hamilton TA, Ellis CN, Voorhees JJ. Topical tretinoin (retinoic acid) improves melasma. A vehicle-controlled, clinical trial. *Br J Dermatol*. 1993;129: 415–421.

Lawrence N, Cox SE, Brody HJ. Treatment of melasma with Jessner's solution versus glycolic acid: a comparison of clinical efficacy and evaluation of the predictive ability of Wood's light examination. *J Am Acad Dermatol*. 1997;36:589–593.

Lim JT, Tham SN. Glycolic acid peels in the treatment of melasma among Asian women. *Dermatol Surg*. 1997;23: 177–179.

Manaloto RM, Alser TM. Erbium:YAG laser resurfacing for refractory melasma. *Dermatol Surg*. 1999;25:121–123.

Torok HM, Jones T, Rich P, Smith S, Tschen E. Hydroquinone 4%, tretinoin 0.05%, fluocinolone acetonide 0.01%: a safe and efficacious 12-month treatment for melasma. *Cutis*. 2005;75(1):57–62.

Tse Y, Levine VJ, McClain SA, Ashinoff R. The removal of cutaneous pigmented lesions with the Q-switched ruby laser and the Q-switched neodymium:yttrium-aluminum garnet laser. A comparative study. *J Derm Surg Oncol*. 1994;20:795–800.

Verallo-Rowell VM, Veralo V, Graupe K, Lopez-VillafuerteL, Garcia Lopez M. Double-blind comparison of azeleic acid and hydroquinone in the treatment of melasma. *Acta Derm Venereol*. 1989;143:58–61.

Victor FC, Gelber J, Rao B. Melasma: a review. *J Cutan Med Surg*. 2004;8(2):97–102.

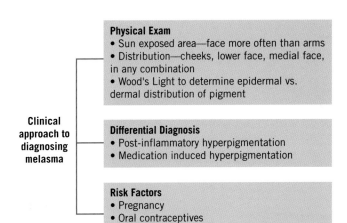

Figure 21.3 *Clinical approach to diagnosing melasma*

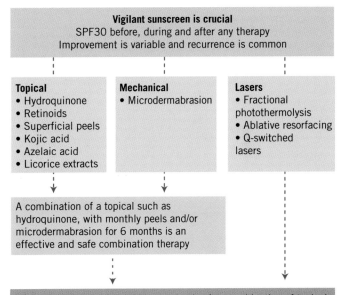

Figure 21.4 *Melasma treatment protocol*

CHAPTER 22 Nevus of Ota

Nevus of Ota, also known as nevus fusoceruleus ophthalmomaxillaris, represents a benign partially confluent macular brown-blue pigmentation of the skin and mucous membranes in the distribution of the first and second branches of the trigeminal nerve. It may be unilateral or bilateral. The ipsilateral sclera is frequently involved.

EPIDEMIOLOGY

Incidence: 0.4–0.8% of Japanese dermatology patients

Age: bimodal distribution at birth and puberty

Race: more common in Asians and blacks than whites

Sex: more females than males seek treatment for this condition. Unknown if there is a sex predilection

Precipitating factors: sporadic, not an inherited disorder

PATHOGENESIS

Hyperpigmentation arises as a result of dermal melanocytes that have not migrated to the epidermis.

PATHOLOGY

Heavily pigmented, elongated, dendritic melanocytes are located among the reticular dermal collagen. Most typically, these melanocytes are found in the upper one-third of the reticular dermis but are also seen in the papillary dermis in some lesions.

PHYSICAL LESIONS

It presents as confluent or partially confluent brown-blue patches in the distribution of the first and second branches of the trigeminal nerve. Gray, black, and purple coloration may be present in some lesions as well. It can be unilateral or bilateral. The magnitude of involvement can vary from local periocular involvement to much of the side of the face. Approximately two-thirds of patients feature ipsilateral scleral involvement.

DIFFERENTIAL DIAGNOSIS

Melasma, café au lait macule, blue nevus, bruising, ochronosis, argyria, photodermatoses, fixed drug eruption, and other medication-related eruptions should be considered in the proper clinical setting.

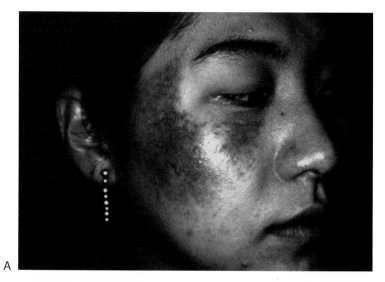

A

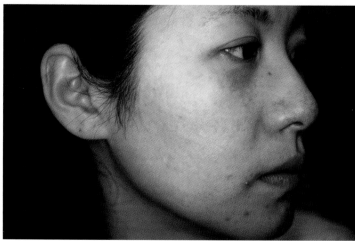

B

Figure 22.1 (A) *Nevus of Ota prior to treatment with Q-switched ruby laser.* **(B)** *Significant clearance after serial treatments with Q-switched ruby laser*

LABORATORY EXAMINATION

Biopsy may be indicated if the diagnosis is in question or to exclude the rare case of melanoma arising in this lesion.

COURSE

There is a bimodal distribution for nevus of Ota, birth and puberty. It remains relatively similar in appearance after initial presentation.

KEY CONSULTATIVE QUESTIONS

- Onset of eruption
- Medication history

MANAGEMENT

There is no medical indication to treat nevus of Ota. Cosmetic appearance, however, is distressing to patients. While cryotherapy and topical bleaching treatments have been utilized, the treatment of choice is Q-switched laser treatment.

TOPICAL TREATMENT

Makeup can camouflage or assist in camouflaging nevus of Ota. Topical medications are less effective than laser.

TREATMENT

- Numerous studies have shown that nevus of Ota is amenable to successful resolution with Q-switched laser therapies including the Q-switched ruby (694 nm), the alexandrite (755 nm), and The Nd:YAG (1064 nm) lasers (Figs. 22.2-22.3).
- Test spot can be performed prior to treatment.
- The Q-switched ruby laser has been shown to be effective at producing 75% or greater clearance at fluences of 5–7 J/cm^2, 4-mm spot size, and a 30 ns pulse width at 3–4 month treatment intervals.
  - In a study of 46 children and 107 adults with nevus of Ota, treatments were more successful in children than in adults.
  - The mean number of treatment sessions to achieve significant clearing or better was 3.5 for the younger age group and 5.9 for the older age group.
  - Additionally, complications were lower in the children than adults, i.e., 4.8% as compared to 22.4%.
  - One retrospective study examined 101 patients 1 year after treatment with Q-switched ruby laser and found that 16.8% displayed hypopigmentation and 5.9% showed hyperpigmentation. One patient who had complete resolution developed recurrence.
- The Q-switched alexandrite laser is also effective for the treatment of nevus of Ota.

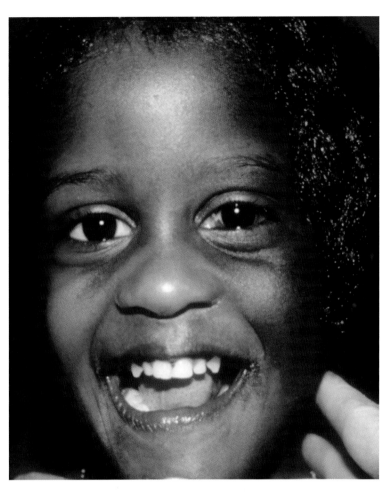

Figure 22.2 *Nevus of Ota. Periorbital blue-gray pigmentation with scleral involvement (Kay K, Jen R, Richard J, Howard B, Alexander S, eds. Color Atlas & Synopsis of Pediatric Dermatology. McGraw-Hill, Inc.; 2002)*

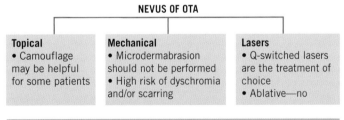

NEVUS OF OTA

Topical	**Mechanical**	**Lasers**
• Camouflage may be helpful for some patients	• Microdermabrasion should not be performed • High risk of dyschromia and/or scarring	• Q-switched lasers are the treatment of choice • Ablative—no

- Multiple treatments with Q-switched lasers are needed
- Improvement moderate to dramatic after multiple treatments
- Q-switched laser treatment of lesions that arise in infancy may respond better to laser therapy than later in life
- If a Q-switched YAG laser is used a combination of 532 nm/1064 nm may result in better clinical improvement than 1064 nm alone

Figure 22.3 *Treatment of nevus of Ota algorithm*

– One study treated 13 patients at fluences ranging between 6 and 8 J/cm^2 at 8-week intervals. The mean number of treatments was about seven. Seven patients achieved 75% or better lightening, three patients achieved between 51 and 75% improvement, one achieved between 25 and 50% improvement, and another achieved less than 25% improvement.

– Two patients experienced transient hyperpigmentation; one experienced transient hypopigmentation.

• The Q-switched Nd:YAG (1064 nm) laser has also proven to be effective.

– Slightly less effective than other Q-switched lasers.

– It is safer for use in dark skin types.

– Less risk of hypopigmentation.

PITFALLS TO AVOID/OUTCOME EXPECTATIONS/COMPLICATIONS/ MANAGEMENT

• Laser treatment for nevus of Ota is frequently successful.

• Given the high proportion of patients with dark skin phototypes, there is the risk of hypopigmentation and hyperpigmentation.

• The risk of such an adverse reaction should be discussed with the patient prior to therapy.

• Additionally, a test site can be treated before performing full treatment of any lesion.

• Q-switched laser treatment can be associated with transient hyperpigmentation.

• Recurrence after treatment is infrequent.

BIBLIOGRAPHY

Chan HH, Leung RS, Ying SY, Lai CF, Kono T, Chua JK, Ho WS. A retrospective analysis of complications in the treatment of nevus of Ota with the Q-switched alexandrite and Q-switched Nd:YAG lasers. *Dermatol Surg.* 2000;26(11):1000–1006.

Chan HH, Ying SY, Ho WS, Kono T, King WW. An in vivo trial comparing the clinical efficacy and complications of Q-switched 755 nm alexandrite and Q-switched 1064 nm Nd:YAG lasers in the treatment of nevus of Ota. *Dermatol Surg.* 2000;26(10):919–922.

Kono T, Chan HH, Ercocen AR, Kikuchi Y, Uezono S, Iwasaka S, Isago T, Nozaki M. Use of Q-switched ruby laser in the treatment of nevus of Ota in different age groups. *Lasers Surg Med.* 2003;32(5):391–395.

Kono T, Nozaki M, Chan HH, Mikashima Y. A retrospective study looking at the long-term complications of Q-switched ruby laser in the treatment of nevus of Ota. *Lasers Surg Med.* 2001;29(2):156–159.

Radmanesh M. Naevus of Ota treatment with cryotherapy. *J Dermatol Treat.* 2001;12(4):205–209.

CHAPTER 23 Post-inflammatory Hyperpigmentation

Post-inflammatory hyperpigmentation (PIH) is a common sequela of inflammatory dermatoses or injury to the skin. It occurs most commonly in darker skin types. Depending on the etiology of the hyperpigmentation, pigment may be deposited in the dermis or epidermis with important implications for treating the pigment changes.

EPIDEMIOLOGY

Incidence: common, especially in darker skin types

Age: all ages

Race: more common in darker skin types

Sex: none

Precipitating factors: any inflammatory disorder or injury to the skin can produce hyperpigmentation. It may also result from laser therapy, dermabrasion, cryotherapy, or chemical peels. It presents more exuberantly and with a greater duration in darker skin phototypes

PATHOGENESIS

Unknown.

DERMATOPATHOLOGY

Basal cell layer pigmentation and dermal melanophages are seen.

PHYSICAL LESIONS

In epidermal PIH, patients display indistinct tan to dark brown macules at sites of previous skin inflammation. In dermal PIH, there is more of a brown-gray hue.

DIFFERENTIAL DIAGNOSIS

Mastocytosis, macular amyloidosis, minocin hyperpigmenation, exogenous ochronosis, melasma, and erythema dyschromicum perstans.

LABORATORY EXAMINATION

None.

COURSE

PIH does not worsen in the absence of further insult or inflammation at the affected site. PIH usually resolves over a period of a few months. In the case of dermal hyperpigmentation, there may not be improvement.

KEY CONSULTATIVE QUESTIONS

- Sun exposure, sunscreen use
- Time of onset
- Recent rashes, injury, or treatment of skin
- Medication use

MANAGEMENT

While there is no medical indication to treat PIH, many patients are as bothered by PIH as they are by the processes that produced the it initially. Furthermore, PIH can endure far longer than the original eruption. There are multiple treatments including topical, laser, and chemical peels (Table 23.1). Perhaps the safest and most effective treatment is time. Normally, epidermal PIH will resolve on its own over a period of months.

TABLE 23.1 ▪ Post-inflammatory Hyperpigmentation Treatment

Therapeutic options	Retinoid/ hydroquinone	Peels/ microdermabrasion	Q-switched laser	Ablative lasers	Fractional resurfacing
Post-inflammatory hyperpigmentation	Needs to be used for weeks to months for improvement	20–70% glycolic acid peels, Jessner peels, combination Jessner TCA/peels and Salicylic acid peels and/or microdermabrasion may help improve more quickly	No	No	No
	Face/upper body improves more quickly than lower half of the body	Risk of paradoxically making post-inflammatory changes *worse* if too much inflammation is created			

SUNPROTECTION

Sunblocks and sunscreens used daily are crucial to prevent worsening, as is sun avoidance. Without their use, other therapies will not be effective.

TOPICAL TREATMENTS

There are a host of topical treatments for PIH that produce mild improvement and may expedite resolution.

- Hydroquinone formulations, particularly with sunscreens
  - Hydroquinone (2–4%) creams are effective, first-line treatment.

– Bleaching creams are contraindicated in pregnant and lactating women.

• Retinoids

– Solage (2% mequinol and 0.01% tretinoin) and Triluma (0.01% fluocinolone acetonide, 4% hydroquinone, and 0.05% tretinoin) provide an exfoliative benefit.

– Triluma should not be used indefinitely due to its corticosteroid content and risk for atrophy.

• Azelaic acid (20%) cream applied twice daily provides slow lightening of pigmentation.

• Kojic acid (1–2.5%) cream

– The exact concentration of kojic acid needed for effective results is unknown.

• If any of these topicals produce significant inflammation or irritation, it is important to discontinue their use to avoid worsening of PIH.

CHEMICAL PEELS

Chemical peels are an effective treatment option for the reduction of PIH.

• Over-the-counter α-hydroxy acid peels are a beneficial adjunct to physician-strength chemical peels. The continual exfoliation achieved from consistent use of the peels will result in mild lightening.

• Glycolic acid peels (20–70%) are administered every 2–3 weeks utilizing increasing strengths as tolerated.

– The treatment endpoint is mild confluent erythema.

– Treated areas must be fully neutralized with sodium bicarbonate or water at the completion of the peel.

– Lightening of superficial PIH may be observed after four to six peels.

– Strict photoprotection for 1 month is essential and must be stressed.

• Jessner peels (resorcinol, lactic acid, and salicylic acid) are administered every 6–8 weeks.

– Treatment endpoint is a light whitening of the skin.

– Strict photoprotection for 2–3 months is advised.

– Multiple treatments are recommended.

– Contraindicated in pregnant and lactating women.

• Combination Jessner/10% trichloroacetic (TCA) peels may also be employed in a similar fashion as the Jessner peel. The Jessner peel results in exfoliation allowing for greater penetration of the TCA peel.

– Multiple peels are generally needed.

– Contraindicated in pregnant and lactating women

– Deeper peels are rarely employed given the risk of PIH exacerbation with healing.

• Caution must be used in treating skin phototypes III–V, particularly with medium-depth peels. Salicylic acid peels are safest for dark skin phototypes (Fig. 23.1).

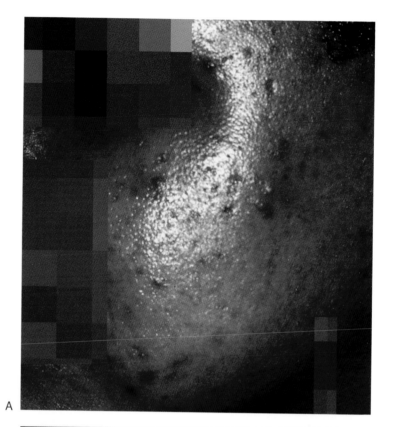

A

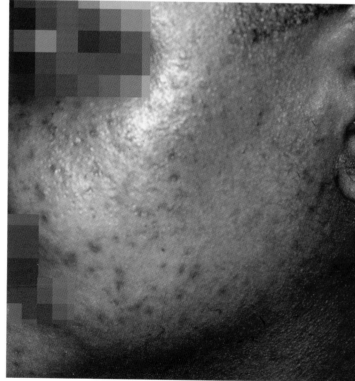

B

Figure 23.1 (A) *Hyperpigmentation on left side of face before treatment.* **(B)** *Improvement after a series of salicylic acid peels and topical application of 4% hydroquinone (photographs courtesy of Pearl E. Grimes, MD)*

LASERS

Laser treatment for PIH does not produce reliable improvement and is not first line therapy. In fact, laser therapy may exacerbate PIH. It is not recommended.

PITFALLS TO AVOID/COMPLICATIONS/ MANAGEMENT/OUTCOME EXPECTATIONS

- It is important to reassure patients that PIH will resolve on its own with time, except if it is a dermal process.
- Laser treatment is unreliable and may produce worsening. It is not recommended.
- It is important to discontinue any topical medications that produce inflammation or irritation to avoid worsening PIH.
- Chemical peels are likely to only lighten and not fully eliminate the PIH. Caution in darker skin phototypes.
- It is better and safer to utilize serial superficial peels rather than a single deeper peel to minimize this risk.
- PIH may not improve despite serial chemical peel use.

BIBLIOGRAPHY

Kilmer SL. Laser eradication of pigmented lesions and tattoos. *Dermatol. Clin.* 2002;20(1):37–53.

Mishima Y, Ohyama Y, Shibata T, et al. Inhibitory action of kojic acid on melanogenesis and its therapeutic effect for various human hyperigmentation disorders. *Skin Res.* 1994;36(2):134–150.

Nakagawa M, Kawai K. Contact allergy to kojic acid in skin care products. *Contact Dermatitis.* 1995;31(1):9–13.

Ngujen QH, Bui TP. Azelaic acid: pharmacokinetic and pharmacodynamic properties and its therapeutic role in hyperpigmentary disorders and acne. *Int J Dermatol.* 1995;34(2):75–84.

CHAPTER 24 Vitiligo

Vitiligo is an acquired idiopathic condition that produces symmetric depigmented patches of the skin. It is particularly distressing and clinically apparent in patients with darker skin phototypes.

EPIDEMIOLOGY

Incidence: about 2% of the world population

Age: can present at any age but most commonly presents in the second to fourth decade

Race: equal

Sex: equal

Precipitating factors: inheritance, trauma, illness, emotional states

PATHOGENESIS

Unknown.

DERMATOPATHOLOGY

There are no melanocytes in basal cell layer.

PHYSICAL LESIONS

Patients display well-demarcated, symmetric, depigmented, chalk-white macules. Common locations include elbows, knees, sacral area, penis, perioral areas, and neck. Hair may also lose pigmentation (Figs. 24.1-24.2).

DIFFERENTIAL DIAGNOSIS

Chemical leukoderma, post-inflammatory hypopigmentation, nevus depigmentosus, nevus anemicus, pityriasis alba, lupus erythematosus, leprosy, and genodermatoses.

LABORATORY EXAMINATION

Wood's lamp examination is helpful in making the diagnosis. In cases of uncertainty, biopsy should be performed of both lesional and nonlesional skin in order to determine if there is an absence of melanocytes in the affected skin. Check TSH for hypothyroidism.

COURSE

Vitiligo can pursue a variable course. After an initial rapid presentation, it tends to stabilize. Typically, it is a chronic

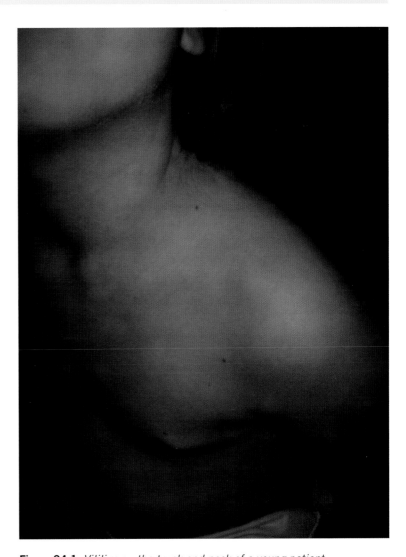

Figure 24.1 *Vililigo on the trunk and neck of a young patient*

disease with periods of partial repigmentation but not resolution. It may improve in the summertime. In some cases, depigmentation becomes extensive.

KEY CONSULTATIVE QUESTIONS

- Age of patient
- Time of onset
- Family history
- Occupation
- Chemical exposures

MANAGEMENT

There are multiple treatment modalities for vitiligo. Unfortunately, treatment is frustrating and often ineffective. Patients understandably are distressed by the appearance of vitiligo and desire treatment. In extensive cases, it produces a striking appearance, particularly for patients with darker skin phototypes.

PREVENTION

Sunscreens and sun avoidance protect vitiliginous skin from burning and are an important component of therapy.

TOPICAL TREATMENT

There are a host of topical treatments for vitiligo. They include

- Corticosteroids
  - Topical
  - Intralesional
- Tacrolimus, pimecrolimus
- Monobenzylether of hydroquinone
  - Produces permanent depigmentation
  - Twice daily over a 1 year period
  - Permanent depigmentation is produced in less than 50% of patients
  - Poor or no depigmentation in nearly half of patients
  - Caution prior to pursuing this permanent treatment
  - Side effects include contact dermatitis, erythema, and pruritus
- Camouflaging makeup to hide depigmented macules

PHOTOTHERAPY

Phototherapy is a mainstay of vitiligo treatment:

- PUVA with topical or oral 5-methoxypsoralen or 8-methoxypsoralen
- Narrow-band UVB

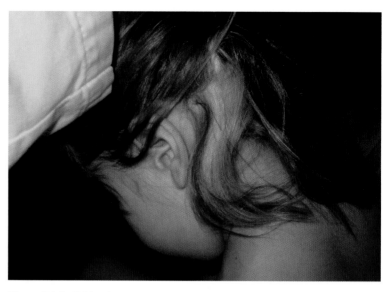

Figure 24.2 *White forelock in the same patient*

ORAL THERAPY

Oral therapies include

- Oral 5- or 8-methoxypsoralen in combination with gradual, limited sun exposure
- Pulse therapy with corticosteroids

SURGICAL TREATMENTS

Autologous skin grafting can be a helpful treatment for vitiligo recalcitrant to other therapies. It is not a first- or second-line treatment. Split-thickness grafts, epidermal blister grafts, cultured melanocyte grafts, single hair grafts, and noncultured epidermal suspension grafts have all been examined. Pain after graft procedures is common, particularly at the harvest site.

- A majority of patients employing the epidermal suction graft technique showed improvement.
- Split-thickness grafting and dermabrasion have also achieved repigmentation within an average of 6 months in one study of 22 patients.
- Single hair grafts are most effective in localized or segmental vitiligo. Success in generalized vitiligo is poor.
- Cultured pure melanocyte supension as well as cultured epidermal grafting after treatment with CO_2 laser have both also been shown successful in treating vitiligo.
  - Results were best in localized cases of vitiligo.

LASER THERAPY

■ Excimer Laser

An excimer laser emits UVB range light at 308 nm, close to the wavelength of narrow-band UVB therapy that has been used to successfully treat vitiligo.

Beginning with a starting dose of 100 mJ/cm^2, with increasing doses in standard phototherapy increments, there was good improvement in recalcitrant vitiligo after 30 weeks of treatments.

- Acral lesions were most refractory to treatment.
- Few adverse effects.
- Best results are produced on the face > neck, extremities, trunk, and genitalia > hands, feet.
- More expensive than many traditional therapies.

PITFALLS TO AVOID/ COMPLICATIONS/ MANAGEMENT/ OUTCOME EXPECTATIONS

- Vitiligo is a difficult disease to treat.
- There are multiple first- and second-line therapies that should be employed before seeking surgical or laser treatments.

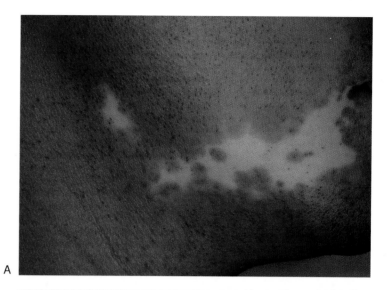

A

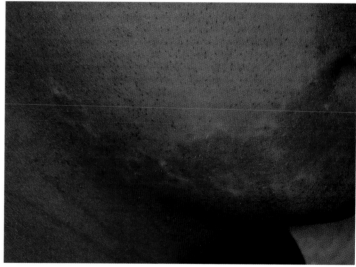

B

Figure 24.3 (A) *Depigmented patch of skin on right mandible.* **(B)** *Significant improvement after multiple 1 mm punch grafts (courtesy of Pearl E. Grimes, MD)*

- It is especially difficult to produce long-term significant cosmetic improvement in extensive cases.
- Frequently, repigmentation may be confined to perifollicular areas creating a "spotty" appearance.
- Patients need to be educated that any therapy may not succeed.
- The excimer laser is not widely available making its use particularly difficult.

BIBLIOGRAPHY

Chen YF, Yang PY, Hu DN, Kuo FS, Hung CS, Hung CM. Treatment of vitiligo by transplantation of cultured pure melanocyte suspension: analysis of 120 cases. *J Am Acad Dermatol.* 2004;51(1):68–74.

Hadi SM, Spencer JM, Lebwohl M. The use of the 308-nm excimer laser for the treatment of vitiligo. *Dermatol Surg.* 2004;30(7):983–986.

Koga M. Epidermal grafting using the tops of suction blisters in the treatment of vitiligo. *Arch Dermatol.* 1988; 124(11):1656–1658.

Na GY, Seo SK, Choi SK. Single hair grafting for the treatment of vitiligo. *J Am Acad Dermatol.* 1998;38(4): 580–584.

Ozdemir M, Cetinkale O, Wolf R, Kotogyan A, Mat C, Tuzun B, Tuzun Y. Comparison of two surgical approaches for treating vitiligo: a preliminary study. *Int J Dermatol.* 2002;41(3):135–138.

Taneja A, Trehan M, Taylor CR. 308-nm excimer laser for the treatment of localized vitiligo. *Int J Dermatol.* 2003; 42(8):658–662.

Toriyama K, Kamei Y, Kazeto T, Yasue T, Suga Y, Inoie M, Tomita Y, Torii S. Combination of short-pulsed CO_2 laser resurfacing and cultured epidermal sheet autografting in the treatment of vitiligo: a preliminary report. *Ann Plast Surg.* 2004;53(2):178–180.

van Geel N, Ongenae K, De Mil M, Haeghen YV, Vervaet C, Naeyaert JM. Double-blind placebo-controlled study of autologous transplanted epidermal cell suspensions for repigmenting vitiligo. *Arch Dermatol.* 2004;140(10): 1203–1208.

SECTION SIX

Vascular Alterations

CHAPTER 25 Angiokeratoma

Angiokeratomas are telengiectasias with keratotic elements. They present in different clinical scenarios including (a) solitary or multiple angiokeratomas occurring predominantly on lower extremities, (b) angiokeratoma of Fordyce affecting the scrotum and the vulva, (c) angiokeratoma of Mibelli, an autosomal dominant disorder affecting dorsum of hands and feet, elbows, and knees, (d) angiokeratoma corporis diffusum associated with Fabry's disease, an X-linked recessive disorder characterized by α-galactosidase-A deficiency and affecting the lower abdomen, buttocks, and genitalia, and (e) angiokeratoma circumscriptum usually grouped on one extremity.

EPIDEMIOLOGY

Age: solitary or multiple angiokeratomas usually affect young adults, angiokeratomas of Fordyce affect middle-aged and elderly individuals. Angiokeratoma of Mibelli and angiokeratoma circumscriptum are usually diagnosed in childhood.

Sex: angiokeratoma of Mibelli and angiokeratoma circumscriptum exhibit female predominance. Otherwise, there is no sex predisposition.

PHYSICAL EXAMINATION

Red to violaceous, well-circumscribed hyperkeratotic papules.

DIFFERENTIAL DIAGNOSES

Solitary lesions can be mistaken for melanoma, acquired hemangioma, seborrheic keratosis, and warts.

LABORATORY DATA

■ Dermatopathology

Marked dilated, thin-walled blood vessels in the papillary dermis, associated with an overlying acanthotic hyperkeratotic epidermis.

COURSE MANAGEMENT

• Lasers: angiokeratomas have been treated successfully with multiple lasers.

 – The pulsed dye laser (PDL) is an effective device for the improvement of the vascular component of angiokeratomas, but frequently some keratosis

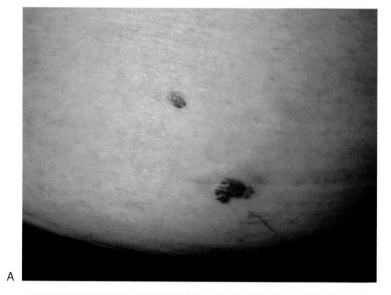

A

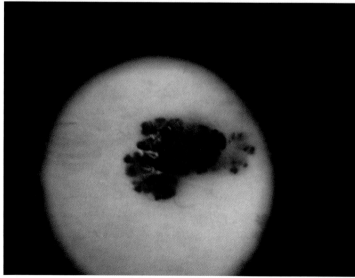

B

Figure 25.1 (A) *Angiokeratomas on the abdomen of a young patient.* **(B)** *Angiokeratoma imaged through an epiluminescence microscope (DermLite)*

remains. The target chromophore is hemoglobin. The Scleroplus PDL (Candela, Wayland, MA) has proven successful at 595 nm, 5–7 mm spot, 9–11 J/cm^2, DCD 30/20. Variable pulsed PDL is also effective. Covering the angiokeratoma with a glass slide, i.e., diascopy is helpful. The endpoint is lesional purpura. Healing occurs over 10–14 days. Multiple treatments may be required (Fig. 25.3).

– Resurfacing lasers such as CO$_2$ and Er:YAG lasers can be utilized for lesional vaporization. Patients generally require local infiltration with 1% lidocaine with or without epinephrine prior to treatment. The Ultrapulse CO$_2$ (Lumenis, Santa Clara, CA) is employed using a 3 mm collimated handpiece, with an energy of 300–500 mJ with nonoverlapping pulses. The various scanned CO$_2$ lasers such as the Sharplan Feathertouch are employed using the 125 mm handpiece, 3 mm scan size at 14–40 W. The treatment endpoint is ablation to achieve lesional flattening and opalescence. Treatment sites should be cleansed with saline soaked gauze between laser passes. Postoperative care requires twice daily washing with soap and water and application of an antibiotic ointment. Healing occurs over 2–6 weeks. Scarring may be observed.

– Other lasers that have been used with variable success include potassium-titanyl-phosphate laser, long-pulse Nd:YAG (1064 nm) laser as well as argon laser and copper vapor laser.

• Other surgical treatments include excision, electrocautery, electrofulgration, or cryosurgery.

PITFALLS TO AVOID

• Patients should be advised that the PDL treatment will cause obvious bruising for up to 14 days.

• Keratotic features may persist after treatment

BIBLIOGRAPHY

Gorse SJ, James W, Murison MS. Successful treatment of angiokeratoma with potassium tritanyl phosphate laser. *Br J Dermatol.* March 2004;150(3):620–622.

Lapins J, Emtestam L, Marcusson JA. Angiokeratomas in Fabry's disease and Fordyce's disease: successful treatment with copper vapour laser. *Acta Derm Venereol.* April 1993;73(2):133–135.

Occella C, Bleidl D, Rampini P, Schiazza L, Rampini E. Argon laser treatment of cutaneous multiple angiokeratomas. *Dermatol Surg.* February 1995;21(2):170–172.

Sommer S, Merchant WJ, Sheehan-Dare R. Severe predominantly acral variant of angiokeratoma of Mibelli: response to long-pulse Nd:YAG (1064 nm) laser treatment. *J Am Acad Dermatol.* November 2001;45(5): 764–766.

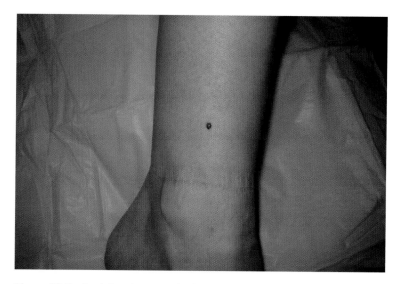

Figure 25.2 *Angiokeratoma on the lower leg*

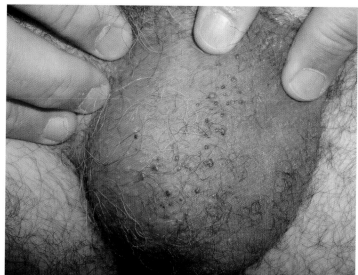

A

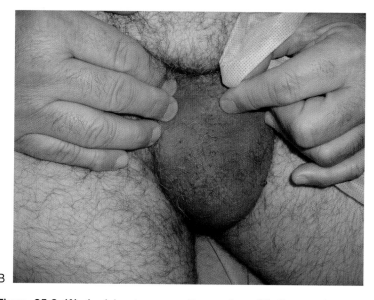

B

Figure 25.3 (A) *Angiokeratomas on the scrotum.* **(B)** *Purpura immediately after treatment with pulsed dye laser at a wavelength of 595 nm with a 5 mm spot, pulse duration of 1.5 ms, and a fluence of 8 J/cm^2. The larger lesions were treated twice.*

CHAPTER 26 Cherry and Spider Angiomas

Cherry angiomas, also known as ruby spots, senile hemangiomas, acquired capillary hemangioma and Campbell de Morgan spots, are very common benign vascular lesions that predominantly affect the trunk. Spider angiomas, also known as nevus araneus, spider telangiectasia, arterial spider, and vascular spider, represent localized telangiectasias radiating from central feeding arterioles. They are common vascular lesions that predominantly affect the face, upper trunk, arms, and hand.

EPIDEMIOLOGY

Incidence: very common

Age: cherry angiomas—middle-aged and elderly people; spider angiomas—all ages

Sex: more common in females

Precipitating factors: cherry angiomas can erupt during pregnancy or with hepatic disease. Spider angiomas are strongly associated with pregnancy, intake of oral contraceptive pills, and hepatocellular disease

PATHOGENESIS

Unknown for both. Association with pregnancy, oral contraceptive use, and liver disease suggest a hormonally-mediated angiogenic mechanism.

PHYSICAL EXAMINATION

Cherry angioma presents as a 1–3 mm bright red to violaceous, smooth, dome-shaped papule. Spider angioma displays a network of dilated capillaries radiating from a central vessel. Both may bleed when traumatized.

PATHOLOGY

Cherry angiomas show loss of rete ridges as well as congested and ectatic capillaries and postcapillary venules in the papillary dermis. Spider angiomas reveal a central ascending arteriole that branches and communicates with multiple dilated capillaries.

DIFFERENTIAL DIAGNOSES

Cherry angiomas can be mistaken for angiokeratoma, glomeruloid hemangioma, pyogenic granuloma, and nodular melanoma. Spider angiomas can be mistaken for

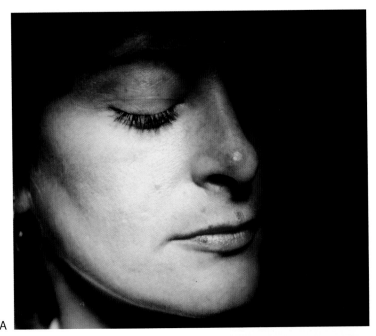

A

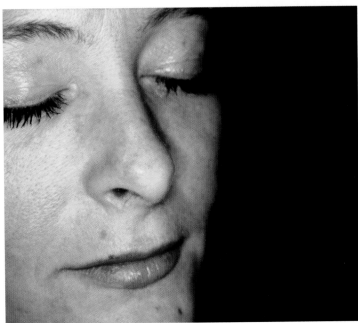

B

Figure 26.1 (A) *Spider angioma, right nose.* **(B)** *Full resolution of spider angioma after a single pulsed dye laser treatment to central vessel and surrounding skin*

generalized essential telangiectasia and hereditary hemorrhagic telangiectasia.

COURSE

Cherry and spider angiomas arising during pregnancy may regress postpartum. Spider angiomas arising in childhood may also resolve spontaneously. Otherwise, both lesions tend to persist.

MANAGEMENT

Although medically insignificant, cherry and spider angiomas are frequently treated for cosmetic purposes. Multiple effective surgical treatment options exist. Depending on the procedure selected, the cost to the patient may vary significantly. Cherry and spider angiomas that present during pregnancy should not be treated until several months after delivery as they may resolve on their own.

- Electrosurgery
  - Electrodessication with coagulation (monopolar setting, 1–2 W followed by gentle curettage with endpoint of lesional flattening and hemostasis) has been the traditional treatment modality for these lesions.
  - It is effective and easily accessible.
  - The potential for scar formation must be considered.
- Laser surgery: different lasers have been used successfully in treatment of cherry and spider angiomas.
  - Pulsed dye laser (PDL) is the most commonly employed laser. A spot size should be selected that matches the vessel diameter. With spider angiomas, the central feeding vessel as well as the surrounding vessels should be treated. Treatment endpoint is a purpuric change representing coagulation (Figs. 26.1-26.2).
  - The potassium-titanyl-phosphate (KTP) 532-nm laser produces a favorable response. Spot size should match the lesion diameter. As with PDL treatment, the vessels should be traced out completely for most effective treatment. Treatment endpoint is lesional clearance or superficial whitening. Erythema can be expected post-treatment, lasting 24–48 h.
  - Carbon dioxide laser (Ultrapulse 3-mm collimated handpiece, 300–400 mJ/pulse, nonoverlapping pulses; Sharplan Feathertouch 125-mm handpiece, 14–40 W, 3 mm scan size, nonoverlapping pulses) has been employed as second line therapy with success. Treatment endpoint is lesional flattening. Potential scar formation must be considered.
- Light therapy
  - Intense pulsed light (IPL) has also been employed with some success. As coagulation is needed for lesional resolution, higher fluences may be required for treatment efficacy.

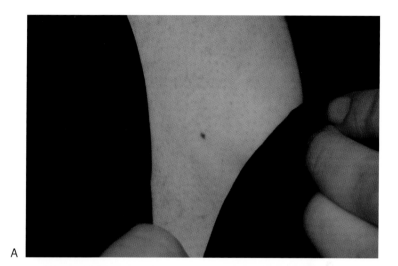

A

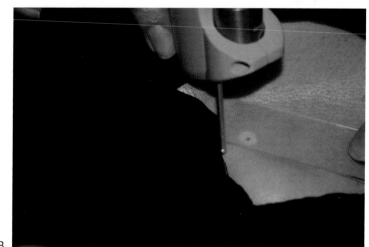

B

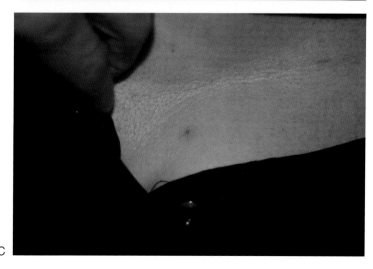

C

Figure 26.2 (A) *Cherry angioma, chest.* **(B)** *Pulsed dye laser treatment to cherry angioma utilizing diascopy.* **(C)** *Purpura immediately post pulsed dye laser treatment.*

- Surgical excision
  - Excision should be reserved for lesions that are resistant to other treatments. A postoperative scar is expected which may be less cosmetically pleasing than the angioma.

PITFALLS TO AVOID

- Patients need to be counseled as to the likelihood of obvious purpura following treatment with PDL that may persist for 10–14 days. Lesions are less likely to be completely treated at subpurpuric fluences.
- Simple electrocautery may be just as effective as PDL at a reduced cost to the patient.
- Compressing the lesion with a glass slide during PDL or KTP treatment is helpful to minimize its size and allowing for greater laser penetration. This reduces the total energy needed for coagulation and increases the treatment success rate.
- Multiple treatments may be required, in particular for large spider angiomas.

BIBLIOGRAPHY

Dawn G, Gupta G. Comparison of potassium titanyl phosphate vascular laser and hyfrecator in the treatment of vascular spiders and cherry angiomas. *Clin Exp Dermatol.* 2003;28(6):581–583.

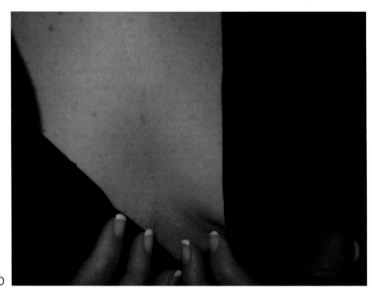

D

Figure 26.2 *(continued)* **(D)** *Complete resolution of cherry angioma after one pulsed dye laser treatment*

CHAPTER 27 Granuloma Faciale

Granuloma faciale (GF) was first described by Wigley in 1945 who labeled the disease "eosinophilic granuloma." Pinkus renamed this disorder granuloma faciale in 1952. GF is an idiopathic chronic cutaneous disorder that usually involves the face, particularly the nose.

EPIDEMIOLOGY

Incidence: uncommon

Age: 30–50 years

Race: primarily seen in Caucasians

Sex: males > females

PATHOGENESIS

Unknown, but may be mediated by immune complex deposition.

PHYSICAL EXAMINATION

Single indurated facial brownish-red papule or plaque. Multiple lesions may be present. Extrafacial sites rarely observed. (Fig. 27.1)

DIFFERENTIAL DIAGNOSES

Cutaneous lupus erythematosus, sarcoidosis, lymphoma, pseudolymphoma, fixed drug eruption, rosacea.

DERMATOPATHOLOGY

Dense, polymorphous inflammatory cell infiltrate in the upper two-thirds of the dermis. The infiltrate is composed of numerous eosinophils, neutrophils, lymphocytes, and histiocytes. A prominent grenz zone is characteristically present. Leukocytoclastic vasculitis is frequently observed.

COURSE

The lesions of GF are usually chronic and only occasionally resolve spontaneously.

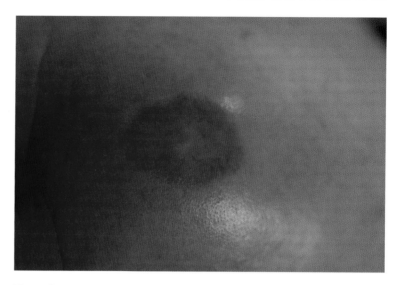

Figure 27.1 *Granuloma faciale on the scalp*

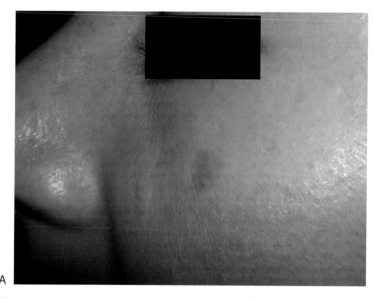

A

Figure 27.2 (A) *Indurated brownish-red plaque on the left cheek of a middle-aged female with granuloma faciale.*

MANAGEMENT

■ Topical Treatment

• Corticosteroids: topical, intralesional

• Tacrolimus ointment (0.1%)

■ Systemic Treatment

• Dapsone

• Antimalarials

• Colchicine

• Clofazamine

• Gold injections

SURGICAL TREATMENT

• Cryosurgery: multiple reports indicating successful clearance. Results are unpredictable (Fig. 27.3)

• Surgical excision

• Dermabrasion

• Electrosurgery

■ Light Treatment

• Topical PUVA therapy

• Laser therapy: different lasers have been used in the treatment of GF with promising results, either as an ablative therapy with carbon dioxide laser or as a selective therapy targeting the prominent vasculature in GF lesions using the Q-switched argon laser, pulsed dye, diode laser, and KTP 532-nm laser (Fig. 27.2).

PITFALLS TO AVOID

• Patients should be aware of the chronic nature of GF.

• GF is often recalcitrant to therapy. Patients should be counseled that successful treatment is often elusive.

BIBLIOGRAPHY

Ammirati CT, Hruza GJ. Treatment of granuloma faciale with the 585-nm pulsed dye laser. *Arch Dermatol.* 1999;135(8):903–905.

Apfelberg DB, Druker D, Maser MR, Lash H, Spence B Jr, Deneau D. Granuloma faciale. Treatment with the argon laser. *Arch Dermatol.* 1983;119(7):573–576.

Chatrath V, Rohrer TE. Granuloma faciale successfully treated with long-pulsed tunable dye laser. *Dermatol Surg.* 2002;28(6):527–529.

Elston DM. Treatment of granuloma faciale with the pulsed dye laser. *Cutis.* 2000;65(2): 97–98.

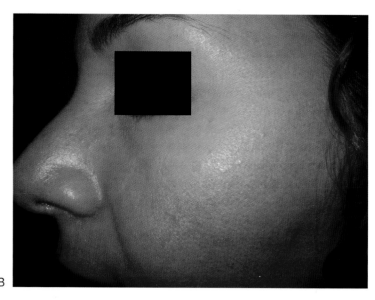

B

Figure 27.2 (B) *Two-year follow-up showing resolution of granuloma faciale after multiple pulsed dye laser treatments*

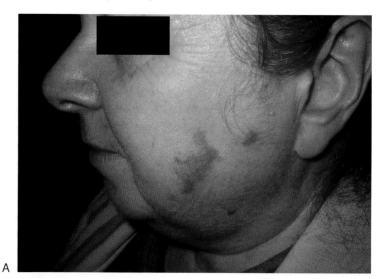

A

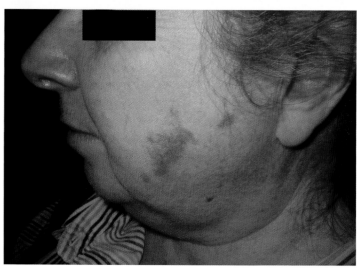

B

Figure 27.3 (A) *Multiple lesions of granuloma faciale on the face.* **(B)** *No significant improvement detected after one treatment with cryotherapy on a 4-month follow-up visit*

Ludwig E, Allam JP, Bieber T, Novak N. New treatment modalities for granuloma faciale. *Br J Dermatol.* 2003;149(3):634–637.

Maillard H, Grognard C, Toledano C, Jan V, Machet L, Vaillant L. Granuloma faciale: efficacy of cryosurgery in 2 cases. *Ann Dermatol Venereol.* 2000;127(1):77–79.

Wheeland RG, Ashley JR, Smith DA, Ellis DL, Wheeland DN. Carbon dioxide laser treatment of granuloma faciale. *J Dermatol Surg Oncol.* 1984;10(9):730–733.

Zacarian SA. Cryosurgery effective for granuloma faciale. *J Dermatol Surg Oncol.* 1985;11(1):11–13.

CHAPTER 28 Infantile Hemangioma

Infantile hemangioma (IH), also known as strawberry, capillary, or cavernous hemangioma, is a benign endothelial proliferation that represents the most common tumor in infancy. It can be classified into superficial hemangioma (SH, 55% of cases), deep hemangioma (DH, 30% of cases), and mixed superficial and deep hemangioma (MH, 15% of cases). They occur most commonly on head and neck areas.

EPIDEMIOLOGY

Incidence: 1–3% are present at birth, 10–12% are present by 1 year of age

Age: majority (80%) become apparent between 2 and 5 weeks of age; 20% are noted at birth

Sex: females are affected 2–4 times more than males

Precipitating Factors: premature infants are more commonly affected

PHYSICAL EXAMINATION

The appearance of the lesions depends on the depth of the hemangioma and the phase of evolution. SH presents as bright red colored plaque. DH presents as a soft dermal or subcutaneous nodule with a bluish-purple color. MH shows features of both SH and DH. Multiple truncal hemangiomas may be observed. Involuting hemangiomas demonstrate a flatter surface with a grayish-purple hue that begins centrally and expands outward. The hemangiomas might become ulcerated and hemorrhagic. Residual fatty tissue, atrophy, telangiectasia, scar formation, and hypertrophy may be observed.

DIFFERENTIAL DIAGNOSIS

Congenital hemangiomas can be confused with a vascular malformation at birth. Hemangiomas are generally present after birth versus vascular malformations, which are generally present at birth.

LABORATORY TESTS

▓ Dermatopathology

Proliferations of plump endothelial cells that may extend from the superficial dermis to the deep subcutaneous tissue, depending on the hemangioma subtype.

▓ Ancillary Tests

- An abdominal ultrasound should be obtained if more than four truncal hemangiomas are noted prior to 4 months of age.
- An EKG and a cardiac ECHO should be considered for any concern of high cardiac output.

COURSE

Hemangiomas characteristically exhibit three phases of evolution: (a) proliferative phase, (b) involuting phase, and (c) involuted phase.

The proliferating phase is characterized by a rapid growth phase that starts at 1–2 months of age and lasts until 6–9 months of age. This growth phase is followed by the involuting phase that usually starts in the second year of life and persists for several years. More than 90% of untreated hemangiomas involute, i.e., attain maximal regression by 9 years of age. Up to 30% of hemangiomas leave post-involution changes including hypopigmentation, scarring, telangiectasia, and fibrofatty tissue.

COMPLICATIONS

Bleeding and ulceration with secondary infection and scarring especially in hemangiomas involving the diaper area are commonly seen. Other serious complications include orbital obstruction and amblyopia with periorbital hemangioma, upper airway obstruction with hemangiomas in the beard distribution, spinal abnormalities with lumbosacral hemangiomas, posterior fossa malformation in large facial hemangioma (PHACE syndrome), and high output cardiac failure with multiple cutaneous hemangiomas associated with visceral involvement.

KEY CONSULTATIVE QUESTIONS

- Onset of lesion
- Number of lesions noted

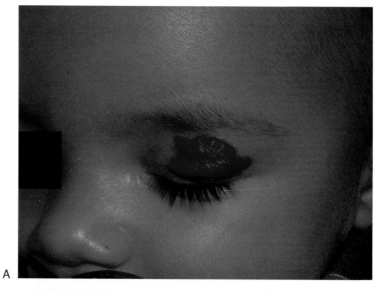

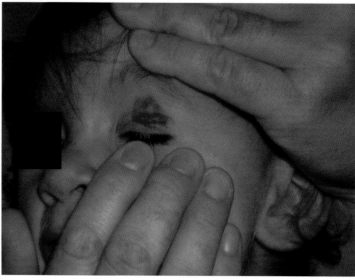

Figure 28.1 (A) *Left upper eyelid hemangioma in its early growth phase, a lesion that may threaten the child's vision.* **(B)** *Marked lightening and flattening of the hemangioma after multiple pulsed dye laser treatments*

- Ulceration noted
- Bleeding noted
- Prior treatments and response

MANAGEMENT

The treatment of IHs is controversial. Given the natural course of IH with spontaneous resolution, many physicians choose to carefully observe the area with no intervention, especially in nonfacial, small and noncomplicated hemangiomas. Early intervention is recommended for (a) all IHs that interfere with the function of vital organs (e.g., periorbital hemangiomas, airway obstruction with hemangiomas in the beard distribution, high-output cardiac failure); (b) large facial hemangiomas that usually involute with permanent disfiguring; (c) ulcerated hemangiomas; and (d) hemangiomas in the diaper area that are very likely to ulcerate causing severe pain.

- Medical treatment

  - Steroids including topical steroid application (class 1 corticosteroid applied twice daily with monitoring every 2 weeks), intralesional steroids (triamcinolone acetonide 10 mg/mL administered monthly), and oral steroids (1.5–2 mg/kg per day of prednisone) are the mainstay of treatment. Patients must be monitored closely, especially with oral steroid use given the risk of systemic complications including growth retardation and glucose alterations. Localized side effects include atrophy and yeast infection.

  - Other treatment options include topical imiquimod (applied daily), interferon alpha (3 million units/m^2/day, SC), and vincrisitine (0.05 mg/kg/day if less than 10 kg, IV), especially in steroid-resistant IH. As interferon alpha is associated with spastic diplegia, patients must be monitored closely.

- Laser treatment

  - Pulsed dye laser (PDL) treatment induces significantly faster regression of the IH. Fluences lower than those of PWS are effective and are associated with lower risk of laser-induced scarring (Figs. 28.1-28.2). PDL has been used extensively in the treatment of IH in three clinical scenarios:

    1. Ulcerated hemangiomas respond effectively to PDL. PDL markedly decreases the associated pain and induces rapid healing of the ulceration (75% within 2 weeks) (Fig. 28.3). Residual scar formation from the ulceration is expected.

    2. SHs can respond well to PDL if started either before or early in the proliferative phase. Multiple treatments, every 4–6 weeks, are required in the proliferative phase. The only exception is a rapidly proliferating facial hemangioma. PDL treatment may induce ulceration of these variants so treatment should be avoided. IH with deeper components (MH, DH) respond less effectively to PDL

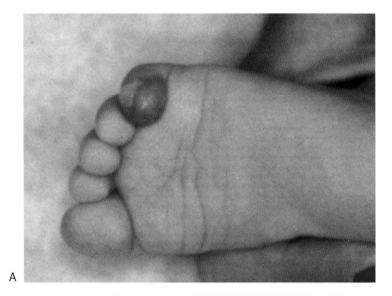

A

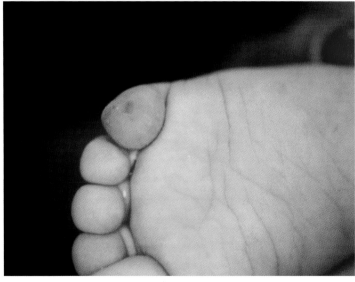

B

Figure 28.2 (A) *Hemangioma on the left fifth toe pad, a location that interfered with the child's ability to ambulate.* **(B)** *Significant clearing and near resolution of the hemangioma after multiple pulsed dye laser treatments*

because of the limitation of penetration of PDL to 1.2 mm in the skin.

3. PDL can help treat the residual erythema and telangiectasias on the surface of involuted hemangiomas.

– Long-pulsed Nd:YAG lasers are useful for photocoagulation of DHs but have a higher incidence of scarring.

• Other interventions include surgical debulking and embolization. The risks and benefits of each surgical approach should be considered carefully before intervention since the scar from spontaneous regression is usually much better than the surgical scar. Embolization is utilized in hemangiomas associated with high-output cardiac failure.

PITFALLS TO AVOID

• Use of excessive PDL fluences without skin cooling can cause scar.

• Parents are understandably anxious about their child's hemangioma. A full discussion of the natural course of hemangiomas is mandatory prior to starting therapy. The option of foregoing treatment and clinically monitoring a patient should be reviewed carefully prior to starting therapy.

• Parents should also have a realistic idea of the limitations of therapy. Large hemangiomas respond less successfully to oral, surgical, and laser therapy. Complicated hemangiomas that may interfere with the child's health should be referred to an appropriate pediatric specialist. Parents must be aware that treatment will provide an improvement only and not full resolution of the hemangioma.

• Parents need to be educated on proper wound care, especially for ulcerated hemangiomas, in order to improve the child's quality of life.

BIBLIOGRAPHY

Batta K, Goodyear HM, Moss C, Williams HC, Hiller L, Waters R. Randomised controlled study of early pulsed dye laser treatment of uncomplicated childhood haemangiomas: results of a 1-year analysis. *Lancet*. 2002; 360(9332):521–527.

Morelli JG, Tan OT, Yohn JJ, Weston WL. Treatment of ulcerated hemangiomas infancy. *Arch Pediatr Adolesc Med*. 1994;148(10):1104–1105.

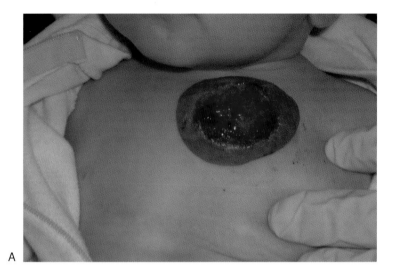

A

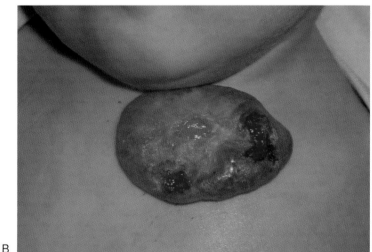

B

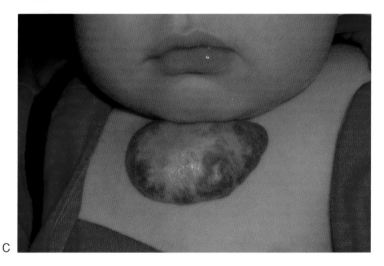

C

Figure 28.3 (A) *Ulcerated hemangioma, isolated nodular type, extremely painful and hemorrhaging, treated twice with PDL 6 J/cm², 7 mm spot size, 590 nm.* **(B)** *At 2 months follow-up, significant healing of the ulceration after a single treatment with pulsed dye laser.* **(C)** *Four months after initial pulsed dye laser treatment and 2 months after second pulsed dye laser treatment, there is complete healing of the ulceration.*

CHAPTER 29 Keratosis Pilaris Atrophicans

Keratosis pilaris atrophicans (KPA) is a group of inherited disorders with three subtypes including (1) keratosis pilaris atrophicans faciei (KPAF), (2) atrophoderma vermiculatum (AV), and (3) keratosis follicularis spinulosa decalvans (KFSD). KPAF and AV present mainly on the face with KFSD often appearing on the eyebrow and AV most commonly seen on the cheeks, sparing the eyebrows and scalp. KFSD can affect the face, scalp, and trunk. Inheritance pattern can be autosomal dominant (KPAF, AV), recessive (AV), or X-linked (KFSD).

EPIDEMIOLOGY

Incidence: very rare; KPAF is the most common subtype

Age: KPAF and KFSD in infancy; AV in childhood

Sex: males are more severely affected in KFSD

PATHOGENESIS

Abnormal follicular keratinization of the upper section of the hair follicle that may later result in atrophic follicular scarring.

PHYSICAL EXAMINATION

Follicular plugging with erythema in early stages. Atrophic follicular scar formation with associated alopecia in later stages.

DIFFERENTIAL DIAGNOSIS

Keratosis pilaris, seborrheic dermatitis (KPAF), atopic dermatitis (KFSD), other etiologies of scarring alopecia (KFSD), acne scarring (AV), Rombo syndrome (AV), and KID syndrome (KFSD).

DERMATOPATHOLOGY

Dilated follicles with follicular hyperkeratosis and inflammation in early stages. Follicular fibrosis and atrophy in later stages.

COURSE

The course is chronic with no spontaneous resolution. With time, the erythematous follicular hyperkeratotic papules involute into depressed atrophic follicular scars with alopecia.

MANAGEMENT

There is no effective treatment for KPA. Multiple treatment options have been tried with variable success.

Patients should be counseled that therapy may not be effective.

- Topical therapy
  - Lactic acid and α-hydroxy acid lotions (10–12%) applied twice daily may improve the textural roughness. However, they may produce irritation.
  - Retinoids (tazarotene, retin-A) applied nightly may improve textural roughness. They may produce irritation.
  - Corticosteroids applied sparingly may show improvement. Risk of facial atrophy limits their use.
- Systemic therapy
  - Other options that have provided variable success include oral retinoids and dapsone.
  - They are most helpful for the inflammatory stage of KPA, but provide minimal improvement in the follicular hyperkeratosis.
  - They require careful monitoring for potential side effects.
- Laser therapy
  - Pulsed dye laser (Scleroplus, Candela, Wayland, MA, 595 nm, 7 mm spot, 6–7.5 J/cm², DCD 40/20 with 10% overlapping passes) can be effective in the treatment of the associated erythema of KPAF but will not significantly improve the textural roughness of KPA (Fig. 29.1).
  - Laser-assisted hair removal with long-pulsed non-Q-switched ruby laser may be an effective treatment in patients with KFSD.

PITFALLS

Patient expectations are generally very high. They must be counseled as to the chronic nature of the condition and minimal response to available therapies.

BIBLIOGRAPHY

Baden HP, Byers HR. Clinical findings, cutaneous pathology, and response to therapy in 21 patients with keratosis pilaris atrophicans. *Arch Dermatol.* 1994;130(4):469–475.

Chui CT, Berger TG, Price VH, Zachary CB. Recalcitrant scarring follicular disorders treated by laser-assisted hair removal: a preliminary report. *Dermatol Surg.* 1999;25(1): 34–37.

Clark SM, Mills CM, Lanigan SW. Treatment of keratosis pilaris atrophicans with the pulsed tunable dye laser. *J Cutan Laser Ther.* 2000;2(3):151–156.

Kunte C, Loeser C, Wolff H. Folliculitis spinulosa decalvans: successful therapy with dapsone. *J Am Acad Dermatol.* 1998;39(5, pt 2):891–893.

Richard G, Harth W. Keratosis follicularis spinulosa decalvans. Therapy with isotretinoin and etretinate in the inflammatory stage. *Hautarzt.* 1993;44(8):529–534.

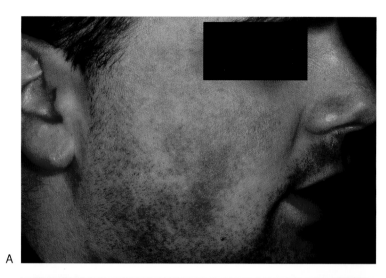

A

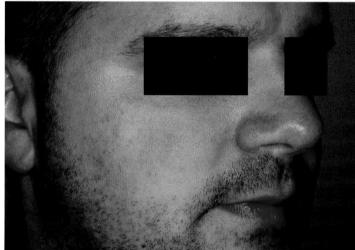

B

Figure 29.1 (A) *Keratosis pilaris atrophicans. Patient is emotionally bothered by persistent erythema.* **(B)** *Marked lightening of erythema 2 years following three pulsed dye laser treatments*

CHAPTER 30 Port-wine Stains

Port-wine stains (PWS) are usually low-flow venule mal-formations. They represent the most common type of vascular malformations and they most commonly affect the head and neck areas.

EPIDEMIOLOGY

Incidence: 3 per 1000 newborns

Age: present at birth in the majority of patients; rarely appear in adolescence or adulthood

Sex: no sex predilection

Race: less common in Asians and African-Americans

Associated syndromes: PWS can be a manifestation of several syndromes including Sturge–Weber syndrome, Klippel–Trenaunay syndrome, Proteus syndrome, and phakomatosis pigmentovascularis

PHYSICAL EXAMINATION

Light pink, well-demarcated macular lesions and patches that darken with age to dark red, usually in a segmental distribution.

DIFFERENTIAL DIAGNOSIS

PWS exhibits characteristic clinical features and is sel-dom misdiagnosed. It can be confused with the macular stage of hemangioma at birth.

DERMATOPATHOLOGY

Dilated thin-walled vessels in the papillary and reticular dermis.

ANCILLARY TESTS

• The parents should be counseled regarding the possi-bility of Sturge–Weber syndrome in lesions located in a facial V1 or V2 dermatomal distribution. An ophthalmo-logic examination to rule out glaucoma and cataract for-mation with continued follow-up is necessary for these patients. A head CT or MRI should be obtained to rule out brain involvement which could affect mental devel-opment.

• Large extremity PWS should raise the consideration of Klippel–Trenaunay syndrome. Leg girth and length should be measured and followed over time.

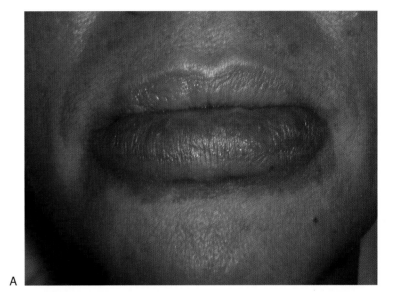

A

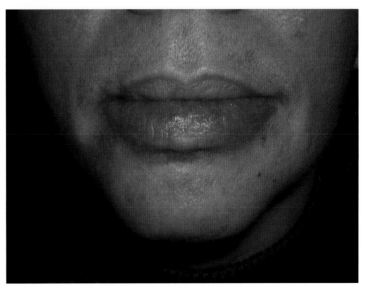

B

Figure 30.1 (A) *Port-wine stain on the lower mucosal and cutaneous lip.* **(B)** *Significant lightening of port-wine stain after three treatments with a combination of pulsed dye laser to the cutaneous lip and vermilion and long-pulsed 1064 nm Nd:YAG laser to the inner mucosal lip and vermil-lion*

COURSE

PWS grows proportionally with the patient and gradually darkens in color from pink to dark red to deep purple. The affected skin thickens and may develop nodularity, blebs, and/or pyogenic granulomas. It may be associated with hypertrophy of underlying soft tissue and bone, particularly in Sturge–Weber syndrome and Klippel–Trenaunay syndrome.

KEY CONSULTATIVE QUESTIONS

• Onset of lesion

• Associated clinical findings

• Is the child meeting developmental milestones?

• Has the child had an eye exam?

• Has the child had a head MRI or CT?

• Past treatments and response

MANAGEMENT

PWS demonstrates progressive vascular dilatation with age, thus making earlier treatment essential for a better response. Treatment can be started as early as 2 weeks of age. Treatment provides a reduction in the number of vessels and does not completely remove the entire lesion. Therefore, the PWS may exhibit some darkening and thickening over time despite intervention. The use of a topical anesthetic has significantly decreased the discomfort associated with the procedure. General anesthesia might be needed for treating large PWS in young children.

• Laser treatment (Figs. 30.1-30.4)

  – Pulsed dye lasers (PDL), specifically with a wavelength of 585 nm and short pulse duration of 0.45 ms remains the treatment of choice for PWS. The most commonly used PDLs include the Scleroplus (Candela, Wayland, MA, variable wavelengths of 585-600 nm, 6-15 J/cm^2, 5-10 mm spot size) and Vbeam (Candela Wayland, MA, 595 nm wavelength, 6-15 J/cm^2, variable pulse duration of 0.45 or 1.5 ms, 7-10 mm spot size). Lower fluences are initially utilized for PWS off the face and in darker skin types. Delivering this PDL with cryogen spray cooling projects the epidermis allowing for the use of higher fluences and more effective blanching of PWS than PDL alone. Cooling also decreases the treatment pain and the incidence of blistering.

  – Resistance to PDL treatment is more common in PWS with deeper and/or more branched vessels. Helpful maneuvers for resistant PWS include increasing the wavelength (up to 600 nm) and increasing the fluences utuilized (15-20 J/cm^2 coupled with cryogen cooling of 40-48 ms). With extreme caution

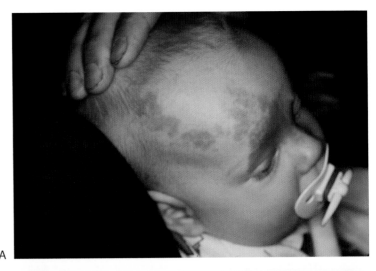

A

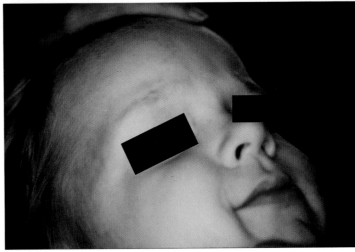

B

Figure 30.2 (A) *Extensive port-wine stain on the right face and forehead of an infant male.* **(B)** *Significant resolution after multiple treatments with pulsed dye laser*

to avoid scarring, it is possible to treat resistant deeper or hypertrohic adult PWS using long-pulsed alexandrite (755 nm) or Nd: YAG lasers (1064 nm at high fluences (NdYag: 50-250 J/cm^2, alexandrite: 45–60 J/cm^2) coupled with adequate cooling.

* Light treatment: intense pulsed light may be effective in treatment of PWS, especially in Asians and in patients with PDL-resistant PWS. A green-yellow waveband and lowest available pulse duration should be used, with skin cooling.

PITFALLS TO AVOID

* Patients should be counseled that PWS display a variable response to treatment. More extensive and thicker lesions respond less well when compared to superficial lesions. Facial PWS responds best. PWS treatment efficacy decreases as one descends from face to feet, with the lower extremities displaying the least treatment benefit.

* Multiple treatment sessions may be required. Bruising is a necessary side effect to obtain efficacious therapy.

* Laser treatment may produce "footprinting" or only partial improvement.

* Treatments should be ceased when the patient is satisfied with lightening, or when no further benefit has been noted, i.e., after two subsequent treatments.

BIBLIOGRAPHY

Bjerring P, Christiansen K, Troilius A. Intense pulsed light source for the treatment of dye laser resistant port-wine stains. *J Cosmet Laser Ther*. 2003;5(1):7–13.

Chiu CH, Chan HH, Ho WS, Yeung CK, Nelson JS. Prospective study of pulsed dye laser in conjunction with cryogen spray cooling for treatment of port wine stains in Chinese patients. *Dermatol Surg*. 2003;29(9):909–915. Discussion 915.

Greve B, Raulin C. Prospective study of port wine stain treatment with dye laser: comparison of two wavelengths (585 nm vs. 595 nm) and two pulse durations (0.5 milliseconds vs. 20 milliseconds). *Lasers Surg Med*. 2004;34(2):168–173.

Ho WS, Ying SY, Chan PC, Chan HH. Treatment of port wine stains with intense pulsed light: a prospective study. *Dermatol Surg*. 2004;30(6):887–890. Discussion 890–891.

Yang M, Yaroslavsky A, Farinelliw, et al. Long-pulsed neodymium: yttrium-aluminum-garnet laser treatment for port-wine stains. *J Am Acad Dermatol*, 2005;52(3): 480–90.

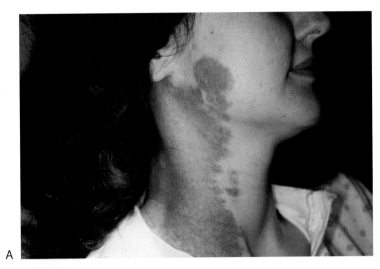

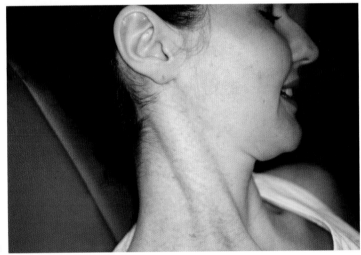

Figure 30.3 (A) *Extensive port-wine stain on the right neck of a young female.* **(B)** *Marked resolution of the port-wine stain after multiple treatments with pulsed dye laser*

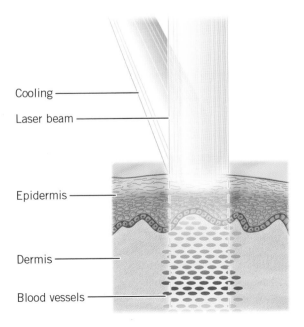

Figure 30.4 *Laser beam of a pulsed dye laser coupled with cooling applied on the skin*

CHAPTER 31 Pyogenic Granuloma

Pyogenic granuloma (PG) can be regarded as a benign vascular tumor or as a reactive vascular process arising at sites of previous trauma or irritation. PG is also known as lobular capillary hemangioma, granuloma telangiectaticum, and granuloma gravidarum when presenting on the gingiva of pregnant women. It commonly occurs in areas of trauma including the face and fingers.

EPIDEMIOLOGY

Incidence: common

Age: most common in children and young adults

Precipitating factors: minor trauma, pregnancy, laser treatment of port-wine stains, isotretinoin.

PATHOGENESIS

Reactive neovascularization suggested by common association with preexisting trauma or irritation and limited growth capacity.

PHYSICAL EXAMINATION

Red to violaceous, dome-shaped, friable papule or nodule, 0.5–1.5 cm in size, with smooth surface that frequently ulcerates. (Figs. 31.1-31.2)

DIFFERENTIAL DIAGNOSES

Nodular amelanotic melanoma, glomus tumor, hemangioma, squamous cell carcinoma (SCC), nodular basal cell carcinoma, wart, bacillary angiomatosis, Kaposi's sarcoma, and metastatic cancer.

DERMATOPATHOLOGY

Well-circumscribed exophytic lobular proliferation of capillaries with flattened and sometimes eroded overlying epidermis, with peripheral epidermal "collarettes".

COURSE

PG usually grows rapidly over the course of weeks or months and then stabilizes. It bleeds frequently with minor trauma and can persist indefinitely if not treated.

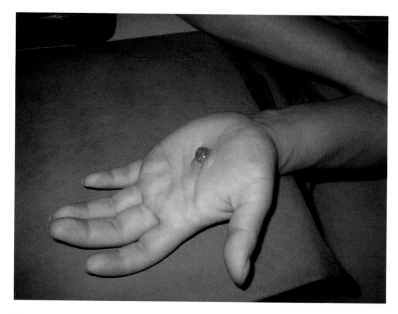

Figure 31.1 *Pyogenic granuloma on the palm of a pregnant woman, bleeding frequently*

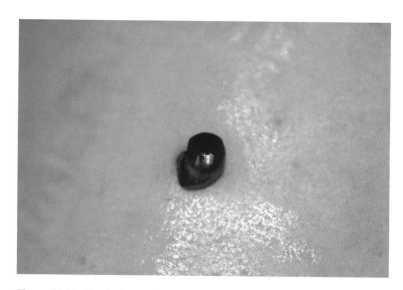

Figure 31.2 *Classic hemorrhagic pyogenic granuloma*

MANAGEMENT

- Laser treatment

  - Pulsed dye laser (Scleroplus 585 nm, Candela Corp., Walyand, MA, 0.45 ms, 5–7 mm, 5.5–8 J/cm², DCD 20-40/20 with diascopy) is a safe and effective device for the treatment of small lesions and for pediatric patients. Serial treatments required. Treatment is well tolerated without anesthesia.

  - Carbon dioxide laser (Ultrapulse Coherent Inc., Palo Aeto, CA, 3 mm handpiece, 300–500 mJ/pulse, nonoverlapping pulses) is effective. Lesional flattening is the clinical endpoint. Intralesional lidocaine 1% is necessary prior to treatment. Postoperative care requires twice daily cleansing with soap and water and application of antibiotic ointment over a 2–6 week healing time. Scar formation is likely. A low recurrence rate is noted.

- Surgical treatment: all treatments may result in scar formation.

  - Shave excision followed by electrodessication of the base is the procedure most commonly employed. Recurrence is common (Figs. 31.3-31.4).

  - Elliptical excision can be performed with low recurrence.

  - Ligation of the base.

  - Cryosurgery.

- Alternative treatment options include

  - Intralesional injection of absolute ethanol.

  - Sclerotherapy with monoethanolamine oleate.

  - Topical alitretinoin (9-cis-retinoic cid) gel, a drug that is used for the treatment of Kaposi's sarcoma.

PITFALLS TO AVOID

- Patients should be aware that recurrence is common after treatment.

- Patients should be informed that all treatments may result in scarring.

- Amelanotic melanoma as well as SCC and other skin cancers can mimic PG. A biopsy should be performed for any suspicious lesions in the appropriate clinical setting.

BIBLIOGRAPHY

Holbe HC, Frosch PJ, Herbst RA. Surgical pearl: ligation of the base of pyogenic granuloma—an atraumatic, simple, and cost-effective procedure. *J Am Acad Dermatol.* September 2003;49(3):509–510.

Maloney DM, Schmidt JD, Duvic M. Alitretinoin gel to treat pyogenic granuloma. *J Am Acad Dermatol.* December 2002;47(6):969–970.

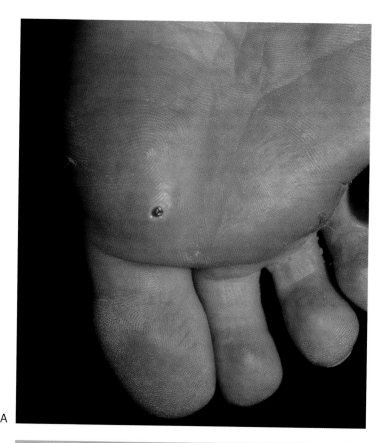

A

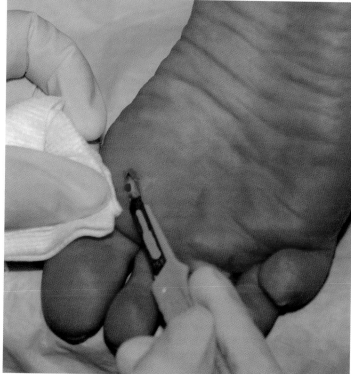

B

Figure 31.3 (A) *Hemorrhagic, painful pyogenic granuloma on the plantar foot.* **(B)** *Shaving the pyogenic granuloma with #15 blade. The specimen was sent for histological confirmation.*

Matsumoto K, Nakanishi H, Seike T, Koizumi Y, Mihara K, Kubo Y. Treatment of pyogenic granuloma with a sclerosing agent. *Dermatol Surg.* June 2001;27(6):521–523.

Raulin C, Greve B, Hammes S. The combined continuous-wave/pulsed carbon dioxide laser for treatment of pyogenic granuloma. *Arch Dermatol.* January 2002;138(1):33–37.

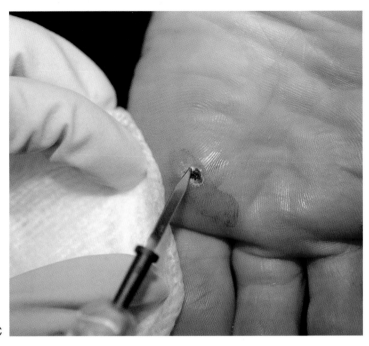

C

Figure 31.3 (*continued*) (**C**) *Electrodessication of the residual pyogenic granuloma*

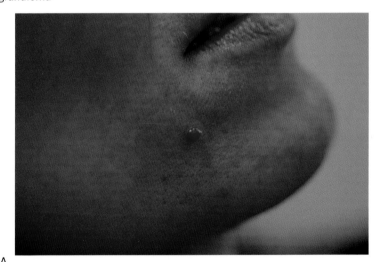

A

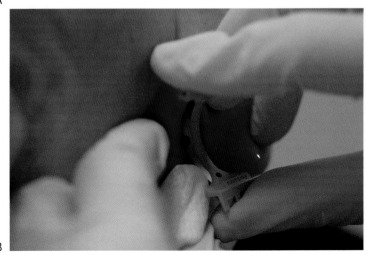

B

Figure 31.4 (**A**) *Biopsy proven pyogenic granuloma on right chin of a young female.* (**B**) *Shave excision of pyogenic granuloma with Derma Blade (Personna Medical, Verona, VA)*

CHAPTER 32 | Lower Extremity Telangiectasias, Reticular and Varicose Veins

Lower extremity telangiectasias, reticular and varicose veins develop as a result of venous system impairment.

EPIDEMIOLOGY

Incidence: very common and the incidence increases with age. Reticular veins can occur in up to 10% of children 10–12 years old. The incidence of varicose veins in the seventh decade is 72% in women and 43% in men.

Age: more common in adults and elderly

Sex: more common in women

Precipitating factors: familial predisposition, pregnancy, static gravitational pressures, dynamic muscular forces, hormonal influences

PATHOPHYSIOLOGY

Venous pathology develops when venous return is impaired for any reason.

It can develop from venous obstruction (thrombotic or nonthrombotic) or from venous valvular incompetence.

PHYSICAL EXAMINATION

Lower extremity telangiectasias are red to violaceous in color and up to 2 mm in diameter. Reticular veins are blue to blue-green in color and up to 4 mm in diameter. Varicose veins are blue to blue-green in color with a diameter greater than 3–4 mm.

LABORATORY DATA

■ Dermatopathology

Dilated vascular channels in the dermis.

■ Vascular Studies

Doppler ultrasound and/or duplex scanning are indicated in the following clinical scenarios:

* Asymptomatic varicosity greater than 4 mm in diameter
* Symptomatic veins
* Reticular, perforating, and/or varicose veins
* Signs of venous insufficiency or stasis changes

- Prior history of deep vein thrombosis, thrombophlebitis
- Prior history of sclerotherapy with recurrences or bad outcome

MANAGEMENT

▦ Sclerotherapy (Figs. 32.1-32.2)

Sclerotherapy is the treatment of choice for lower leg telangiectasias and reticular veins. It should be repeated at 8–12 week intervals. Patients may require two to six sclerotherapy sessions to achieve the greatest treatment benefit.

Sclerosing agents

An ideal sclerosing agent causes complete local endothelial destruction of the vessel wall with secondary fibrosis and lumen obliteration, with no systemic toxicity. Sclerosing agents are classified into three groups depending on their mechanism of action of inducing endothelial injury. These include hyperosmotic agents, detergents, and chemical irritants (Tables 32.1-32.2). The most commonly used sclerosant agents in the US are hypertonic saline (HS) and sodium tetradecyl sulfate (STS). Both HS and STS are FDA approved and have lowest incidence of allergenicity and fewest complications. Sodium morrhuate is also FDA approved.

Sclerotherapy technique for telangiectasias and reticular veins

- Fill the sclerosant agent into 3 cc disposable syringes with disposable 30-gauge 1/2 in. needles.
- Swab the site to be treated with alcohol to better visualize the vessels.
- Treat larger vessels first.
- Bend the needle at a 30–45° angle.
- Stretch the skin overlying the vessels being treated.
- Insert the needle slowly in the vessel wall. You may use the air bolus technique by injecting less than 0.5 cc of air in the vessel or the puncture-fill technique relying on the feel associated with vessel wall perforation while

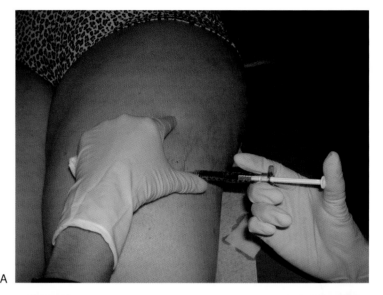

A

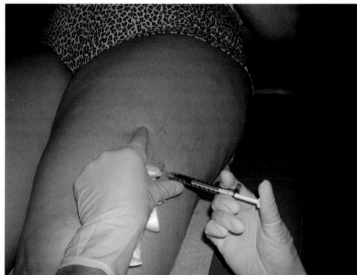

B

Figure 32.1 **(A)** *Sclerotherapy of spider veins. The needle is bent at a 45° angle and the vessel is canalized.* **(B)** *Immediate blanching of the spider veins seen after injecting 0.4 cc of 23.4% sodium chloride*

TABLE 32.1 ▪ **Sclerosing Agents**

Sclerosant class	Sclerosant types	Mechanism
Hyperosmotic agents	Hypertonic saline (10–30%) Hypertonic saline (10%) dextrose (25%) (Sclerodex)	Dehydration
Detergents	Sodium tetradecyl sulfate (Sotradechol", Thromboinject") Polidocanol (Aethoxysclerol, Aetoxisclerol, Sclerovein) Sodium morrhuate (Scleromate) Ethanolamine oleate	Surface tension change
Chemical irritants	Polyiodide iodide (Varigloban, Variglobin, Sclerodine) Glycerin (72%) with 8% chromium potassium alum (Chromex)	Corrosives

injecting. The empty vein technique, performed by elevating the leg and gently kneading the vein prior to injection, allows for thrombus reduction and need for smaller sclerosant volumes. When treating reticular and varicose veins, aspirate a small amount of blood to confirm intravascular location.

- Inject the sclerosant very slowly to ensure sufficient contact of the sclerosant with the vessel endothelial wall and to prevent distention and rupture. Inject less than 0.5 cc per injection at 3 cm intervals.

- Apply small circular band aids, taped cotton balls or rolls at the injection sites for compression.

Foam sclerotherapy

A treatment modification can be made for larger vessels by vigorously foaming an air-sclerosant solution just prior to injection to induce a solution that displaces blood and remains for an extended time in the target vessel without being flushed. Theoretically, lower sclerosant concentrations can be used with a lower incidence of pigmentation and matting (Table 32.3). A solution of either 0.25–3.0% sotradechol or 0.5–1.0% polidocanol is prepared by a back and forth motion using a three-way stop-lock until a foamed emulsion is created. The foam sclerosant is injected in a manner similar to that with other sclerotherapy techniques.

Postoperative care

- Compression increases the efficacy of sclerotherapy and decreases the incidence of hyperpigmentation. Elastic compression stockings (15–60 mmHg) are highly recommended immediately following sclerotherapy and up to 2–3 weeks after the procedure, especially post-treatment of larger caliber vessels. Fashion hose (15–18 mmHg) and Class I hose (20–30 mmHg) are the most commonly used graduated compression hose used post-sclerotherapy of telangiectasias and reticular veins.

- Encourage walking to avoid thromboembolic diseases.

- Avoid sun exposure to minimize post-treatment hyperpigmentation.

Complications (Table 32.3)

- Post-sclerotherapy hyperpigmentation (PSH): The incidence of PSH can be up to 30% depending on the technique used, the size of the treated vessels, the type of sclerosing agent, and the solution concentration. Post-sclerotherapy compression decreases the incidence of PSH. PSH is caused by perivascular

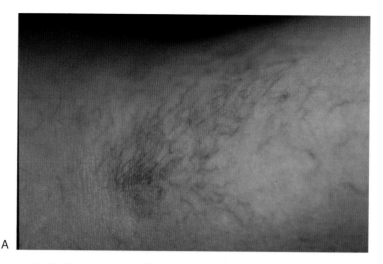

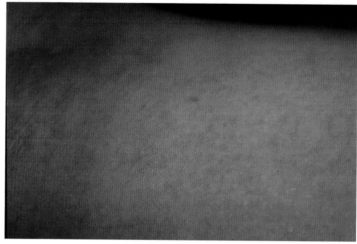

Figure 32.2 (A) *Spider veins, prior to treatment with sclerotherapy.* **(B)** *Marked resolution of the spider veins after sclerotherapy treatment*

TABLE 32.2 ■ Recommended Sclerosant Concentration

Sclerosant/recommended concentration	Telangiectasias	Reticular veins	Varicose veins	Dose limitation
Hypertonic saline	11.7–23.4%	23.4%	Not commonly used	6–10 mL of 18–30% solution
Sodium tetradecyl sulfate	0.1–0.3 %	0.3–0.5%	0.5–3%	10 mL of 3% solution

TABLE 32.3 ■ Complications of Sclerotherapy

Sclerosant	Allergenicity	Cramping	Pain	Hyperpigmentation	Telangiectatic matting	Skin necrosis
Hypertonic saline	−	+	+	+	+	+
Sodium tetradecyl sulfate	+ Anaphylaxis (rare)	−	+	+	+	+

deposition of hemosiderin rather than melanin and follows the course of the treated site. The pigmentation usually resolves in 6–12 months. It can improve with the use of intense pulsed light (IPL).

- Telangiectatic matting (TM): The incidence of TM can be up to 16%. It consists of a network of blush-like, fine (<0.2 mm) telangiectatic vessels surrounding a previously treated area, occurring within days to months after sclerotherapy. They usually resolve within 3–12 months. Predisposing factors include pregnancy, obesity, hormonal therapy, and family history of telangiectasias. TM can improve with pulsed dye laser or IPL. Ways to avoid this complication include
  - Lower injection pressure
  - Lower sclerosant volume (up to 1.0 mL per injection site)
  - Lower sclerosant concentration
  - Limiting blanching (up to 1–2 cm)
- Skin necrosis and ulceration: Necrosis can occur secondary to extravasation of the sclerosing agent into the tissue, regardless of the technique used or the sclerosant type. To minimize extravasation, the surgeon should stop the injection when encountering
  - Even slight resistance to injection
  - Bleb formation
  - Increased pain reported by the patient

If extravasation is recognized immediately, the surgeon can inject normal saline at the site or apply 2% nitroglycerin paste.

- Other complications include pain and cramping (common), allergic reactions (rare), superficial thrombophlebitis (up to 1%), and thromboembolic reactions (very rare).

■ Laser and Intense Pulsed Light (IPL) Therapies (Figs. 32.3–32.4)

Lasers and IPL sources have been used successfully in the treatment of lower extremity telangiectasias and reticular veins, especially when coupled with longer pulse duration and cooling devices. They are considered second-line treatment after sclerotherapy. Wavelengths in the range of 500–1100 nm are most effective, with shorter wavelengths (e.g., PDL, KTP) being used for red superficial blood vessels and longer wavelengths (e.g.,

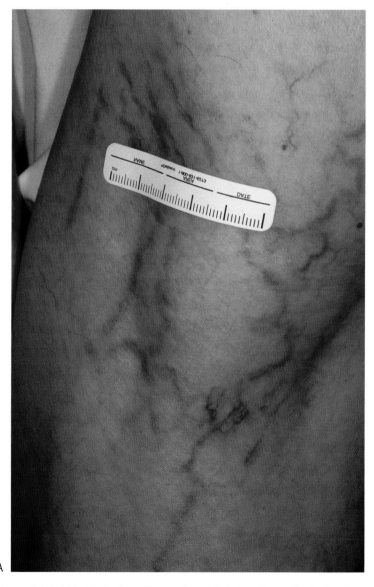

A

Figure 32.3 (A) *Marked erythema immediately after pulsed dye laser treatment to lower extremity spider veins.*

1064 Nd:YAG laser) for bluish deeper blood vessels. Indications for laser/IPL treatments include

- Needle phobic patients
- Vessels resistant to sclerotherapy
- Vessels located below the ankle
- Telangiectatic matting (TM)
- Propensity for post-sclerotherapy hyperpigmentation or TM

Ambulatory Phlebectomy, Endovascular Techniques, Surgical Ligation/Stripping

Multiple treatment options exist for varicose veins including: ambulatory phlebectomy, endovascular laser ablation, endovascular radiofrequency obliteration, as well as surgical ligation and stripping procedures. Ambulatory phlebectomy can be used for large varicosities. Endovenous occlusion can be achieved with radiofrequency (RF) or laser sources. Either a laser fiber or an RF catheter is inserted into the saphenous vein at or just below the knee. Laser systems include 810 nm diode, 940 nm diode, 980 nm diode, and 1320 nm Nd:YAG lasers. These devices spare the need for general anesthesia and extended recovery time associated with vein stripping and ligation. There is little downtime, with patients resuming normal activities on the same day of the procedure.

BIBLIOGRAPHY

Barrett JM, Allen B, Ockelford A, Goldman MP. Microfoam ultrasound-guided sclerotherapy of varicose veins in 100 legs. *Dermatol Surg.* 2004;30(1):6–12.

Kahle B, Leng K. Efficacy of sclerotherapy in varicose veins—prospective, blinded, placebo-controlled study. *Dermatol Surg.* 2004;30(5):723–728.

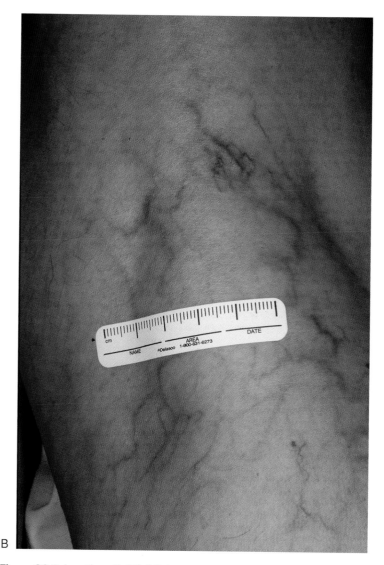

B

Figure 32.3 (*continued*) (B) *Mild reduction in spider veins after a single pulsed dye laser treatment*

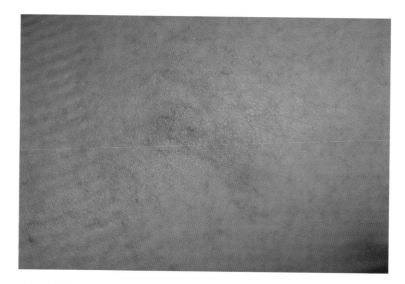

Figure 32.4 *Post-inflammatory changes after laser leg vein treatment*

CHAPTER 33 Facial Telangiectasias

Facial telangiectasias are dilated vessels appearing superficially in the dermis mostly on the alae nasi. Telangiectasias are also common in scars and various skin lesions.

EPIDEMIOLOGY

Incidence: very common

Age: most common in adults and elderly people

Sex, race: no sex or race predisposition

Precipitating factors: chronic actinic damage, rosacea, and topical steroid use are the most common precipitating factors. Other less common etiologies include hereditary hemorrhagic telengiectasia Figure 33.1, Cockayne syndrome, ataxia telengiectasia, Bloom's syndrome, Rothmund–Thomson syndrome, scleroderma, CREST syndrome, lupus, and radiation dermatitis

PHYSICAL EXAMINATION

Telangiectasias consist of fine, tiny, erythematous linear vessels, typically 0.2–2 mm in diameter, coursing along the surface of the skin, which blanch easily upon pressure.

DERMATOPATHOLOGY

Dilated thin-walled vessels in the upper dermis.

COURSE

Facial telangiectasias are usually chronic in nature with no spontaneous resolution.

MANAGEMENT

Facial telangiectasias are frequently treated for cosmetic purposes. Multiple effective treatment options exist.

• Laser treatment: multiple effective options are available. Patients must be aware that over time they are likely to develop more telangiectasias.

  – Pulsed dye lasers (PDL) are the treatment of choice for facial telangiectasias (Figs. 33.2-33.4).

    ○ The traditional PDL with a short pulse duration of 0.45 or 1.5 ms provides the most effective treatment for facial telangiectasias. However, post-treatment purpura occurs which generally lasts 7–14 days.

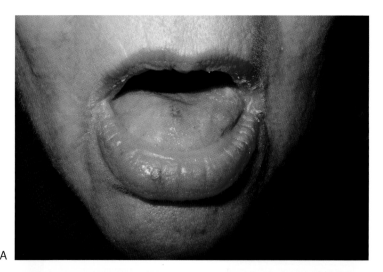

A

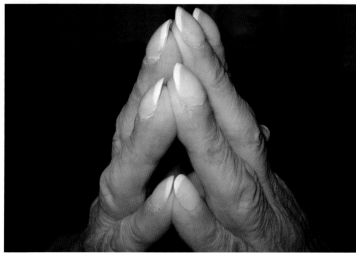

B

Figure 33.1 (A) *A patient with Osler–Weber–Rendu syndrome, also known as hereditary hemorrhagic telangiectasia. Note the telangiectasias on the tongue and the lower lip.* **(B)** *The same patient with clubbing secondary to pulmonary arteriovenous malformation with right-to-left shunting*

- A variable-pulse 595 nm PDL, i.e., V-beam laser (Candela Corp., Wayland, MA) with stuttered pulse durations (i.e., 0.45, 1.5, 3, 6, 10, 20, 30, 40 ms) can provide a reduced purpura treatment of facial telangiectasias, but is somewhat less effective and usually requires multiple treatments.

  - Commonly, subpurpuric fluences of less than 10 J/cm^2 at pulse duration of 10 ms, with a 7 mm spot size are utilized.

  - Better efficacy of the variable-pulse PDL in treating facial telangiectasias can be achieved by utilizing purpuric fluences or by pulse stacking with sub-purpuric pulses (stacked 2–4 subpupuric pulses at a 1.5 Hz repetition rate, 7.5 J/cm^2, 10 ms pulse duration, 10 mm spot size, DCD of 30/20).

  - Facial edema, erythema, and discomfort can occur after extensive treatment with the purpura-free variable-pulse PDL. However, these undesired effects are generally better tolerated when compared to a purpura-inducing laser treatment.

- The variable pulse width 1064 nm Nd:YAG laser has proven to be effective in the treatment of facial telangiectasias. Shorter pulse widths with higher fluences might be necessary for effective treatment of smaller vessels but have an increased risk of blister and scar formation.

- Frequency-doubled 532 nm Nd:YAG laser also called, potassium-titanyl-phosphate (KTP) laser, provides effective absorption of hemoglobin with a pulse duration of 1–50 ms making it ideally suited to treat superficial vessels without purpura formation. Tracing of individual vessels is a useful technique for patients with a countable number of discrete, visible vessels.

- Flashlamp (intense pulsed light) treatment

  - Intense pulse light (IPL) provides another effective, purpura-free method for reducing facial telangiectasias and erythema (Figs. 33.5-33.6). For example, fluences of 30–40 J/cm^2 with 20-ms pulse duration are effective with the Starlux Lux G handpiece (Palomar Medical Technologies, Burlington, MA). The treatment endpoint is immediate vessel clearance or selective vessel darkening. Multiple treatments may be required for the greatest treatment benefit.

- Other treatment options include electrosurgery, cryotherapy, and infiltration of sclerosing agents. These are less selective, often less effective, and more likely to result in scarring than laser or IPL treatment.

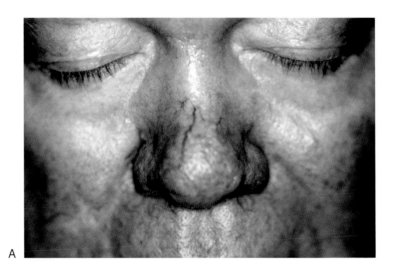
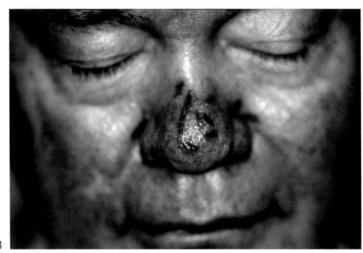
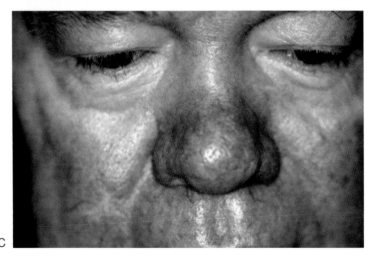

Figure 33.2 (A) *Middle-aged male with multiple facial telangiectasias.* **(B)** *Purpura observed immediately after pulsed dye laser treatment.* **(C)** *Significant reduction in telangiectasias after a single pulsed dye laser treatment*

PITFALLS TO AVOID

- Treatment typically is well-tolerated.

- Obvious post-treatment purpura for 7–14 days with purpuric settings is expected.

- Purpura can be avoided by utilizing nonpurpuric settings at the expense of decreased efficacy.
- Facial edema, erythema, and discomfort can occur after extensive treatment with the purpura-free variable-pulse PDL.
- Telangiectasias will recur over years.
- Caution in darker skin types.

BIBLIOGRAPHY

Alam M, Dover JS, Arndt KA. Treatment of facial telangiectasia with variable-pulse high-fluence pulsed-dye laser: comparison of efficacy with fluences immediately above and below the purpura threshold. *Dermatol Surg.* July 2003;29(7):681–684. Discussion 685.

Alam M, Omura NE, Dover JS, Arndt KA. Clinically significant facial edema after extensive treatment with purpura-free pulsed-dye laser. *Dermatol Surg.* September 2003;29(9):920–924.

Bjerring P, Christiansen K, Troilius A, Dierickx C. Facial photo rejuvenation using two different intense pulsed light (IPL) wavelength bands. *Lasers Surg Med.* 2004;34(2):120–126.

Jasim ZF, Woo WK, Handley JM. Long-pulsed (6-ms) pulsed dye laser treatment of rosacea-associated telangiectasia using subpurpuric clinical threshold. *Dermatol Surg.* January 2004;30(1):37–40.

Mark KA, Sparacio RM, Voigt A, Marenus K, Sarnoff DS. Objective and quantitative improvement of rosacea-associated erythema after intense pulsed light treatment. *Dermatol Surg.* June 2003;29(6):600–604.

Misirlioglu A, Gideroglu K, Akan M, Akoz T. Using silicone gel sheet for the treatment of facial telangiectasias with sclerotherapy. *Dermatol Surg.* March 2004;30(3):373–377.

Rohrer TE, Chatrath V, Iyengar V. Does pulse stacking improve the results of treatment with variable-pulse pulsed-dye lasers? *Dermatol Surg.* February 2004;30(2, pt 1):163–167. Discussion 167.

Sarradet DM, Hussain M, Goldberg DJ. Millisecond 1064-nm neodymium:YAG laser treatment of facial telangiectases. *Dermatol Surg.* January 2003;29(1):56–58.

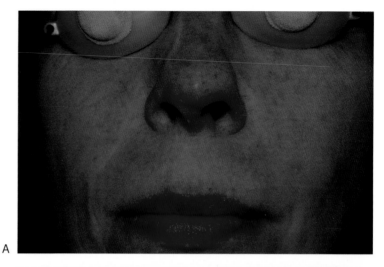

A

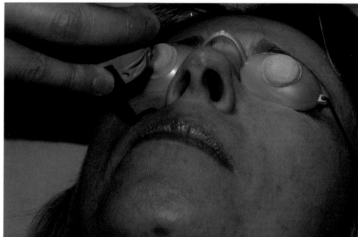

B

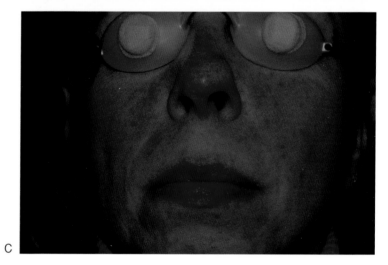

C

Figure 33.3 (A) *Female with centrofacial telangiectasias and erythema prior to pulsed dye laser therapy.* **(B)** *Pulsed dye laser treatment at a wavelength of 595 nm, 10 ms pulse duration, 7 J/cm², 7 mm spot size.* **(C)** *Appropriate clinical endpoint of erythema and slight edema at sites of treatment. No purpura was produced*

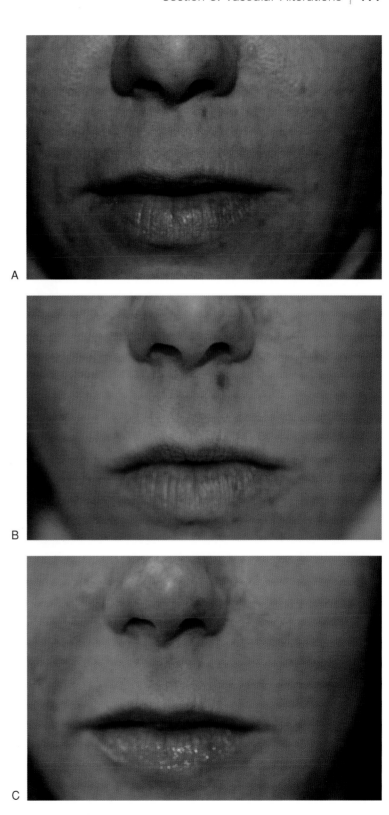

Figure 33.4 (A) *Telangiectasias prior to pulsed dye laser treatment. The setting was 10 mm spot, 595 nm, 8 J/cm², 6 ms pulse duration.* **(B)** *Immediately post-treatment.* **(C)** *Ten days after pulsed dye laser treatment*

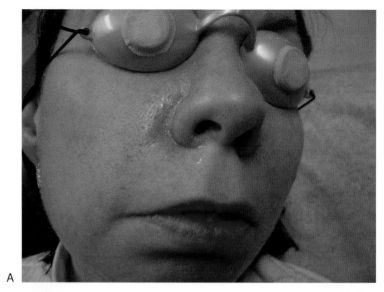

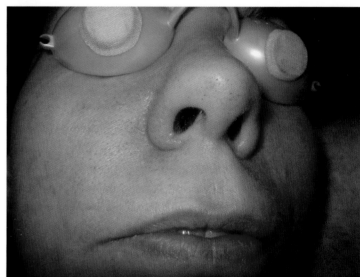

Figure 33.5 (A) *Nasal alae telangiectasias prior to intense pulse light treatment.* **(B)** *Immediate post-treatment erythema and vessel disappearance after intense pulse light treatment*

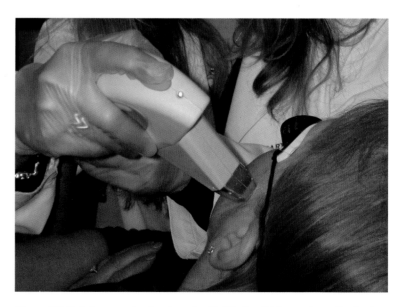

Figure 33.6 *Intense pulse treatment with Starlux (Palomar Inc., Burlington, MA) of facial telangiectasias. The handpiece is in full contact with the skin*

CHAPTER 34 Venous Lakes

Venous lakes are benign vascular lesions that result from dilated venules. They commonly affect the lips, face, and ears.

EPIDEMIOLOGY

Incidence: common

Age: most commonly observed in the elderly

Precipitating factors: may be related to sun exposure

PHYSICAL EXAMINATION

Venous lakes consist of dark blue to violaceous, elevated, soft, and easily compressible lesions.

DIFFERENTIAL DIAGNOSES

Pyogenic granuloma, melanoma.

DERMATOPATHOLOGY

Dilated thin-walled venules in the superficial dermis. Thrombosis may be observed.

EPILUMINESCENCE MICROSCOPY (ELM)

ELM reveals erythematous globules with no pigmentary network. It is helpful in differentiating this vascular lesion from a melanocytic lesion.

COURSE

They usually persist for years and can bleed after trauma.

MANAGEMENT

Venous lakes are frequently treated for cosmetic purposes. Multiple treatment options exist.

- Light treatment
  - Lasers (Figs. 34.1-34.3)
    - Pulsed dye laser (Scleroplus, Candela Corp., Wayland, MA, 585 nm, 0.45 ms, 3–7 mm spot, 4.5–8.5 J/cm^2, DCD 30-40/20, with diascopy).
    - Aura KTP laser (Laserscope, San Jose, CA, 532 nm, 1 mm spot, 10 ms, 14–16 J/cm^2 with diascopy).

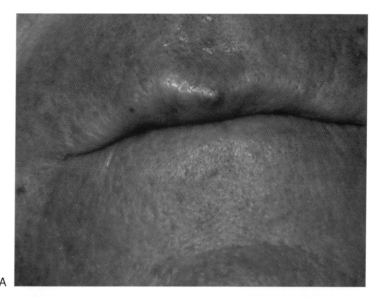

A

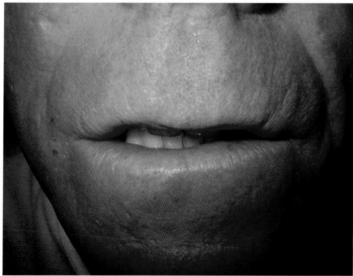

B

Figure 34.1 **(A)** *Venous lake on the upper lip.* **(B)** *Five-month follow-up demonstrating complete resolution of the venous lake after a single treatment with an 800-nm diode laser at energy settings of 45 J/cm2 (one pulse) and 50 J/cm2 (one pulse). A 30 ms pulse duration was utilized*

○ Versapulse HELP-G laser (Coherent Inc., Palo Alto, CA, 532 nm, 4 mm spot, 9.5–12 J/cm², 10–30 ms) has been used successfully in the treatment of venous lakes. Repeat treatments are generally required, spaced 3–6 weeks apart. Treatment endpoint is lesional whitening.

○ Diode laser (LightSheer XC, 800 nm, 30 ms, 40–50 J/cm² with diascopy) can also be effective.

○ Argon laser (0.5–1.0 mm spot, 0.5–1.0 W, continuous beam) and carbon dioxide laser have been successfully employed when alternate therapies fail.

– Intense pulse light (IPL) can also be effective.

• Sclerotherapy: In one study, intralesional injections with 1% polidocanol have been shown to be effective in clearing two venous lakes after two sessions of sclerotherapy. An inconspicuous scar was noted to occur in one patient.

• Electrosurgery, surgical excision, cryotherapy are other alternate treatment options.

PITFALLS

• May require several treatments.

• All therapeutic modalities may produce scar.

BIBLIOGRAPHY

Ah-Weng A, Natarajan S, Velangi S, Langtry JA. Venous lakes of the vermillion lip treated by infrared coagulation. *Br J Oral Maxillofac Surg.* 2004;42(3):251–253.

Jay H, Borek C. Treatment of a venous-lake angioma with intense pulsed light. *Lancet.* 1998;351(9096):112.

2. Kuo HW, Yang CH. Venous lake of the lip treated with a sclerosing agent: report of two cases. *Dermatol Surg.* 2003;29(4):425–428.

3. Majamaa H, Hjerppe M. Treatment of venous-lake angiomas with a carbon dioxide laser. *J Eur Acad Dermatol Venereol.* 2003;17(3):352–353.

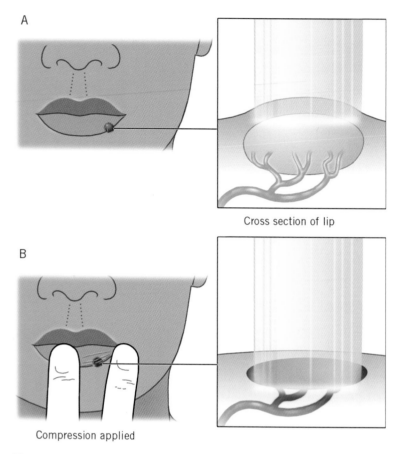

Cross section of lip

Compression applied

Figure 34.2 *Clinical efficacy of pulsed dye laser for a venous lake with compression of the vessels during treatment versus no compression*

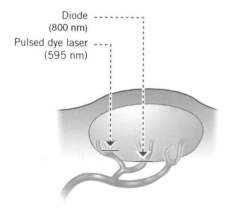

Diode
(800 nm)
Pulsed dye laser
(595 nm)

Laser penetration: pulsed dye vs diode vs long pulsed YAG

Figure 34.3 *Pulsed dye laser does not penetrate deep enough. Compression is needed. Diode laser penetrates deeper and therefore is more effective than PDL*

CHAPTER 35 Warts

Viral warts are caused by human papillomaviruses (HPV). Various types of HPV-induced warts exist including common warts (70% of all warts), palmoplantar warts, plane warts, and genital warts.

EPIDEMIOLOGY

Incidence: common

Age: children and adults

Precipitating factors: skin trauma, immunosuppression (HIV and transplant patients), genetic predisposition (epidermodysplasia verruciformis, EDV)

PATHOGENESIS

HPVs are non-enveloped double-stranded DNA viruses that produce infection and induction of hyperproliferation when the virus enters proliferating basal epithelial cells. Avoidance of host immune surveillence occurs. Exact mechanisms of infection, latency, and reactivation of HPV are unknown.

PHYSICAL EXAMINATION

Warts present as single or multiple hyperkeratotic, exophytic, skin-colored papules, nodules or plaques. They can have finger-like projections (filiform warts) or can be flat-topped (plane warts). Black punctate dots representing thrombosed capillaries are frequently observed. They most frequently present on fingers, dorsal hands, plantar surfaces, and pressure areas.

DIFFERENTIAL DIAGNOSES

Hypertrophic actinic keratosis, seborrheic keratosis, squamous cell carcinoma, and acral amelanotic melanoma. Plantar warts can also be mistaken for corns or calluses.

DERMATOPATHOLOGY

The epidermis features hyperkeratosis, acanthosis, papillomatosis, with tiers of parakeratosis, valleys of hypergranulosis and koilocytosis. The dermis features dilated capillary loops and hemorrhage.

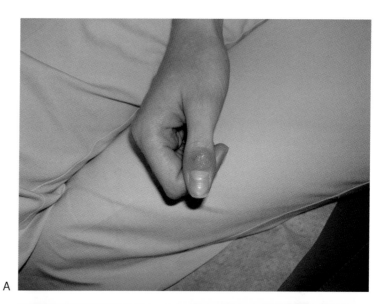

A

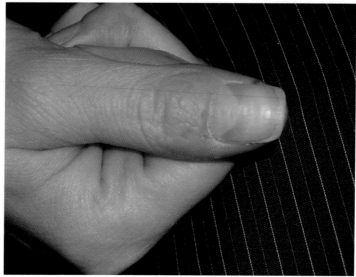

B

Figure 35.1 **(A)** *Verruca vulgaris on the left thumb immediately post-treatment with pulsed dye laser, 590 nm wavelength, 7 mm spot size, 10 J/cm², with pulse stacking.* **(B)** *Five-month follow-up with complete resolution of the wart after single pulsed dye laser treatment.*

COURSE

They generally resolve spontaneously in immunocompetent patients, but this may take years. They tend to persist and resist treatment in immunosuppressed patients. Autoinoculation by scratching may occur.

MANAGEMENT

There is no current specific antiviral therapy for HPV. Treatment options are multiple and they either induce local physical destruction of the warts or stimulate the immune response against HPV infection. Squamous cell carcinoma can arise from some lesions, i.e., condylomas and EDV, and require continuous monitoring. Histological evaluation should be considered for warts that are unresponsive to multiple treatment modalities to rule out malignant change.

■ Topical Treatment

Patients should be educated as to the viral, infectious, and recurrent nature of HPV despite therapeutic intervention. Patients must also be informed of the need for repetitive treatments for all treatment modalities employed. Multiple effective topical treatments exist.

- Localized tissue destruction: salicylic acid, 5% cantharone, trichloracetic acid, 0.5% podophyllotoxin, and tretinoin are commonly employed daily. Localized wart occlusion with duct tape has demonstrated efficacy. Surrounding normal tissue may demonstrate temporary maceration during treatment.

- Viral cell division alteration: intralesional bleomycin (0.4 mg/mL) in normal preserved saline; 5-fluorouracil cream.

- Immune modulation: imiquimod commonly applied twice weekly.

■ Surgical Treatment

Lasers (Table 35.1)
- Pulsed dye laser (PDL) (Figs. 35.1–35.3)
  - PDL is the most commonly employed laser. It may induce a therapeutic response by vascular absorption of laser light producing thermal necrosis of wart

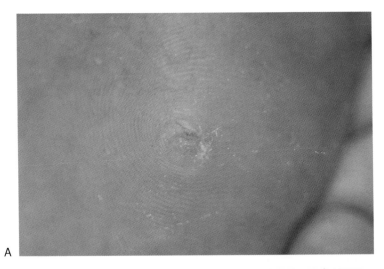

A

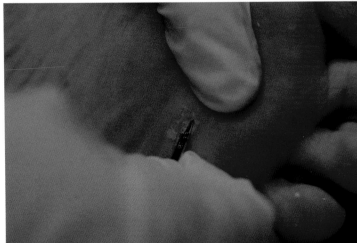

B

Figure 35.2 (A) *Plantar verruca with characteristic thrombosed capillaries.* **(B)** *Paring of wart with #15 blade prior to pulsed dye therapy*

TABLE 35.1 ■ Laser Treatment of Warts

	PDL	CO$_2$
Efficacy	Variable	Effective
Average number of sessions	Two to five	One to three
Anesthesia needed	No	Variable
Scarring risk	Very low	Yes
Dyschromia risk	Low	Moderate
Infection risk	Slight	Slight
Pain	Minimal to moderate	Minimal to high

tissue. Clinical improvement is variable. PDL is generally utilized after failure of first-line therapies.

– PDL protocol

  ○ Protective laser masks, gloves, and gowns as well as use of a smoke evacuator are recommended to avoid transmission of the wart virus.

  ○ The hyperkeratotic portion of the wart should be pared prior to treatment. Bleeding is to be avoided, as this will minimize laser light absorption by the wart.

  ○ High fluences (585–590 nm, 8–15 J/cm^2) and multiple pulses (three to ten per site) are required for effective treatment. Diascopy with pulses should be considered. Laser pulses should be delivered as close to 1 Hz as possible to obtain cumulative heating of the wart.

  ○ Treat until lesional purpura is apparent.

  ○ Repetitive treatments spaced 3 weeks apart are generally optimal. Longer intervals between treatment sessions may facilitate wart regrowth and shorter intervals may prevent complete healing.

- Carbon dioxide laser (CO$_2$)

  – CO$_2$ laser treatment is generally reserved for recalcitrant, widespread, painful, or hyperkeratotic warts.

  – Advantages: high success rate usually after one or two sessions, no bleeding

  – Disadvantages: unknown hazard of HPV in laser plume, risks of dyschromia, recurrence and infection; prolonged healing time of weeks to months; residual scarring that can be painful; risk of permanent nail dystrophy with periungual treatment.

  – CO$_2$ protocol

    • Protective laser masks, gloves, and gowns as well as use of a smoke evacuator are recommended to avoid transmission of the wart virus.

    • Draw a 1.0 cm margin around the wart.

    • Administer intralesional infiltrative anesthesia or a digital block (1% lidocaine with or without 1:100,000 epinephrine).

    • Vaporize the wart and a 1.0 cm margin until the surface is charred (Ultrapulse CW defocused, 15–20 W; Sharplan superpulsed mode, 1–2 mm spot, 5–15 W).

    • Remove the char by rubbing a saline-soaked gauze pad. Allow the area to dry.

    • Revaporize the wart as above with char removal between passes until tissue separation occurs and normal tissue is observed.

Non-laser surgical modalities

- Cryotherapy with liquid nitrogen is the most commonly employed surgical treatment modality employed. Treatment benefit is dependent on ice crystal-induced cell death.

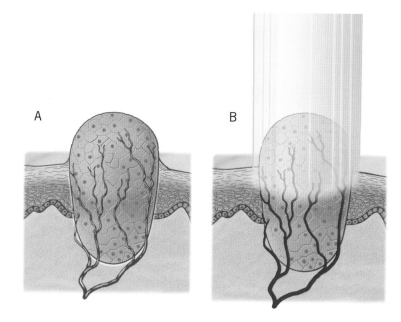

Figure 35.3 *Mechanism of action of pulsed dye laser treatment of verruca. The verruca is characterized by a rich vascular supply.* **(A)** *The pulsed dye laser selectively targets the vascular component of the verruca.* **(B)** *The laser light is selectively absorbed by the blood leading to coagulation of the vessels*

- Treatment may be delivered via a cryosurgical unit (Brymill Cryogenic Systems, Ellington, CT) or via a cotton-tipped applicator, dipstick, or forceps.

- A single or double 5–15 s freeze–thaw cycle may be delivered depending on the treatment site and lesion thickness. Thicker lesions and plantar lesions require more aggressive treatment. Multiple treatment sessions are generally required.

- Treatment may induce temporary or permanent hyperpigmentation and hypopigmentation, blistering and scar formation.

• Electrodessication and curettage and surgical excision have also been employed with variable response.

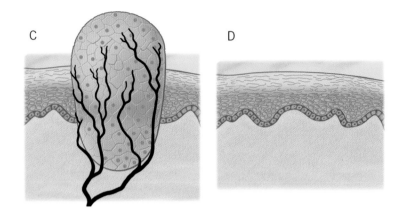

Figure 35.3 (*continued*) (**C**) *and resolution of the wart* (**D**).

PITFALLS TO AVOID

• Be very aware of the depth of destruction with CO_2 laser. As you go below the papillary dermis, the risk of scarring and dyschromia increases.

• Patients must be aware that scar formation is likely and may be painful. Painful scarring is most common on pressure-bearing areas.

• Recurrences most frequently occur at the wound edge. A 1.0-cm margin minimizes this risk.

BIBLIOGRAPHY

Kopera D. Verrucae vulgaris: flashlamp-pumped pulsed dye laser treatment in 134 patients. *Int J Dermatol.* 2003;42(11):905–908.

Kuflik EG. Specifc indications for cryosurgery of the nail unit. Myxoid cyts and periungual verucae. *J Dermatol Surg Oncol* 1986;18:702–706.

Ozluer SM, Chuen BY, Barlow RJ, Markey AC. Hypertrophic scar formation following carbon dioxide laser ablation of plantar warts in cyclosporin-treated patients. *Br J Dermatol.* 2001;145(6):1005–1007.

Serour F, Somekh E. Successful treatment of recalcitrant warts in pediatric patients with carbon dioxide laser. *Eur J Pediatr Surg.* 2003;13(4):219–223.

Shumer SM, O'Keefe EJ. Bleomycin in the treatment of recalcitrant warts. *J Am Acad Dermatol.* 1983;9:91.

SECTION
SEVEN

Benign Growths

CHAPTER 36 Angiofibroma

Angiofibroma is a descriptive term for multiple different lesions with the same histopathology including fibrous papules, pearly penile papules, adenoma sebaceum, periungual fibromas, and Koenen's tumor. This chapter will focus on facial angiofibroma. Generally, an angiofibroma presents as a 1–5 mm skin-colored to erythematous dome-shaped papule on the face. When it presents as multiple lesions on the face, it can be associated with tuberous sclerosis or multiple endocrine neoplasia type I (MEN I).

EPIDEMIOLOGY

Incidence: common

Age: dependent on etiology, may present in children or adults

Race: none

Sex: equal

Precipitating factors: Tuberous sclerosis, MEN I

PATHOGENESIS

Unknown.

PATHOLOGY

A symmetric, well-circumscribed papule with a normal epidermis. The papillary and reticular dermis feature a proliferation of varying degrees of normal blood vessels within a fibrotic stroma. The collagen fibers are arranged perpendicularly to the epidermis and concentrically around the vessels and hair follicles. Stellate-shaped fibroblasts may be seen.

PHYSICAL LESIONS

Firm skin-colored to erythematous papules (1–5 mm) on the nose, chin, and cheeks arranged bilaterally.

DIFFERENTIAL DIAGNOSIS

Acne, rosacea.

LABORATORY EXAMINATION

In the setting of multiple angiofibromas, tuberous sclerosis and MEN I must be investigated. This is best performed by referral to pediatric specialists.

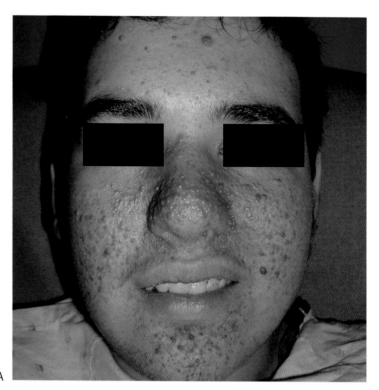

A

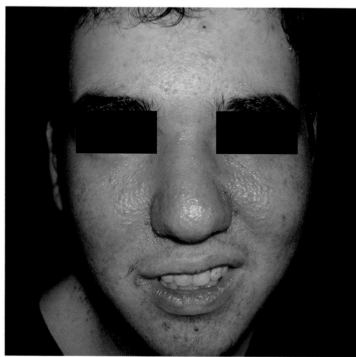

B

Figure 36.1 (A) *Multiple angiofibromas on a 16-year-old male with tuberous sclerosis.* **(B)** *Improvement 2 months after single treatment with CO_2 laser.*

COURSE

Multiple facial angiofibromas typically present in childhood and are associated with tuberous sclerosis.

KEY CONSULTATIVE QUESTIONS

- Number of lesions
- Any family history of similar lesions
- Family history of cancers
- Any central nervous system disorders
- Evaluate for tuberous sclerosis and MEN I in the appropriate clinical setting, such as multiple angiofibromas

MANAGEMENT

There is no medical indication to treat angiofibromas. Their cosmetic appearance, however, may be striking and understandably concerning to some individuals. There are multiple therapeutic modalities available for treatment. None is ideal.

■ Treatment

Dermabrasion
- Best for multiple lesions
- Recurrence is common

Shave excision
- Mark the lesion with a surgical pen prior to applying local anesthesia as the lesion may blanch after the anesthetic is injected.
- Shave off the lesion flush to the surrounding skin with a scalpel or blade.
- Alternatively, punch excision, elliptical excision, or electrodessication can be employed.
- Recurrence is common.

Pulsed dye laser (PDL)
- Reduces the erythematous color of angiofibromas, rendering lesions less cosmetically apparent.
- Especially helpful to treat multiple lesions early. Early treatment may impair and minimize the growth.
- Can be followed by "maintenance" treatments to minimize recurrent erythema.

Continuous wave CO_2 laser (Fig. 36.1)
- In the setting of multiple facial angiofibromas, CO_2 lasers produced long-term improvement in 77% of 13 patients studied. Adverse effects included persistent hypertrophic scarring in three of 13 patients treated. Significant relapse was seen in one patient.
- Combination therapy with PDL showed improvement in three of four patients treated.

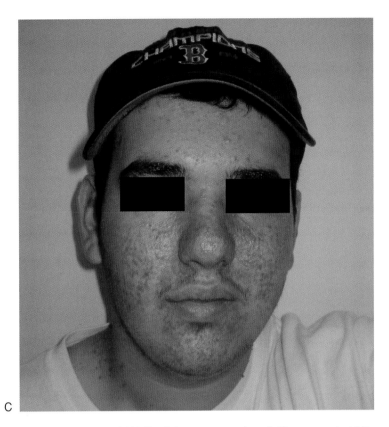

C

Figure 36.1 (*continued*) (C) *Partial recurrence of angiofibromas noted 13 months after treatment*

• In a retrospective study of 10 patients treated with CO_2 laser, recurrence was more common than resolution. Improvement seen at 6 months was usually not sustained to 24 months. Nonetheless, despite the high rate of recurrence, patient satisfaction with the results was good, even in those with recurrent lesions.

PITFALLS TO AVOID/COMPLICATIONS/ MANAGEMENT/OUTCOME EXPECTATIONS

• There are several methods to improve angiofibromas. None is completely optimal.

• Treatment of angiofibromas may be frustrating with high rates of recurrence.

• It is important to educate the patient that each of the procedures has a risk of recurrence after treatment.

• PDL may be most effective in that it reduces the erythematous appearance of the lesions and thus renders them less clinically apparent. Side effects are uncommon.

• Ablative therapies carry a risk of scarring and have a significant risk of recurrence.

• The benefits of ablative therapy must be considered against the likelihood of recurrence and the possibility of such adverse side effects as postprocedure morbidity, the risk of scarring, and the risk of pigmentary changes.

• The side effects of treatment may outweigh its benefits in some cases.

• Dermabrasion can produce pigmentary changes and scarring.

BIBLIOGRAPHY

Bittencourt RC, Huilgol SC, Seed PT, Calonje E, Markey AC, Barlow RJ. Treatment of angiofibromas with a scanning carbon dioxide laser: a clinicopathologic study with long-term follow-up. *J Am Acad Dermatol*. 2001;45(5): 731–735.

Boixeda P, Sanchez-Miralles E, Azana JM, Arrazola JM, Moreno R, Ledo A. CO_2, argon, and pulsed dye laser treatment of angiofibromas. *J Dermatol Surg Oncol*. 1994;20(12):808–812.

Kaufman AJ, Grekin RC, Geisse JK, Frieden IJ. Treatment of adenoma sebaceum with the copper vapor laser. *J Am Acad Dermatol*. 1995;33(5, pt 1):770–774.

Papadavid E, Markey A, Bellaney G, Walker NP. Carbon dioxide and pulsed dye laser treatment of angiofibromas in 29 patients with tuberous sclerosis. *Br J Dermatol*. 2002;147(2):337–342.

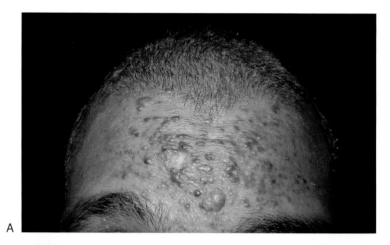

A

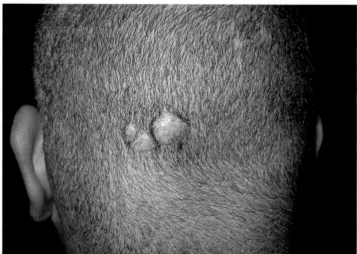

B

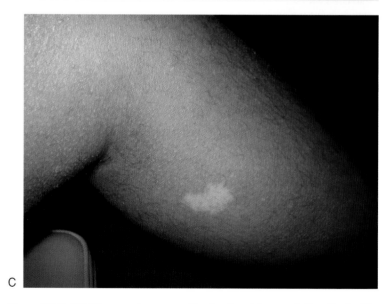

C

Figure 36.2 (A) *Fibrous plaques on the forehead in an adult patient with tuberous sclerosis.* **(B)** *Fibrous plaques on the scalp.* **(C)** *Ash leaf macule on the leg of the same patient*

| **CHAPTER 37** | Becker's Nevus |

Becker's nevus is a sharply demarcated tan to brown macule or a slightly raised verrucous plaque that most commonly appears on the chest, upper back, and shoulders. It typically presents unilaterally and features overlying hypertrichosis. It is a benign smooth muscle hamartoma.

EPIDEMIOLOGY

Incidence: 0.5% of males

Age: childhood to teenage years; rarely congenital

Race: all races

Sex: males > females (6:1)

Precipitating factors: none

PATHOGENESIS

Unclear.

PATHOLOGY

There is papillomatosis, hyperkeratosis, acanthosis, and basal layer hyperpigmentation. A smooth muscle hamartoma is frequently present in the dermis. There is an increase in the melanin content of keratinocytes with little or no change in the number of melanocytes.

PHYSICAL LESIONS

They appear most often on the upper trunk as well-demarcated unilateral tan to light brown macules or slightly elevated verrucous plaques with geographic borders and hypertrichosis.

DIFFERENTIAL DIAGNOSIS

Congenital nevus, café au lait macule, and epidermal nevus.

LABORATORY EXAMINATION

None.

COURSE

It presents in childhood as a unilateral tan macule. Over time, it may develop into a plaque and display a darker brown hue. Hair growth, which becomes darker and coarser

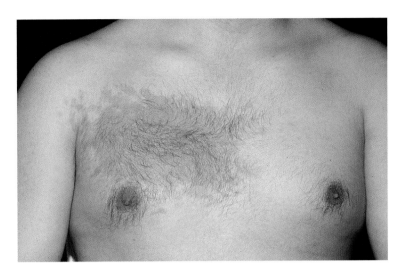

Figure 37.1 *Becker's nevus. A slightly raised light-tan plaque with sharply defined and highly irregular border and hypertrichosis on the chest of a 35-year-old male patient. Klaus W, Richard J, Dick S, eds. Fitzpatrick's Color Atlas & Synopsis of Clinical Dermatology. 5 ed. McGraw-Hill, Inc.; 2005*

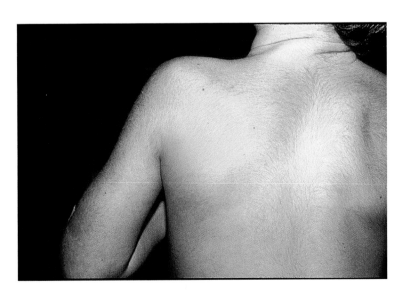

Figure 37.2 *Becker's nevus. Large brown plaque that becomes noticeable at puberty with increased pigment followed by hair growth. From Kay K, Jen R, Richard J, Howard B, Alexander S, eds. Color Atlas & Synopsis of Pediatric Dermatology. McGraw-Hill, Inc.; 2002*

over time, follows pigmentary changes. There can also be slow extension of these lesions.

KEY CONSULTATIVE QUESTIONS

Is the pigment of the lesion or its excess hair growth more cosmetically troubling?

MANAGEMENT

There is no medical indication to treat Becker's nevus. The cosmetic appearance, however, may displease some individuals—most often females who note its hypertrichosis. Treatment options are multiple, but not always effective including camouflage makeup, electrolysis, waxing, laser therapy, and surgical excision. Surgical excision is impractical for larger lesions. Laser therapies can be tailored for hair removal or pigment resolution (Fig. 37.4).

■ Laser Treatment

- A test site is recommended before initiating any laser therapy to assess for efficacy and side effects.
- Pigment: Q-switched ruby (694 nm, 6.5 mm spot, 3.0–4.5 J/cm^2), Q-switched Nd:YAG (532 nm, 3 mm spot, 1.0–1.5 J/cm^2 or 1064 nm, 3 mm spot, 4.0–5.0 J/cm^2), and Q-switched alexandrite (755 nm, 3 mm spot, 2.5–3.5 J/cm^2) lasers have been reported effective in treating the pigmentation of a Becker's nevus (Fig. 37.3).
  - In general, response is poor. Multiple treatments are usually required for efficacy.
  - There is a high rate of repigmentation. This is likely due to deep hair follicle melanocytes.
- Hair removal: long-pulsed alexandrite (10–40 J/cm^2, pulse duration 2–20 ms) and ruby (30–60 J/cm^2, pulse duration 40–100 ms) and pulsed diode (804 nm, 35–45 J/cm^2, pulse duration 5–30 ms) lasers can produce hair reduction but are less effective with long-term pigment lightening.
- Ablative therapy: Erbium: YAG laser (2940 nm) was more effective than long-pulsed Nd:YAG laser (1064 nm) in side by side comparison treatment of a Becker's nevus on a young male. Both therapies produced erythema that cleared within 15 days. The lesion showed clinical and histological clearance 2 years after treatment.
  - It is important to note that there is a high risk of texture change associated with ablative therapy.
- Intense pulsed light has demonstrated mixed success in improving pigmentation and hair loss.

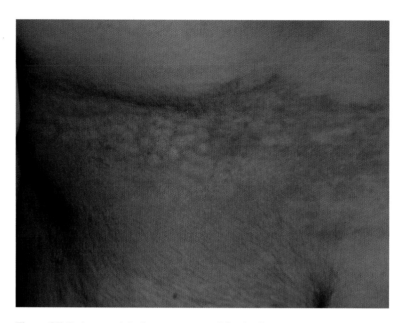

Figure 37.3 *Incomplete improvement of Becker's nevus on upper buttock after three treatments with Q-switched ruby laser*

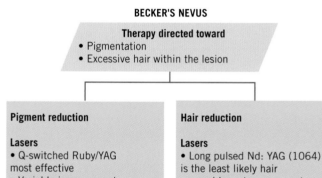

BECKER'S NEVUS

Therapy directed toward
- Pigmentation
- Excessive hair within the lesion

Pigment reduction

Lasers
- Q-switched Ruby/YAG most effective
- Variable improvement
- Risk uneven pigment reduction creating poor cosmetic result
- Ablative lasers have higher risk of side effects

Surgical
- Serial excision should only be pursued in lesions of limited size

Hair reduction

Lasers
- Long pulsed Nd: YAG (1064) is the least likely hair removal laser to cause post inflammatory changes. Long–pulsed ruby, alexandrite and diode lasers are more likely to cause hypopigmentation in a Becker's nevus

- Permanent hair reduction is an effective safe option for improving a Becker's nevus. A long pulsed Nd: YAG laser should be used.
- Laser reduction of the pigmented component is less effective and may produce worse cosmetic appearance
- Any improvement with lasers and pigment reduction may be temporary with future recurrence

Figure 37.4 *Becker's nevus treatment diagram*

PITFALLS TO AVOID/COMPLICATIONS/ MANAGEMENT/OUTCOME EXPECTATIONS

- Treatment of Becker's nevus is often ineffective and recurrences are common.
- Laser hair removal can improve overlying hypertrichosis.
- Post-inflammatory hypo and hyperpigmentation are a risk.
- Patients with dark skin phototypes (types IV and V) should be treated cautiously and at lower fluences, as their threshold response occurs at lower energies.
- Laser treatment should be limited to nontanned individuals to avoid temporary spotty hypopigmentation.
- Surgical excision is dependent on the size and location of a lesion and is usually not a good option.

BIBLIOGRAPHY

Kopera D, Hohenleutner U, Landthaler M. Quality-switched ruby laser treatment of solar lentigines and Becker's nevus: a histopathological and immunohistochemical study. *Dermatology.* 1997;194(4):338–343.

Nanni CA, Alster TS. Treatment of a Becker's nevus using a 694-nm long-pulsed ruby laser. *Dermatol Surg.* 1998; 24(9):1032–1034.

Trelles MA, Allones I, Velez M, Moreno-Arias. Becker's nevus: Erbium:YAG versus Q-switched neodymium:YAG. *Lasers Surg Med.* 2004;34(4):295–297.

Tse Y, Levine VJ, McClain SA, Ashinoff R. The removal of cutaneous pigmented lesions with the Q-switched ruby laser and the Q-switched neodymium: yttrium-aluminum-garnet laser. A comparative study. *J Dermatol Surg Oncol.* 1994;20(12):795–800.

CHAPTER 38 Epidermal Inclusion Cyst

The epidermal inclusion cyst (EIC), also known as seba-ceous cyst and epidermoid cyst, is the most common cyst of the skin. It ranges in size from a few millimeters to a few centimeters and originates from the follicular infundibulum. Its contents are a cheesy, malodorous mix-ture of degraded lipid and keratin. It often ruptures, with associated pain and inflammation, requiring surgical removal.

EPIDEMIOLOGY

Incidence: very common

Age: young adults to middle-aged adults

Race: none

Sex: equal

Precipitating factors: develop spontaneously on glabrous skin

PATHOGENESIS

There may be an association with trauma to the hair follicle.

PATHOLOGY

Within the dermis or subcutaneous fat, there is a well-demarcated cyst containing laminated keratin debris. The cyst wall is a true epidermis featuring a granular cell layer. In ruptured cysts, there is a foreign body granulo-matous reaction with multinucleated giant cells.

PHYSICAL LESIONS

EICs are smooth, round, firm, mobile skin-colored cysts with a central pore (Fig. 38.1). They range in size from a few millimeters to a few centimeters. They typically present on hair-bearing skin, such as the upper trunk, neck, face, and scalp, but can present on the palms and soles follow-ing injury to the epithelium. After rupture, these cysts develop a strong inflammatory reaction as a result of the spillage of cyst contents into the dermis. In this setting, the cysts become red, inflamed, tender, and enlarged.

DIFFERENTIAL DIAGNOSIS

Pilar cysts (especially on the scalp), dermoid cysts, branchial cleft cysts, nodular fibromas, and dermal tumors may cause confusion with EICs. Of these lesions, only EICs feature central pores.

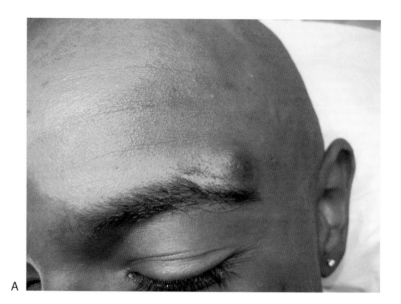

A

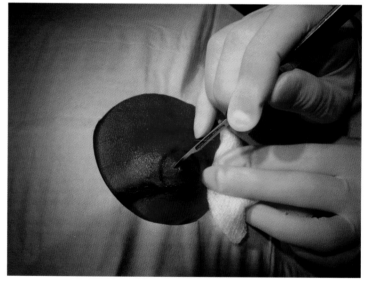

B

Figure 38.1 (A) *Epidermal inclusion cyst on left lateral supraorbital area.* **(B)** *Elliptical excision around epidermal inclusion cyst punctum.*

LABORATORY EXAMINATION

In the event of uncertainty of diagnosis, a biopsy can be performed to rule out neoplasm.

COURSE

They present from young adulthood to middle age. It is not unusual for these cysts to become inflamed and cause pain and discomfort to the patient.

KEY CONSULTATIVE QUESTIONS

- Is the lesion recurrently inflamed and painful?
- Would the patient prefer a surgical scar rather than keeping the cyst?

MANAGEMENT

There is no medical indication to treat EICs if they are not symptomatic. The cosmetic appearance, however, may displease some individuals. In these instances, surgical excision is the treatment of choice. Ruptured EICs can produce recurrent pain and discomfort for some patients. For these lesions, the mainstays of therapy include intralesional steroid injection and surgical excision.

TREATMENT

Surgical excision is the treatment of choice for EICs.

- Noninflamed EICs
  - Typically, a small elliptical-shaped excision or a small punch biopsy is performed over the cyst around the central pore (Figs. 38.1-38.2).
  - The cyst sac is then identified.
  - Careful dissection and removal of the sac are performed.
  - It is important to note that short of full removal of the entire sac wall, there is a likelihood of recurrence.
- Inflamed EICs
  - In the event of an inflamed, infected, or newly ruptured cyst, surgical removal should await a decrease in the surrounding inflammation.
  - Inflamed EICs are more difficult to excise as they become more firmly adherent to the surrounding dermal structures.
  - Drainage of contents is important prior to treating larger inflamed cysts.
  - Intralesional corticosteroids, warm compresses, and antibiotics (in the event of infection) can aid in decreasing inflammation.
  - When the inflammation has subsided, surgical excision can proceed.

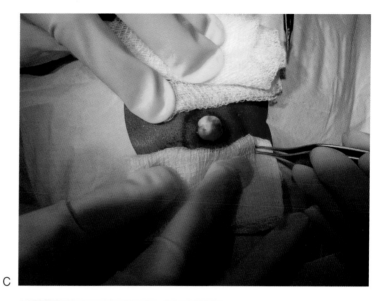

C

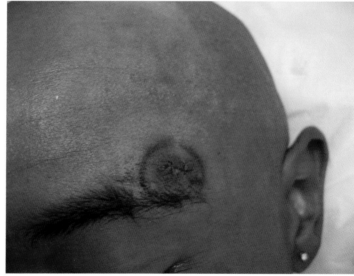

D

Figure 38.1 *(continued)* **(C)** *Cyst sac being "delivered" from excision site.* **(D)** *Postprocedure sutures at site of excision*

PITFALLS TO AVOID/COMPLICATIONS/ MANAGEMENT/OUTCOME EXPECTATIONS

- It is important to discuss with the patient that while surgical excision of an EIC is a routine surgical procedure, the scar left from the surgery may be more cosmetically disturbing than the EIC itself.

- However, recurrently inflamed EICs should be excised to provide relief to the patient.

BIBLIOGRAPHY

Krull EA. Surgical gems: The "little" curet. *J Dermatol Surg Oncol.* 1978;4:656–57.

McGavran MH, Binnington B. Keratinous cysts of the skin. Identification and differentiation of pilar cysts from epidermal cysts. *Arch Dermatol.* 1966;94(4):499–508.

Wade CL, Haley JC, Hood AF. The utility of submitting epidermoid cysts for histologic examination. *Int J Dermatol.* 2000;39:314–315.

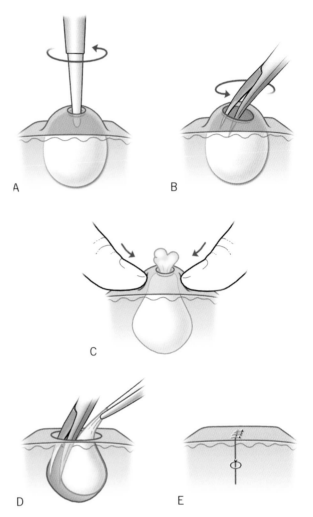

Figure 38.2 (A) *Removal of cyst with punch biopsy,* **(B)** *dissection of cyst from surrounding skin,* **(C,D)** *extrusion of cyst sac, and* **(E)** *suture closure*

CHAPTER 39 Epidermal Nevus

Epidermal nevus (EN) is a benign hamartomatous growth. It presents as a group of verrucous, closely grouped, skin-colored to brown papules often in a linear arrangement following the lines of Blaschko (Fig. 39.1). It is most frequently congenital. There are several variations of EN including localized nevus unius lateris, systematized EN, EN syndrome, and ILVEN (Figs. 39.1-39.2).

EPIDEMIOLOGY

Incidence: 0.1% of live births

Age: usually congenital but may arise in childhood or at puberty

Race: none

Sex: none

Precipitating factors: usually sporadic

PATHOGENESIS

EN is created by overproduction of keratinocytes from undifferentiated basal keratinocytes.

PATHOLOGY

Papillomatosis, acanthosis, epidermal hyperplasia, and hyperkeratosis along with elongated rete ridges are present. In some lesions, epidermolytic hyperkeratosis may be present. If this finding is made in the setting of multiple epidermal nevi, genetic counseling should be offered in order to educate patients as to the risk of epidermolytic hyperkeratosis in offspring.

PHYSICAL LESIONS

It appears as multiple, well-defined, closely grouped linear, yellow, pink or brown verrucous papules on any site of the body. EN often follows the lines of Blaschko on the trunk and travels longitudinally on the extremities. Size can vary from a few millimeters to multiple centimeters.

DIFFERENTIAL DIAGNOSIS

Nevus sebaceous, seborrheic keratosis, verruca vulgaris, lichen striatus, melanocytic nevus.

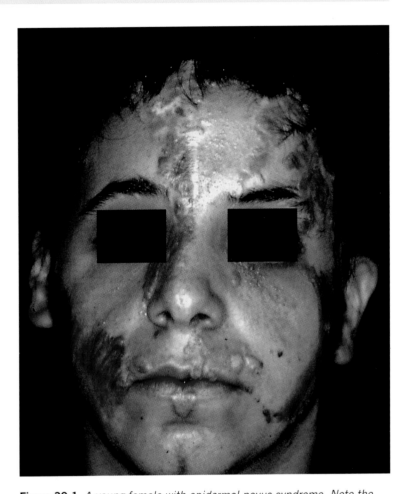

Figure 39.1 *A young female with epidermal nevus syndrome. Note the extensive nature of these lesions even after several surgical procedures*

LABORATORY EXAMINATION

Biopsy may be indicated to distinguish from nevus sebaceous or lichen striatus. Rarely, basal cell and squamous cell carcinoma may arise in EN.

COURSE

They present at birth or childhood as macules intially. Eighty percent of ENs appear within the first year of life. At puberty, they tend to enlarge, darken and become more verrucous.

KEY CONSULTATIVE QUESTIONS

- Age of onset
- CNS difficulties
- Skeletal defects
- Pruritus
- Family history

MANAGEMENT

In patients with multiple ENs, a thorough examination for systemic abnormalities with pediatric specialists is indicated. There is no medical indication to treat EN. The cosmetic appearance, however, may displease some individuals or parents of children with disfiguring growths. There are multiple treatment modalities for EN including surgery, dermabrasion, topical therapy, and laser therapy (Fig. 39.4). Patients should be counseled that results are variable and often unsatisfying. The physician needs to consider whether treatment will produce a superior outcome to nonintervention. The most aggressive forms of therapy, laser and surgical excision, carry a high risk of scar. Laser ablation also risks pigmentary alteration. Finally, all treatments may fail to completely remove ENs.

SURGERY

- Full-thickness surgical excision of EN is curative
  - Surgery leaves a scar
    ○ Cosmesis is variable
    ○ Possibility of hypertrophic or keloidal scarring
  - Surgical outcome is best in smaller lesions
  - Excision may be difficult for young children to tolerate
- Shave biopsies and curettage may be too superficial
  - Recurrences are frequent

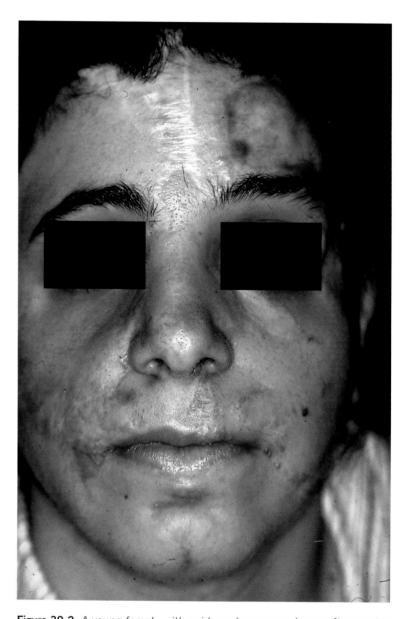

Figure 39.2 *A young female with epidermal nevus syndrome after greater than 30 subsequent surgical procedures including flaps and skin grafts (photographs courtesy of Richard Bennett, Muba Taher, and Mathew Avram)*

CRYOTHERAPY/ELECTROCAUTERY

Cryotherapy, electrocautery, and dermabrasion have limited efficacy, a high rate of recurrence, and risk of pigmentary alteration and scarring.

TOPICAL TREATMENTS

The following topical therapies have, at best, limited success: corticosteroids, tretinoin, anthralin, 5-fluorouracil, podophyllin, calcipotriol, and 5% 5-fluorouracil and 0.1% tretinoin in combination.

LASER TREATMENT

Laser therapy can be effective in treating EN. Prior to treatment, a test site should be performed.

* CO_2 laser (Fig. 39.5)
  – CO_2 laser can vaporize EN with good control of the depth of treatment.
  – Does not treat deeper than the papillary dermis.
  – One study examined the efficacy of short-pulsed CO_2 laser treatment of three young women with multiple ENs. Utilizing a pulse energy of 500 mJ, a 3 mm spot size, and 7 W of power, all but one of the ENs cleared without recurrence. The follow-up time was 10–13 months.
* Erbium:YAG laser
  – Erbium:YAG is also effective, particularly for more superficial lesions. Do not treat deeper than the papillary dermis.
  – In one study, six patients with superficial ENs were treated with an energy of 0.4–0.45 J/cm^2, a 2 mm spot size with four passes. All patients experienced clearance with a follow-up of 6–60 months.
  – Another study showed a 25% recurrence rate within 1 year of treatment with an erbium:YAG laser at two settings:
    ○ Variably pulsed erbium:YAG: 5 mm handpiece, 7.0–7.5 J/cm^2 pulse energy, 500 μs pulse duration.
    ○ Dual-mode erbium:YAG laser: 2 mm handpiece, 6.3 J/cm^2 pulse energy, 350 μs pulse duration.
* Combined CO_2 laser/erbium:YAG laser

For combined CO_2 and erbium:YAG laser, there is a narrow margin between successful treatment and harmful side effects such as scarring and post-inflammatory hyperpigmentation. Recurrences are not uncommon.

* Intense pulsed light

Intense pulsed light was reported as minimally effective for treatment of EN with an average clearance of less than 25%. There were two to four treatments at 4- and 8 week intervals.

* Q-switched lasers

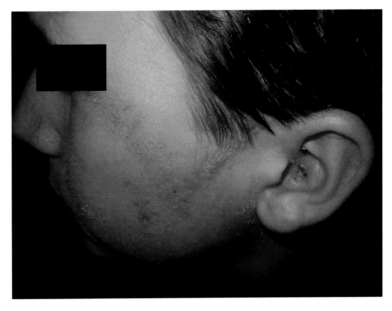

Figure 39.3 *An extensive epidermal nevus on the left face and left ear*

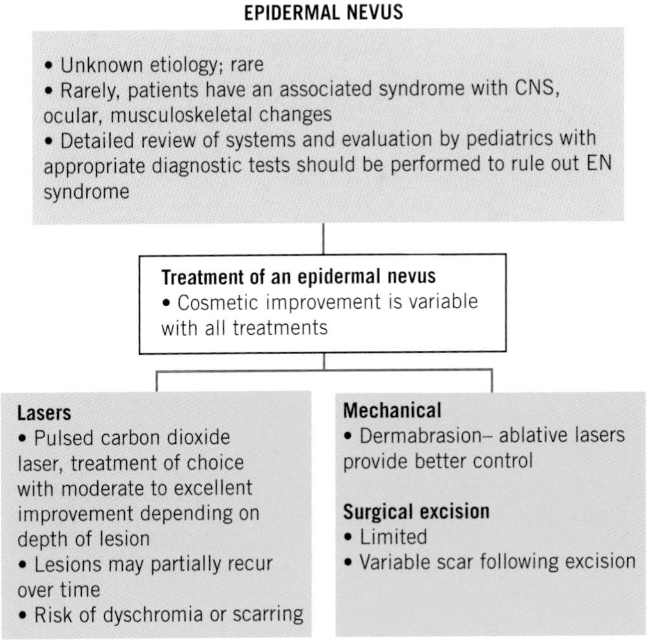

EPIDERMAL NEVUS

* Unknown etiology; rare
* Rarely, patients have an associated syndrome with CNS, ocular, musculoskeletal changes
* Detailed review of systems and evaluation by pediatrics with appropriate diagnostic tests should be performed to rule out EN syndrome

Treatment of an epidermal nevus
* Cosmetic improvement is variable with all treatments

Lasers
* Pulsed carbon dioxide laser, treatment of choice with moderate to excellent improvement depending on depth of lesion
* Lesions may partially recur over time
* Risk of dyschromia or scarring

Mechanical
* Dermabrasion– ablative lasers provide better control

Surgical excision
* Limited
* Variable scar following excision

Figure 39.4 *Epidermal nevus treatment diagram*

Q-switched alexandrite (755 nm) and frequency-doubled Q-switched Nd:YAG (532 nm) lasers are both effective for thin ENs.

PITFALLS TO AVOID/COMPLICATIONS/MANAGEMENT/OUTCOME EXPECTATIONS

- EN is a benign lesion that does not require treatment.
- It is important to inform patients that treatment may only be partially successful.
- Surgical excision may produce scarring.
- There is always the risk that treatment will produce an inferior result to nonintervention. Adverse side effects as described above must be explained in detail to patients.

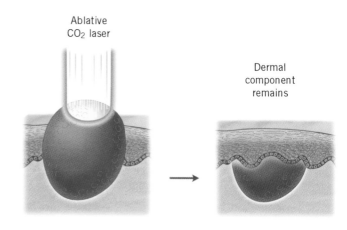

Figure 39.5 *Effect of ablative CO2 laser on removing an epidermal nevus. With the dermal component remaining, there is a risk of recurrence.*

BIBLIOGRAPHY

Boyce S, Alster TS. CO$_2$ laser treatment of epidermal nevi: long-term success. *Dermatol Surg.* 2002;28(7):611–614.

Pearson IC, Harland CC. Epidermal naevi treated with pulsed erbium:YAG laser. *Clin Exp Dermatol.* 2004;29(5): 494–496.

Herman AR, Scott RA. Systematized epidermal nevus treated with isotretinoin. *J Drugs Dermatol.* 2002;1(2): 195–196.

Kim JJ, Chang MW, Schwayder T. Topical tretinoin and 5-fluorouracil in the treatment of linear verrucous epidermal nevus. *J Am Acad Dermatol.* 2000;43(1, pt 1):129–132.

Lee BJ, Mancini AJ, Renucci J, Paller AS, Bauer BS. Full-thickness surgical excision for the treatment of inflammatory linear verrucous epidermal nevus. *Ann Plast Surg.* 2001;47(3):285–292.

Mitsuhashi Y, Katagiri Y, Kondo S. Treatment of inflammatory linear verrucous epidermal naevus with topical vitamin D3. *Br J Dermatol.* 1997;136(1):134–135.

Moreno Arias GA, Ferrando J. Intense pulsed light for melanocytic lesions. *Dermatol Surg.* 2001;27(4):397–400.

Park JH, Hwang ES, Kim SN, Kye YC. Er:YAG laser treatment of verrucous epidermal nevi. *Dermatol Surg.* 2004;30(3):378–381.

Zvulunov A, Grunwald MH, Halvy S. Topical calcipotriol for treatment of inflammatory linear verrucous epidermal nevus. *Arch Dermatol.* 1997;133(5):567–568.

CHAPTER 40 | Lipoma

Lipoma is a benign tumor of mature fat. It presents as a soft subcutaneous flesh-colored tumor that freely moves against overlying skin. Most often, it presents as a solitary lesion on the trunk, neck, and proximal extremities (Fig. 40.1). Infrequently, individuals may present with multiple lipomas, rarely as a part of an inherited syndrome.

EPIDEMIOLOGY

Incidence: very common

Age: can present at any age but most commonly in the fourth decade

Race: none

Sex: equal

Precipitating factors: most frequently, there is no precipitating factor. Multiple lipomas can be associated with syndromes such as Dercum's disease, familial multiple lipomatosis, Madelung's disease, Gardner's syndrome, Bannayan–Zonana and Proteus syndrome

PATHOGENESIS

Unknown.

PATHOLOGY

Well-circumscribed, lobulated tumor of uniform, mature adipocytes in the subcutaneous fat, often with a thin surrounding fibrous capsule and eccentric nuclei.

PHYSICAL LESIONS

A lipoma presents as a soft, freely mobile flesh-colored oval or round subcutaneous nodule with a normal overlying epidermis. Its size can vary greatly from millimeters to many centimeters. It is nontender unless presenting as part of Dercum's disease, as an angiolipoma or if impinging on a nerve.

DIFFERENTIAL DIAGNOSIS

Epidermal inclusion cyst, pilar cyst, hibernoma, angiolipoma, and other fatty tumors including liposarcoma must be considered. If the lesion is greater than 10 cm or fixed, malignancy should be considered.

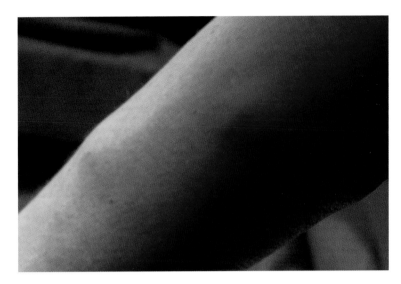

Figure 40.1 *A middle-aged female with two lipomas on her arms*

LABORATORY EXAMINATION

In normal circumstances, no workup is indicated. In the event of rapid or extensive growth, however, biopsy may be indicated if malignancy is suspected. Caution is indicated in the event of excising a lipoma located in the midline saccrococcygeal region. It may represent spinal dysraphism. In this circumstance, consider radiologic and neurosurgical evaluation. Do not perform a biopsy.

COURSE

They tend to grow slowly to a certain size and do not involute without intervention.

KEY CONSULTATIVE QUESTIONS

* Number and location of lipomas
* Family history of similar lesions
* History of keloids/hypertrophic scarring
* Associated pain
* Recent lesional growth

MANAGEMENT

There is no medical indication to treat lipomas unless they produce pain or constriction of movement or demonstrate accelerated growth. Many patients, however, request treatment for cosmesis. Surgical removal, via excision or liposuction, is the mainstay of therapy. If the lesion is located in the midline saccrococcygeal region, consider spinal dysraphism.

TREATMENT

* Surgical excision: best for small lipomas (Figs. 40.2-40.3)
  - Depending on the size of the lipoma, a small elliptical excision is performed over the tumor. Once the lipoma is encountered, it is dissected from its surrounding tissue.
  - After removal, a layered closure with subcutaneous sutures is generally required to repair the cavity produced by the procedure.
  - Recurrence is common due to the difficulty of distinguishing tumor from normal subcutaneous fat.
  - Surgical excision is preferred for smaller lipomas and is less expensive than liposuction.
* Liposuction: best for large lipomas
  - A small incision is created within the center of the lipoma after regional anesthesia and liposuction of the lipoma is performed.

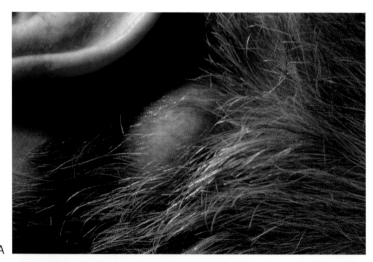

A

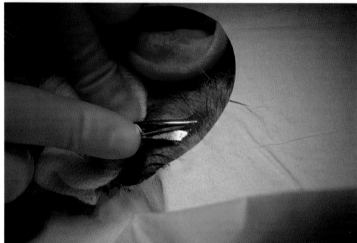

B

Figure 40.2 (A) *Lipoma on scalp prior to surgical excision.* **(B)** *Scissors are used to dissect lipoma from the surrounding skin structures*

– The entire tumor is not necessarily removed. Rather, portions of the lipoma are removed until the affected area lies flush with the surrounding skin.

– Postprocedure fibrosis can ensure a persistent flattened contour of the remaining lipoma tissue.

– The advantage of liposuction over excision is that it produces a smaller scar.

– It is more expensive than standard excision.

PITFALLS TO AVOID/COMPLICATIONS/ MANAGEMENT/OUTCOME EXPECTATIONS

• The physician should inform the patient that all surgical interventions produce some degree of scarring.

• Scarring may bother patients more than the lipoma itself.

• Additionally, removal of large lipomas frequently results in a post-operative skin depression.

• Recurrence is common, especially with liposuction.

BIBLIOGRAPHY

Harrington AC, Admot J, Chesser RS. Infiltrating lipomas of the upper extremities. *J Dermatol Surg Oncol.* 1990; 16:834–836.

Salasche SJ, McCollough ML, Angeloni VL, Grabski WJ. Frontalis-associated lipoma of the forehead. *J Am Acad Dermatol.* 1989;20:462–468.

Sanchez MR, Golomb FA, Moy JA, Potozkin JR. Giant lipoma: case report and review of the literature. *J Am Acad Dermatol.* 1993;28:266–268.

Truhan AP, Garden JM, et al. Facial and scalp lipomas: case reports and study of prevalence. *J Dermatol Surg Oncol.* 1985;11:91.

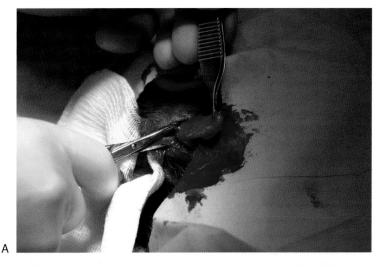

A

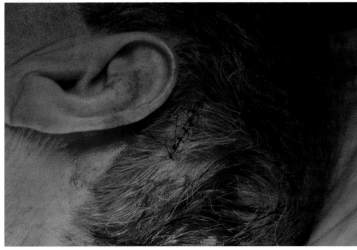

B

Figure 40.3 **(A)** *Extraction of intact lipoma.* **(B)** *Sutures at site of excision*

CHAPTER 41 Milium

Milia are benign superficial white-yellow keratinaceous cysts that typically present on the eyelids, forehead, and face but may present anywhere (Fig. 41.1). They occur at all ages and are very common.

EPIDEMIOLOGY

Incidence: very common

Age: any age; most common in newborns and adults

Race: none

Sex: equal

Precipitating factors: These are most frequently sporadic lesions but they can be associated with subepidermal blistering diseases such as porphyria cutanea tarda, epidermolysis bullosa acquisita, varicella zoster virus, bullous pemphigoid, and bullous lichen planus. They are also associated with skin trauma such as abrasions, burns, dermatologic surgery, CO_2 resurfacing, and radiation therapy. They may also occur following treatment with topical 5-fluorouracil, topical corticosteroids, and microdermabrasion

PATHOGENESIS

Milia are believed to be retention cysts derived from vellus hair follicles. Milia secondary to trauma or bullous diseases arise from ectopic hair follicles.

PATHOLOGY

They represent small epidermoid cysts and feature characteristic stratified squamous epithelium with laminated keratin debris. A granular layer is present in the cyst wall.

PHYSICAL LESIONS

Milia present as 1–4 mm superficial white-yellow cysts that most commonly appear on the eyelids, cheeks, and foreheads.

DIFFERENTIAL DIAGNOSIS

Their clinical appearance is characteristic.

LABORATORY EXAMINATION

None.

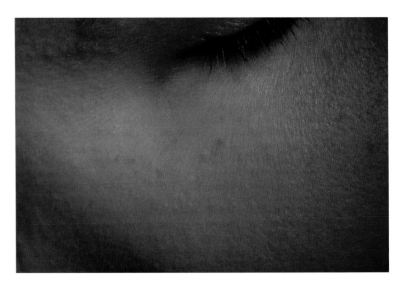

Figure 41.1 *Small milia on face of a 37-year-old female*

COURSE

They can present at any age and do not resolve without intervention.

KEY CONSULTATIVE QUESTIONS

Is there any history of blistering or trauma?

MANAGEMENT

There is no medical indication to treat milia. The cosmetic appearance, however, may displease some individuals.

TREATMENT

- Incision and expression: treatment of choice (Fig. 41.2)
  - Anesthesia is not required.
  - Incision with a scalpel or lancet.
  - Followed by expression of the keratinaceous debris with a comedone extractor.
  - The procedure is fast, simple, and effective.
- Topical medications
  - Topical tretinoin can be effective for multiple milia.
  - This may be more practical and palatable than multiple incision and expression procedures.
- Other treatments
  - Ablative lasers can be effective but are far more expensive with a higher rate of side effects and recovery time.

PITFALLS TO AVOID/COMPLICATIONS/ MANAGEMENT/OUTCOME EXPECTATIONS

Treatment of milia is straightforward. Incision and expression is fast, simple, and successful. It remains the treatment of choice. In cases of multiple milia, topical tretinoin is a good choice, particularly if the lesions are small (Fig. 41.1). Laser plays no practical role in the treatment of milia.

BIBLIOGRAPHY

Olup-Dmovsek, Vedlin B. Use of Er:YAG laser for benign skin disorders. *Lasers Surg Med.* 1997;21(1):13–19.

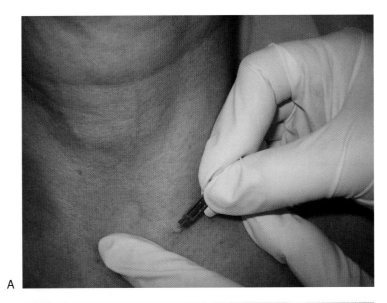

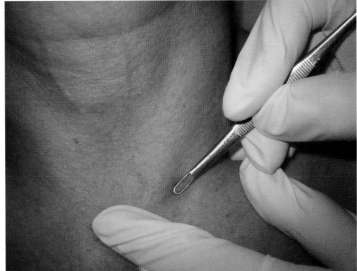

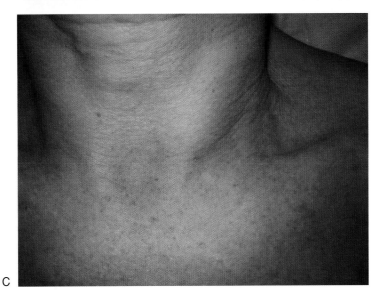

Figure 41.2 (A) *Lancet piercing a milium on the left lower anterior neck of a patient.* **(B)** *Comedone extractor extruding keratinaceous debris from milium.* **(C)** *Postprocedure resolution of milium after comedone extraction*

CHAPTER 42 Neurofibroma

Neurofibromas (NFs) are benign, soft, pink, neuromes-enchymal tumors that can be solitary or multiple (Figs. 42.1-42.2). Solitary tumors are not associated with systemic findings. Multiple NFs are associated with neurofibromatosis types I and II, both neurocutaneous disorders with important systemic manifestations including malignancies.

EPIDEMIOLOGY

Incidence: common

Age: young adults

Race: none

Sex: equal

Precipitating factors: multiple NFs are seen in association with neurofibromatosis I and II. There are no precipitating factors for solitary NFs.

PATHOGENESIS

The pathogenesis of solitary lesions is unknown.

PATHOLOGY

NF displays a well-circumscribed, unencapsulated dermal collection of small nerve fibers and loosely arranged spindle cells possessing wavy nuclei in an eosinophilic matrix. Mast cells are commonly seen. Mitoses are absent (Fig. 42.3).

PHYSICAL LESIONS

NFs present as pink to brown soft, flaccid, pedunculated nodules. The ability to easily invaginate the lesion with pressure, known as "buttonholing," is a characteristic physical finding. They range in size from a few millimeters to a few centimeters.

DIFFERENTIAL DIAGNOSIS

Dermal nevi, congenital nevi, dermatofibromas, neuromas, and fibromas.

LABORATORY EXAMINATION

A solitary NF does not merit a workup. Biopsy may be indicated of a clinically atypical NF. Multiple NFs merit referral to neurologic, ophthalmologic, and orthopedic

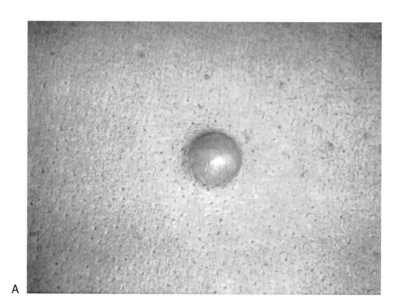

A

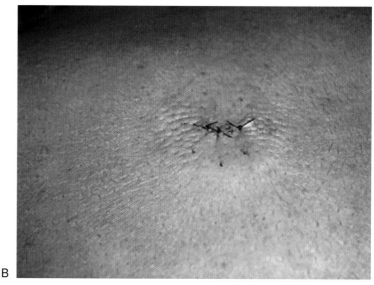

B

Figure 42.1 (A) *Solitary neurofibroma pre-op.* **(B)** *Solitary neurofibroma following simple excision. This is the treatment of choice for solitary neurofibromas. It is also a good option for removal of several neurofibromas*

specialists to assess for neurofibromatosis I or II. Complete skin and eye examination of the patient and immediate relatives is indicated as well. Skin examination should assess for axillary freckling, café au lait macules, plexiform NFs, juvenile xanthogranulomas, and Lisch nodules.

COURSE

They tend to grow indolently and painlessly.

KEY CONSULTATIVE QUESTIONS

- Number of lesions
- Family history
- CNS abnormalities
- Scoliosis
- Eye abnormalities
- Bone defects
- Loss of hearing

MANAGEMENT

There is no medical indication to treat NFs unless they produce pain or are cosmetically disfiguring. Many patients, however, request treatment for improvement of cosmetic appearance. While there are many methods for removing NFs, surgical excision is the most common and efficient means of removal.

TREATMENT

- Surgical excision
  - Elliptical excision is an effective, inexpensive treatment and is particularly appropriate for a fewer number of lesions. As with any surgery, scar will result.
- Laser ablation: not first-line therapy
  - Carbon dioxide (CO_2) laser resurfacing can be utilized for facial lesions.
  - A cutting technique can be utilized to excise tumors.
    - NF margins are marked. Local anesthesia is administered.
    - CO_2 treatment in a focused continuous wave beam, 15–30 W is performed along the marked margin.
    - Re-incise along the margin until the desired depth is obtained.
    - Tissue undermining and hemorrhage control can be obtained utilizing the same laser parameters with the handpiece held away from the wound to defocus the beam. Wound closure is performed in a standard fashion.
  - A vaporization technique may be utilized to flatten and remove tumors.

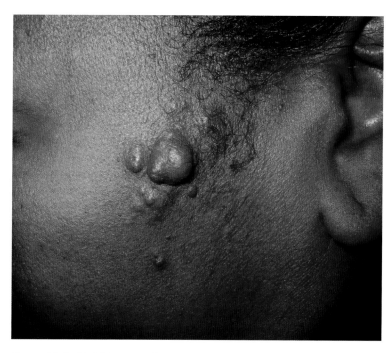

Figure 42.2 *Multiple neurofibromas on the left face*

○ Local anesthesia is administered.

○ CO_2 treatment with a defocused beam and 3–6 W is performed to the level of adjacent normal skin.

○ It may be necessary to manually extract large residual dermal tumor once visualized. Char should be debrided between passes with a wet gauze and dried fully prior to continuing treatment.

– Several sessions of treatment may be required for numerous NFs.

– Post-inflammatory hyperpigmentation, atrophic scarring, hypertrophic scarring, and incomplete removal have been reported as side effects. A test site should be considered.

PITFALLS TO AVOID/COMPLICATIONS/ MANAGEMENT/OUTCOME EXPECTATIONS

• The physician should inform the patient that any surgical or laser intervention produces some degree of scarring.

• Removal of NFs via laser ablation may produce post-inflammatory hyperpigmentation and/or scarring. Recurrence is common.

• CO_2 laser incisional treatment can lead to decreased tensile wound strength during the wound healing phase when compared to standard surgical excision due to laser thermal damage at the wound margin. Sutures should be left in for an additional week to assist in wound healing.

• CO_2 laser vaporization treatment should be limited to facial NFs, given an increased risk of scar formation with use on nonfacial sites.

BIBLIOGRAPHY

Becker DW Jr. Use of the carbon dioxide laser in treating multiple cutaneous neurofibromas. *Ann Plast Surg.* 1991;26(6):582–586.

Katalinic D. Laser surgery of neurofibromatosis 1 (NF 1). *J Clin Laser Med Surg.* 1992;10(3):185–192.

Neville HL, Seymour-Dempsey K, Slopis J, Gill BS, Moore BD, Lally KP, Andrassy RJ. The role of surgery in children with neurofibromatosis. *J Pediatr Surg.* 2001;36(1):25–29.

Roenigk RK, Ratz JL. CO_2 laser treatment of cutaneous neurofibromas. *J Dermatol Surg Oncol.* 1987;13(2): 187–190.

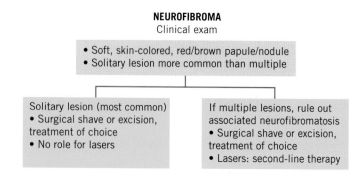

Figure 42.3 *Neurofibroma diagram*

CHAPTER 43 Seborrheic Keratosis

Seborrheic keratosis (SK) is a very common benign warty, keratotic skin growth that first presents in the fourth decade. The color ranges from pink to tan to brown. Lesions can be solitary or multiple (Fig. 43.1). Over time, patients develop anywhere from a few to hundreds of SKs. Many patients request removal of SKs, particularly when multiple or large, due to their unsightly appearance.

EPIDEMIOLOGY

Incidence: very common

Age: usually in fourth decade and become more numerous in middle age and beyond

Race: more common in Caucasians

Sex: equal

Precipitating factors: family history with likely autosomal dominant inheritance

PATHOGENESIS

Unknown.

PATHOLOGY

While there are several histologic variants, typically SKs are well-circumscribed epidermal growths that rise above the surface of the surrounding skin. All feature hyperkeratosis, papillomatosis, and acanthosis. The epidermis contains basaloid cells that show squamous differentiation. Squamous eddies may be present.

PHYSICAL LESIONS

There are many clinical variants of SKs. They range in size from a few millimeters to a few centimeters and most commonly occur on the face, neck, and trunk. They typically first present as well-demarcated tan or light brown macules. With time, they rise to become plaques and develop a warty and stuck-on appearance. Horn cysts become apparent within the lesions. They can occur anywhere on hair-bearing skin and are not seen on the palms and soles.

DIFFERENTIAL DIAGNOSIS

Lentigines, verruca, acrochordons, condyloma acuminatum, acrokeratosis verruciformis, Bowen's disease, nevus, epidermal nevus, lentigo maligna, melanoma, and squamous cell

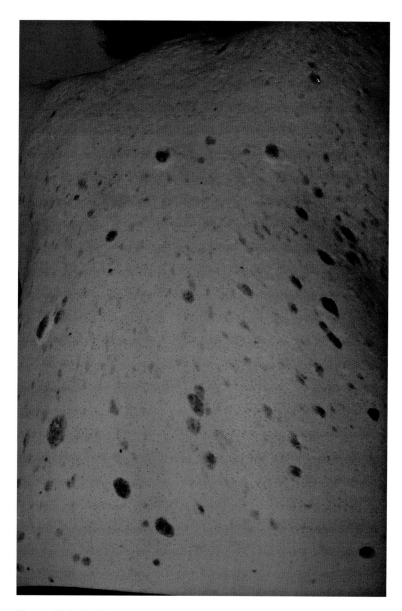

Figure 43.1 *Multiple seborrheic keratoses on back of elderly male*

carcinoma. The clinical appearance and presence of horn cysts in SKs makes the diagnosis straightforward.

LABORATORY EXAMINATION

None; skin biopsy if suspect malignancy.

COURSE

They present in the fourth decade and persist for years. Over time, they become larger, more pigmented and feature a more verrucous appearance. They typically become more numerous with age. Infrequently, they can regress spontaneously.

KEY CONSULTATIVE QUESTIONS

- Family history of skin cancer
- History of bleeding
- Time of onset
- Was there a rapid onset of numerous SKs?

MANAGEMENT

There is no medical indication to treat SKs, unless they are irritated. Still, the cosmetic appearance bothers many patients. There are multiple modalities for treating SKs including cryotherapy, electrodessication, curettage, Q-switched and ablative laser therapy. Most often, the traditional methods of treating SKs are most appropriate.

TRADITIONAL TREATMENTS

- Cryotherapy
  - Light cryotherapy is a quick, inexpensive, and effective method of treating SKs
  - If the lesion does not resolve, re-treatment is necessary
  - No postprocedure care is needed
  - Prolonged cryotherapy may produce hypopigmentation
  - Slight discomfort
- Currettage and light cautery
  - Electrodessication of SKs is another quick and effective method of treatment
  - Curretting the lesion after electrodessication can ensure removal
  - Light, quick electrodessication of the base may also enhance efficacy and prevent recurrence
  - Postprocedure wound care is needed
  - Slight discomfort associated with local anesthesia

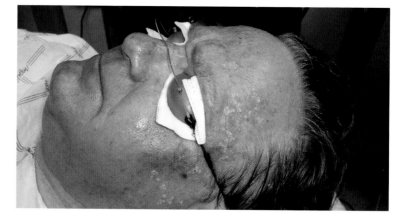

Figure 43.2 *Post-treatment whitening of seborrheic keratoses after treatment with a 755 nm Q-switched alexandrite laser with a fluence of 10 J/cm² and a 3 mm spot size. The procedure was performed after fractional resurfacing, which explains the blue dye remnants apparent on his face*

• Shave excision

  – Shave excision can effectively remove SKs

LASER TREATMENTS

Laser is not a first-line treatment for SKs. Rather, it should be considered an alternative treatment and only used in the correct clinical setting.

• Melanin targeting lasers for thin SKs

  – Q-switched ruby (694 nm) and Q-switched alexandrite (755 nm), and the long-pulsed 532 nm lasers can effectively treat thin SKs (Fig. 43.2)

  – Sometimes ineffective, especially as thickness increases; repeat treatments may be required

  – Risk of hypopigmentation

  – Expensive compared to traditional therapies, but may be more tolerable to a patient with multiple lesions

• Ablative lasers

  – CO_2 and erbium:YAG lasers can ablate SKs

  – Repigmentation of SKs occurs infrequently after treatment

  – Expensive compared to traditional therapies

PITFALLS TO AVOID/COMPLICATIONS/ MANAGEMENT/OUTCOME EXPECTATIONS

• SKs can be treated with a number of different and effective modalities.

• The physician should educate the patient that any therapy has possible adverse effects such as pigmentary changes, scarring, and recurrence.

• Traditional therapies such as light cryotherapy or curettage are simple, quick, and effective (Fig. 43.3).

• Laser therapy is an alternative treatment at a higher expense.

BIBLIOGRAPHY

Kilmer SL. Laser eradication of pigmented lesions and tattoos. *Dermatol Clin.* 2002;20(1):37–53.

Mehrabi D, Brodell RT. Use of the alexandrite laser for treatment of seborrheic keratoses. *Dermatol Surg.* 2002; 28(5):437–439.

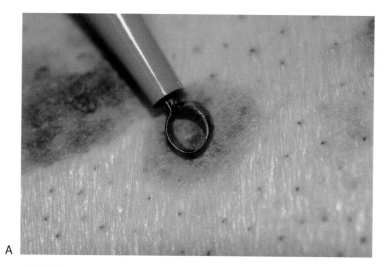

A

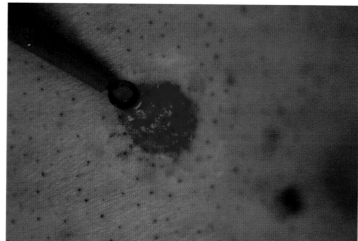

B

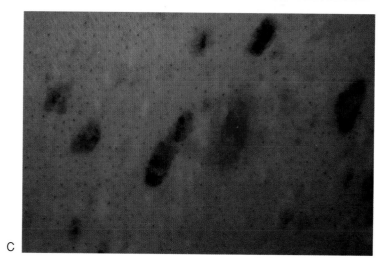

C

Figure 43.3 (A) *Curettage of seborrheic keratosis.* **(B)** *Immediately after curettage of seborrheic keratosis.* **(C)** *Post-inflammatory erythema 1 month after curettage of seborrheic keratosis*

CHAPTER 44 Syringoma

Syringomas are benign appendageal neoplasms of eccrine duct derivation that present most frequently in females on the face, especially around the eyes (Fig. 44.1). They may also be seen on the chest, umbilicus, axillae, and vulva.

EPIDEMIOLOGY

Incidence: common

Age: usually present at puberty

Race: none

Sex: female > male

Precipitating factors: more common in Down's syndrome

PATHOGENESIS

Unknown.

PATHOLOGY

These benign symmetric, well-circumscribed dermal tumors are composed of multiple small ducts with two layers of cuboidal epithelium, often with a "tail" giving a "tadpole," or comma-like appearance in the upper dermis. Some of these ducts are dilated possessing an eosinophilic cuticle. There is a dense fibrous eosinophilic stroma.

PHYSICAL LESIONS

Skin-colored to yellow, 1–3 mm firm papules. They are seen most frequently around the eyes, especially the lower eyelid. Typically, they are multiple and symmetric. They are also seen on the chest, umbilicus, axillae, and genitalia (Fig. 44.2). Acral lesions are seen in eruptive syringomas.

DIFFERENTIAL DIAGNOSIS

Milia, sebaceous hyperplasia, basal cell carcinoma, trichoepithelioma, fibrous papule.

LABORATORY EXAMINATION

Biopsy may be indicated if basal cell carcinoma is suspected. No other laboratories are indicated.

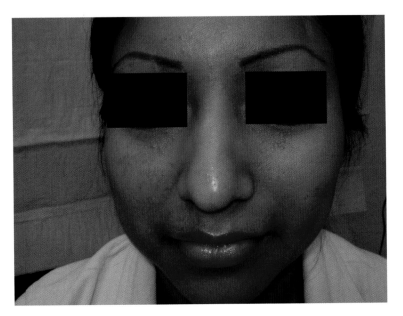

Figure 44.1 *Syringomas on forehead and infraorbital areas on face*

COURSE

They present at puberty and do not resolve without intervention.

KEY CONSULTATIVE QUESTIONS

Time of onset

MANAGEMENT

There is no medical indication to treat syringomas. Many patients, however, request treatment for cosmetic appearance. Syringomas are therapeutically challenging. Although there are multiple treatment modalities available, none is completely successful in complete or permanent removal of syringomas. Often, the side effects of treatment will bother patients more than the syringomas themselves. Ideally, the treatment of syringomas should produce destruction of the tumor with minimal scarring and no recurrence. There are no effective topical medications.

TREATMENT

- Surgical excision: best reserved for solitary lesions.
  - Scar will be produced
- Electrocautery: can be successful (Fig. 44.3).
  - Localized anesthesia with 1% lidocaine with or without epinephrine may be employed.
  - Low energy setting electrocautery performed at 1–2 W with the electrode placed in the center of the syringoma.
  - Clinical endpoint is lesional flattening.
  - Light settings are advised to avoid pigmentary changes or scarring.
  - Gentle curretage is recommended to ensure that effective removal of the syringoma has been obtained.
- Carbon dioxide (CO_2) laser is an effective means of improving these lesions. The goal is to flatten rather than remove the lesions.
  - Limited to patients with skin phototypes I–III.
  - Individual lesions or multiple syringomas with the same cosmetic unit may be treated.
  - CO_2 treatment in a defocused mode, 3–6 W, 3 mm spot, 0.1–0.2 s may be employed.
  - Multiple passes are performed with removal of residual char between passes with saline-soaked gauze pads. Lesions are treated to the level of adjacent normal skin.
  - Lesional recurrence is common. Post-inflammatory hyperpigmentation and scarring may occur.

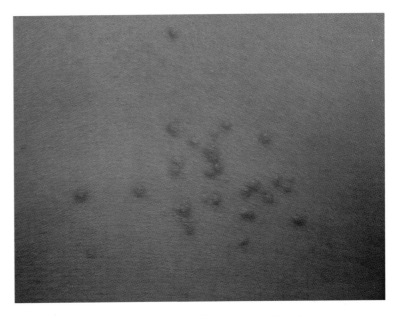

Figure 44.2 *Multiple syringomas on the chest of a female*

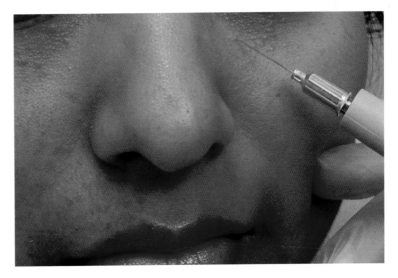

Figure 44.3 *Infraorbital syringomas being treated with low setting electrocautery on a young female. The treatment was not effective.*

• Other treatments: include cryosurgery and dermabrasion. There is little data with which to judge their efficacy and side effect profile.

PITFALLS TO AVOID/COMPLICATIONS/MANAGEMENT/OUTCOME EXPECTATIONS

• Although there are multiple treatment modalities, they are often resistant to therapy. Recurrence is common (Figs. 44.3-44.4).

• Caution should be exercised with each of the above-listed modalities.

• Patients must also be informed that the side effects of treatment may be more cosmetically undesirable than the syringomas themselves. These side effects include scarring, hyperpigmentation, recurrence, and erythema.

• When treating syringomas, care should be taken to not overtreat the lesions. It is not necessary to completely eliminate the lesions, as some dermal fibrosis is expected with healing, with residual lesions becoming less apparent over time.

• Great care should be given to the treatment of patients with skin phototypes IV and higher to avoid temporary and permanent pigmentary changes.

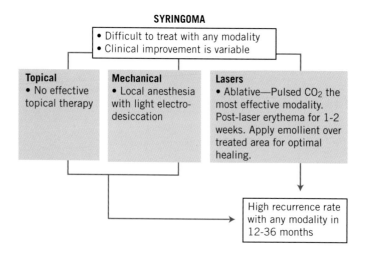

Figure 44.4 *Diagram of syringoma treatment*

BIBLIOGRAPHY

Frazier CC, Camacho AP, Cockerell CJ. The treatment of eruptive syringomas in an African American patient with a combination of trichloroacetic acid and CO_2 laser destruction. *Dermatol Surg.* 2001;27(5):489–492.

Kang WH, Km NS, Kim YB, Shim WC. A new treatment for syringoma. Combination of carbon dioxide laser and trichloroacetic acid. *Dermatol Surg.* 1998;24(12): 1370–1374.

Karam P, Benedetto AV. Syringomas: new approach to an old technique. *Int J Dermatol.* 1996;35(3):219–220.

Sajben FP, Ross EV. The use of the 1.0 mm handpiece in high energy, pulsed CO_2 laser destruction of facial adnexal tumors. *Dermatol Surg.* 1999;25(1):41–44.

Wang JI, Roenigk HH Jr. Treatment of multiple facial syringomas with the carbon dioxide (CO_2) laser. *Dermatol Surg.* 1999;25(2):136–139.

CHAPTER 45 Dermatosis Papulosa Nigra

Dermatosis papulosa nigra (DPNs) are very common benign brown warty papules that appear in African-Americans and other patients with dark skin phototypes, usually on the cheeks, neck, and upper chest (Fig. 45.1). DPNs are a type of seborrheic keratosis. Many patients request removal of DPNs, particularly when multiple or large, due to their unsightly appearance.

EPIDEMIOLOGY

Incidence: very common in African-Americans and Asians

Age: second decade to middle age

Race: more common in African-Americans and Asians

Sex: females > males (2:1)

Precipitating factors: strongly associated with family history

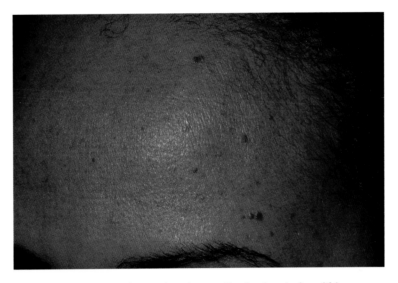

Figure 45.1 *Dermatosis papulos nigra on the forehead of an African-American female*

PATHOGENESIS

Unknown.

PATHOLOGY

All feature hyperkeratosis, papillomatosis, and acanthosis as seen in seborrheic keratoses. No squamous eddies are present.

PHYSICAL LESIONS

They present in a symmetric fashion as small brown smooth sessile papules on the face, neck, and upper trunk of African-Americans and Asians. They range from 1 to 5 mm and are often pedunculated.

DIFFERENTIAL DIAGNOSIS

Seborrheic keratosis, lentigo, verruca, acrochordon, melanocytic nevus, angiofibroma, and adnexal tumors are all in the differential diagnosis.

LABORATORY EXAMINATION

None.

COURSE

They present during teenage years. Over time, they become larger and more numerous, peaking in middle age. They do not regress spontaneously.

KEY CONSULTATIVE QUESTIONS

Family history of DPNs.

MANAGEMENT

There is no medical indication to treat DPNs, unless they are irritated. Still, the cosmetic appearance bothers many patients particularly when numerous. There are multiple modalities for treating DPNs including cryotherapy, electrodessication, gradle scissor removal, curettage, and ablative laser therapy. Primary consideration before treatment should be the effective removal of the DPNs without producing pigmentary change. Test site treatment is highly recommended to avoid pigmentary changes.

TREATMENTS

- Cryotherapy

  - Light cryotherapy is a quick, inexpensive, slightly painful, and effective method of treating DPNs.

  - If the lesion does not resolve, re-treatment is necessary.

  - No postprocedure care or anesthesia is needed.

  - Caution: prolonged cryotherapy can produce hypopigmentation by destroying melanocytes. Hyperpigmentation can also occur.

    ○ Only *light cryotherapy* should be employed.

- Light electrodessication and curettage

  - Light electrodessication of DPNs is another quick and effective method of treatment.

  - With light electrodessication, the lesion will turn white.

  - Curetting the lesion after electrodessication can ensure removal.

  - Light, quick electrodessication of the base after curetting may also enhance efficacy and prevent recurrence.

    ○ Only *light electrodessication* should be employed to avoid scarring or pigmentary alteration.

- Shave or snip excision

  - Shave and snip excision, using gradle scissors, can effectively remove DPNs.

  - Light, quick electrodessication of the base after either snip or shave excision can enhance efficacy and prevent recurrence.

    ○ Only *light electrodessication* should be employed.

LASER TREATMENTS

- Melanin targeting lasers for thin DPNs
  - Q-switched ruby (694 nm), Q-switched alexandrite (755 nm), pulse dye lasers (585 nm), 510 nm pigmented lesion dye laser and long-pulsed 532 nm laser can effectively treat thinner DPNs.
  - Spot size should be less than the size of the lesion.
  - Repeat treatments may be required.
  - Risk of hypopigmentation and hyperpigmentation should be explained carefully to patient.
  - Expensive compared to traditional therapies.
- Ablative lasers
  - CO_2 and erbium:YAG lasers can ablate these epidermal lesions.
  - Superpulsed mode of CO_2 laser is slightly more effective than the continuous mode.
  - Expensive compared to traditional therapies.
  - Risk of hypopigmentation and hyperpigmentation should be explained carefully to the patient.

PITFALLS TO AVOID/COMPLICATIONS/ MANAGEMENT/OUTCOME EXPECTATIONS

- Any therapy has possible adverse effects such as pigmentary changes, scarring, and recurrence.
- DPNs can be treated with a number of different and effective modalities.
- Traditional therapies such as light cryotherapy, scissor excision, or curettage are simple, quick, and effective.
- Laser therapy is more expensive and carries a higher potential for hyper or hypopigmentation. Test spot may be appropriate.

BIBLIOGRAPHY

Kilmer SL. Laser eradication of pigmented lesions and tattoos. *Dermatol Clin.* 2002;20(1):37–53.

SECTION EIGHT

Cutanenous Carcinomas

CHAPTER 46 Basal Cell Carcinoma

Basal cell carcinoma (BCC) is a slow-growing malignant skin tumor that presents in distinct histologic subtypes including nodular, superficial, micronodular, infiltrating, and morpheaform. Nodular BCC is the most common type occurring predominantly on the head and neck regions.

EPIDEMIOLOGY

Incidence: the most common skin cancer in Caucasians with approximately 800,000 cases/year diagnosed in the US

Age: most common in patients over 40

Race: most common in Caucasians

Sex: higher incidence in males

Precipitating factors: chronic ultraviolet radiation and fair skin are the most significant predisposing factors. Other factors include ionizing radiation, arsenic exposure, immunosuppression, PUVA, and genetic predisposition

PATHOGENESIS

The most common altered gene in BCC is the *PTCH* tumor suppressor gene with a resultant altered Hedgehog signaling pathway leading to unregulated cell proliferation and altered cell differentiation. Mutations in the *p53* tumor suppressor gene are also frequently observed leading to cellular immortality and resistance to apoptosis.

PHYSICAL EXAMINATION

Pink or erythematous translucent papule, nodule, or plaque with a pearly border and overlying telangiectasias. The center may become ulcerated and covered by a crust. Morpheaform BCC exhibits a scar-like appearance with ill-defined borders. They most commonly present in photodistributed areas.

DIFFERENTIAL DIAGNOSES

Dermal melanocytic nevi, sebaceous hyperplasia, squamous cell carcinoma (SCC).

LABORATORY DATA

■ Dermatopathology

Lobules, nests, or cords of neoplastic basaloid cells with peripheral palisading, clefting, and mucinous stroma.

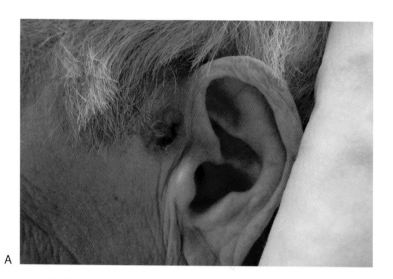

A

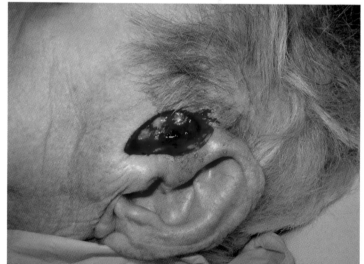

B

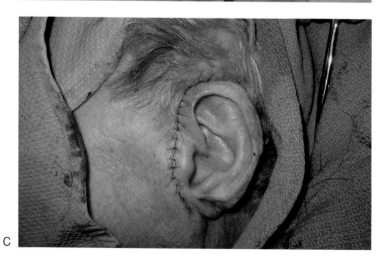

C

Figure 46.1 (A) *Nodular basal cell carcinoma on the left preauricular area.* **(B)** *Clearance of basal cell carcinoma after Mohs surgery.* **(C)** *Primary closure of the Mohs defect with dog-ear repair*

COURSE

Locally invasive and slow growing over months and even years. Metastasis is an exceedingly rare occurrence.

KEY CONSULTATIVE QUESTIONS

Excessive sun-exposure and other predisposing factors; prior history of BCC or SCC; personal and family history of skin cancer; immunosuppression.

MANAGEMENT

There are multiple methods for treating BCC. Treatment selection should be based upon the age, health, and preferences of the patient after a full discussion of treatment options, risks, and benefits. Given the locally destructive nature of BCC, histologic confirmation of complete removal is optimal. Surgical excision and histologic evaluation remain the treatment of choice in most cases. Tumors fixed to underlying bone, especially the scalp, merit radiologic workup prior to surgical excision or Mohs micrographic surgery. Topical therapies require close follow-up for any evidence of treatment failure or recurrence. Patient education regarding the benefits of sun avoidance, sunscreen use, and regular self-examinations are important preventive measures.

■ First-line Therapies

- Mohs micrographic surgery is the treatment of choice for high-risk anatomical locations (i.e., "mask" area of the face), locations where tissue conservation is crucial for functional or cosmetic reasons, recurrent tumors, ill-defined clinical margins, histologically aggressive subtypes, tumors in immunosuppressed patients, tumors larger than 2 cm, irradiated skin, and perineural invasion on biopsy. Mohs micrographic surgery has the highest cure rate of any treatment of BCC (Fig. 46.1)
- Excisional surgery : generally with 4-mm margins (Fig. 46.2)
- Electrodessication and curettage
- Cryotherapy
- Radiotherapy

■ Alternate Therapies

- Topical imiquimod–FDA approved for treatment of superficial BCC
- Topical 5-fluorouracil—primarily reserved for treatment of superficial BCC
- Photodynamic therapy
- Intralesional interferon
- Carbon dioxide laser—may be effective for superficial BCC and patients with multiple shallow tumors such as in basal cell nevus syndrome

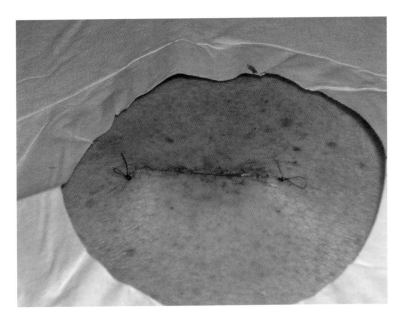

Figure 46.2 *Repair after a surgical elliptical excision of a basal cell carcinoma utilizing running subcuticular suture to optimize the cosmetic results*

PITFALLS TO AVOID

- Poor cosmesis following surgical repair, infection, hypertrophic scarring, pain, nerve damage, and recurrence are all common pitfalls of BCC surgical therapy and should be fully discussed with the patient prior to treatment.

- Non-surgical therapies may provide better cosmesis but significantly higher rates of recurrence. Furthermore, non-surgical interventions do not provide the opportunity for histologic confirmation of complete removal.

BIBLIOGRAPHY

Rowe DE, Carroll RJ, Day CL Jr. Long term recurrence rates in previously untreated (primary) basal cell carcinoma: implications for patient follow-up. *J Dermatol Surg Oncol.* 1989;15:315–328.

Wolf DJ, Zitelli JA. Surgical margins for basal cell carcinoma. *Arch dermatol.* 1987;123:340–344.

CHAPTER 47 Squamous Cell Carcinoma

Squamous cell carcinoma (SCC) most commonly originates from keratinocytes in sun-damaged skin either de novo or from a preexisting actinic keratosis or SCC in situ (also known as Bowen's disease), predominantly affecting the head, neck, and arms. It can also arise in non-sun-exposed skin most commonly from chronic leg ulcers and burn scars.

EPIDEMIOLOGY

Incidence: it is the second most common skin cancer in Caucasians and the most common skin cancer in darkly pigmented skin. Approximately 150,000 cases/year are diagnosed in the US

Age: most common in patients over 55 years

Race: mainly affects Caucasians

Sex: higher incidence in males

Precipitating factors: chronic ultraviolet radiation and fair skin are the most significant predisposing factors. Other factors include immunosuppression, human papilloma virus infection, ionizing radiation, arsenic exposure, genetic disorders (epidermodysplasia verruciformis, albinism, xeroderma pigmentosum, epidermolysis bullosa), PUVA exposure, smoking, and chronic inflammation (ulcers, burn scars, discoid lupus)

PATHOGENESIS

The most common altered gene in SCC is the *p53* tumor suppressor gene, resulting in keratinocyte immortalization and unregulated cell proliferation.

PHYSICAL EXAMINATION

Hyperkeratotic skin-colored to erythematous papule, plaque, or nodule (Figs. 47.1-47.2). It can be ulcerated, friable, or exophytic. It most commonly presents within sun-damaged skin.

DIFFERENTIAL DIAGNOSES

Keratoacanthoma (Fig. 47.3), hypertrophic actinic keratosis, basal cell carcinoma (BCC).

LABORATORY DATA

■ Dermatopathology

Proliferation of atypical keratinocytes with variable differentiation of the epidermis and variably sized nests and islands invading the dermis. Foci of keratinization are noted in well-differentiated variants. Perineural involvement may be observed.

COURSE

SCC tends to be more aggressive than BCC, with a reported 2–3% incidence of metastasis. Mucocutaneous SCC has a higher rate of metastasis, as high as 11%. More aggressive forms of SCC are observed in immunosuppressed patients or SCC that arises within previously irradiated sites, scars, burns, and areas of inflammation. There is a higher metastatic potential for SCC arising on the ear and the lip.

KEY CONSULTATIVE QUESTIONS

Evaluate for past history of blistering sunburns and chronic sun exposure. Determine if other predisposing factors are present such as personal and family history of skin cancer and immunosuppression.

MANAGEMENT

Preventative measures such as sun avoidance and daily sunscreen use are critical for long-term prevention. Treatment selection should be based upon the age, health, and preferences of the patient after a full discussion of treatment options, risks, and benefits. Given the metastatic potential of SCC, histologic confirmation of complete removal is advised. Surgical excision and histologic evaluation remain the treatment of choice in most

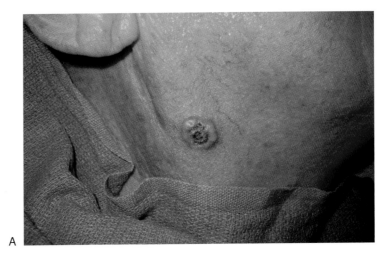

A

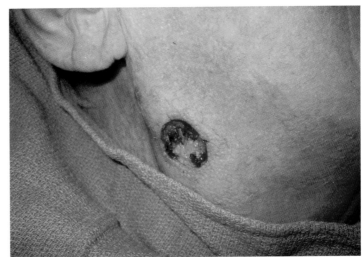

B

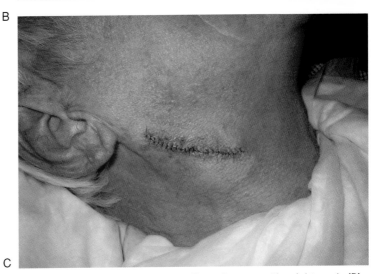

C

Figure 47.1 (A) *Invasive squamous cell carcinoma on the right neck.* **(B)** *Clearance of squamous cell carcinoma after Mohs surgery.* **(C)** *Primary closure of the Mohs defect with dog-ear repair*

cases. Tumors fixed to underlying bone, especially the scalp, merit radiologic workup prior to surgical excision or Mohs micrographic surgery. Prior to treatment, lymph node palpation is appropriate for large SCC, SCC in immunosuppressed patients, and high-risk SCCs. Topical therapies require close follow-up for any evidence of treatment failure or recurrence.

■ First-line Therapies

- Mohs micrographic surgery is the treatment of choice for high-risk anatomical locations (i.e., "mask" area of the face), locations where tissue conservation is crucial for functional or cosmetic reasons, recurrent tumors, ill-defined clinical margins, histologically aggressive subtypes, tumors in immunosuppressed patients, tumors larger than 2 cm, irradiated skin, and perineural invasion on biopsy (Figs. 47.1-47.4). Cure rates of SCC depend on size, histologic grade, perineural invasion, and immunosuppression. Larger lesions, less differentiated variants with perineural involvement, and lesions in immunocompromised patients demonstrate lower cure rates.

- Excisional surgery: 4 mm margins are generally recommended.

- Electrodessication and curettage

- Cryotherapy

- Radiotherapy

■ Alternate Therapies

- Topical 5-fluorouracil—limited to SCC in situ

- Topical imiquimod—limited to SCC in situ

- Intralesional interferon

- Photodynamic therapy—most effective for SCC in situ

- Carbon dioxide laser—highly effective for actinic cheilitis. May be used for SCC in situ

PITFALLS TO AVOID

Poor cosmesis following surgical repair, infection, hypertrophic scarring, pain, nerve damage, and recurrence are all common pitfalls of SCC treatment and should be fully discussed with the patient prior to treatment. Non-surgical therapies may provide better cosmesis but significantly higher rates of recurrence. Furthermore, non-surgical interventions do not provide the opportunity for histologic confirmation of complete removal. This is particularly crucial given the potential of metastatic spread with SCC.

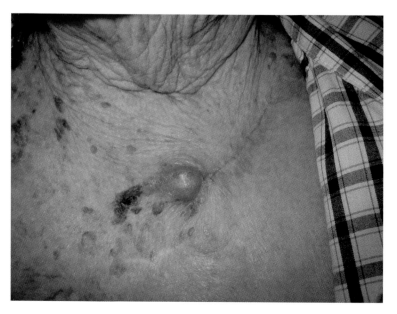

Figure 47.2 *Recurrent squamous cell carcinoma on the chest of an elderly woman*

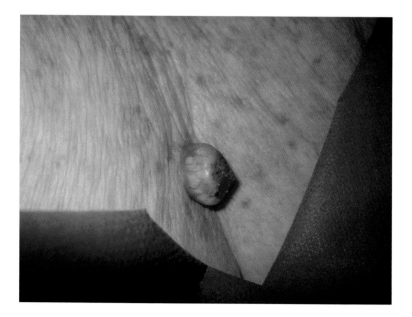

Figure 47.3 *Giant keratoacanthoma on the chest. Many authors regard keratoacanthomas as variants of well-differentiated squamous cell carcinoma*

BIBLIOGRAPHY

Preston DS, Stern RS. Nonmelanoma cancers of the skin. *N Engl J Med.* 1992;327:1649–1662.

Rowe DE, Carroll RJ, Day CL Jr. Prognostic factors for local recurrence, metastasis, and survival rates in squamous cell carcinoma of the skin, ear, and lip. Implications for treatment modality selection. *J Am Acad Dermatol.* 1992;26:976–990.

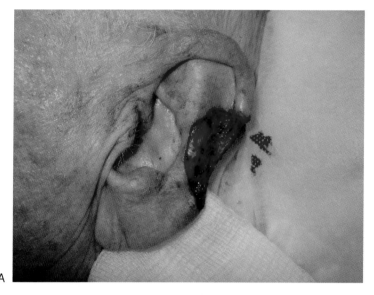

A

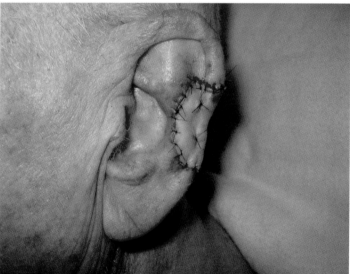

B

Figure 47.4 **(A)** *Defect on the ear after Mohs excision of a squamous cell carcinoma.* **(B)** *The Mohs defect is repaired with a full-thickness skin graft*

SECTION NINE

Inflammatory Disorders

CHAPTER 48 | Lichen Planus

Lichen planus (LP) is a common inflammatory disease involving the skin and mucous membranes (Figs. 48.1-48.2). Many clinical variants exist, which include ulcerative, bullous, annular, linear, lichen planopilaris, and hypertrophic LP.

EPIDEMIOLOGY

Incidence: about 0.5%

Age: 30–60 years

Race: all races are affected equally in most variants

Sex: higher incidence in females

Precipitating factors: most commonly idiopathic; medications may induce a LP-like eruption

PATHOGENESIS

Primarily a T-helper cell-mediated reaction.

PHYSICAL EXAMINATION

Most commonly, primary lesions consist of multiple violaceous, polygonal, flat-topped, grouped papules and plaques that are usually pruritic. Their surface is shiny or transparent and may exhibit small gray-white punctate or reticular fine white lines known as Wickham's striae. The lesions favor the oropharynx, flexural wrists, dorsal hands, medial thighs, shins, trunk, and genitalia. Postinflammatory hyperpigmentation is common.

DIFFERENTIAL DIAGNOSIS

Psoriasis, lichen simplex, lichenoid graft-versus-host disease, chronic cutaneous lupus erythematosus, lichenoid drug eruption.

LABORATORY DATA

◼ Serology

Given the association with hepatitis B and C, hepatitis serologies should be investigated.

◼ Dermatopathology

Pathology reveals lichenoid interface dermatitis, hyperkeratosis, hypergranulosis, saw-tooth acanthosis, associated with colloid or civatte bodies.

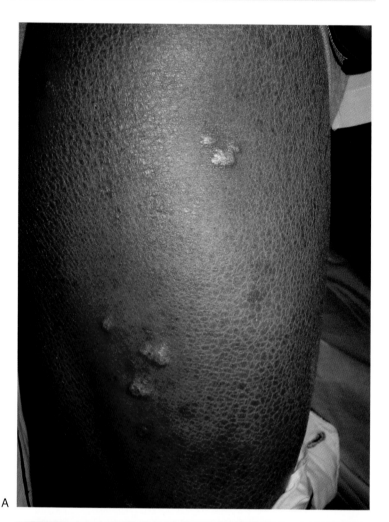

A

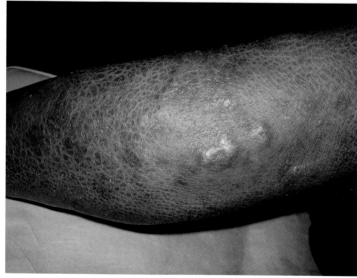

B

Figure 48.1 *Hypertrophic lichen planus on the thigh* **(A)** *and the legs* **(B)** *of 4 years duration resistant to topical and intralesional steroid therapy. The patient improved markedly after 1 month treatment with acetretin.*

COURSE

Spontaneous remission of cutaneous LP occurs within 1 year of onset in the majority of patients. Oral LP persists for many years. Squamous cell carcinoma (SCC) may arise from these lesions, predominantly from the oral variant.

MANAGEMENT (Figs. 48.1-48.2)

■ Topical Treatment

• Corticosteroids, topical and intralesional

• Immunomodulators, such as tacrolimus

• Cyclosporine retention mouthwash for oral LP

■ Systemic Treatment

• Corticosteroids

• Retinoids: isotretinoin and acitretin. Acitretin is the only systemic treatment that has been evaluated in a double-blind, placebo-controlled study

• Griseofulvin, metronidazole, antimalarials, methotrexate, cyclosporine, and mycophenolate mofetil

■ Light Treatment

• Narrow-band UVB

• PUVA

• 308-nm UVB excimer laser for oral LP (Fig. 48.2)

• CO_2 laser for oral LP: variable results with increased risks of side effects

• Extracorporeal photophoresis

PITFALLS TO AVOID

• Patients should be aware of the chronic nature of this disease and its resistance to treatment

• SCC arising in oral LP should be excluded in persistent lesions

BIBLIOGRAPHY

Cribier B, Frances C, Chosidow O. Treatment of lichen planus. An evidence-based medicine analysis of efficacy. *Arch Dermatol.* 1998;134(12):1521–1530.

Laurberg G, Geiger JM, Hjorth N, Holm P, Hou-Jensen K, Jacobsen KU, Nielsen AO, Pichard J, Serup J, Sparre-Jorgensen A, et al. Treatment of lichen planus with acitretin. A double-blind, placebo-controlled study in 65 patients. *J Am Acad Dermatol.* 1991;24(3):434–437.

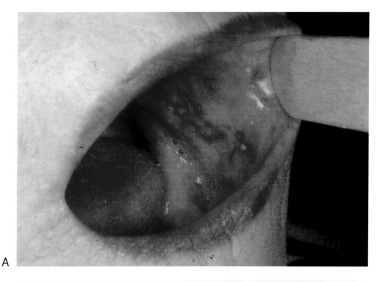

A

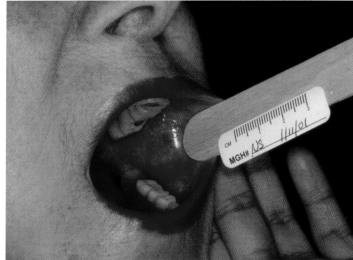

B

Figure 48.2 (A) *Oral lichen planus at baseline.* **(B)** *Two-month follow-up after 18 treatments with 308 nm excimer laser administered weekly (courtesy of Charles Taylor, MD)*

Loh HS. A clinical investigation of the management of oral lichen planus with CO_2 laser surgery. *J Clin Laser Med Surg.* 1992;10(6):445–449.

Trehan M, Taylor CR. Low-dose excimer 308-nm laser for the treatment of oral lichen planus. *Arch Dermatol.* 2004;140(4):415–420.

CHAPTER 49 Morphea

Morphea is localized scleroderma confined to the skin. It most commonly affects the trunk but also occurs on the face and extremities. The four clinical variants include plaque-type morphea, generalized morphea, linear morphea (en coup de sabre), and pansclerotic morphea of children (morphea profunda).

EPIDEMIOLOGY

Incidence: rare

Age: most commonly occurs in the second to fifth decade. Linear scleroderma and morphea profunda are more common in children

Race: slightly more common in Caucasians

Sex: females more than males (2–3:1)

Precipitating factors: *Borrelia* can trigger morphea in some cases, predominantly in Europe

PATHOGENESIS

Overproduction of collagen (types I, II, III) and glycosaminoglycans by skin fibroblasts and vascular damage. Probable T-cell mediated phenomenon.

PHYSICAL EXAMINATION

Ill-defined pink to violaceous, indurated 2–15 cm plaques that transform to smooth sclerotic ivory-colored plaques with a light violaceous border and a shiny surface. Postinflammatory hyperpigmentation is prevalent (Fig. 49.1). Linear morphea presents with a linear erythematous inflammatory streak which may progress to form a scar-like band involving underlying fascia, muscle, and tendons.

DIFFERENTIAL DIAGNOSES

Acrodermatitis chronica atrophicans, eosinophilic fasciitis, lichen sclerosus et atrophicus, scleredema.

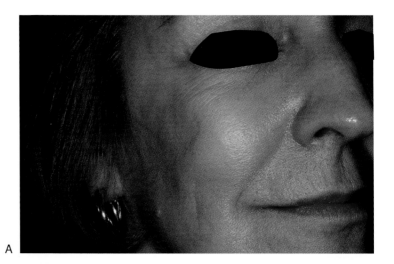

A

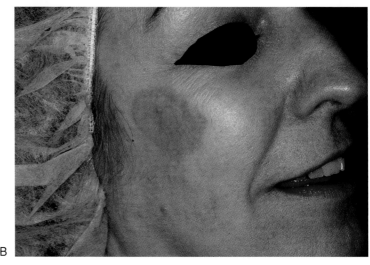

B

Figure 49.1 (A) *Morphea with significant epidermal, dermal, and subcutaneous atrophy.* **(B)** *Elevation of the atrophic plaque of morphea after a single autologous fat transfer. The associated telangiectasias were subsequently treated with the pulsed dye laser with substantial improvement.*

LABORATORY DATA

◼ Serology

Check for Borrelia antibodies

◼ Dermatopathology

Homogenization of dermal collagen bundles with normal or atrophic overlying epidermis.

COURSE

Course is variable. Many patients remit spontaneously but others have a progressive course.

MANAGEMENT

Treatment for this condition can be frustrating due to frequent treatment failure. Patients should be counseled that therapy may not be effective.

- Topical treatment
  - Corticosteroids
  - Calcipotriene
- Systemic treatment
  - Corticosteroids
  - D-penicillamine
  - Vitamin D3
  - Methotrexate
- Light treatment
  - Ultraviolet A-1 phototherapy
  - Pulsed dye laser (585 nm, 5 J/cm^2 twice monthly), reported to be effective in single case report
- Subcision: subcision with a Nokor 18G needle may help to elevate the bound-down skin. It is most effective for linear morphea and facial hemiatrophy. Subcision is performed under local infiltrative anesthesia to the affected site with 1% lidocaine with 1:100,000 epinephrine. The Nokor needle is introduced at a 45° angle into the skin utilizing a sweeping motion to release any tethered areas. Multiple entrance sites should be performed for optimal benefit. Firm pressure is applied to the treatment sites for hemostasis.
- Soft tissue augmentation: various fillers have been employed with variable success to augment the sclerotic sites. They are most commonly utilized for linear morphea and facial hemiatrophy. Temporary fillers currently recommended given the unpredictable course of morphea. Autologous fat transfer can provide significant augmentation of the affected sites (Fig. 49.1). Repeat injections generally required.

PITFALL TO AVOID

Patients must be aware of the unpredictable nature of morphea, therefore the unpredictable nature of the treatment.

REFERENCES

Eisen D, Alster TS. Use of 585 nm pulsed dye laser for the treatment of morphea. *Dermatol Surg*. July 2002;28(7):615–616.

CHAPTER 50 Psoriasis

Psoriasis is a common chronic inflammatory disease of the skin. The lesions are usually nonpruritic. They are symmetric in distribution and favor elbows, knees, scalp, retroauricular skin, and intertriginous areas. Many clinical variants exist and include plaque, pustular, guttate, inverse, and erythrodermic psoriasis, with the plaque variant being the most common type (Figs. 50.1-50.2). Nails and mucous membranes can be affected. Psoriasis is associated with psoriatic arthritis in at least 5% of patients.

EPIDEMIOLOGY

Incidence: about 1.5–2% of the world's population

Age: can occur at any age. Two peaks of onset, the second and sixth decades. Onset earlier in women. Uncommonly affects children

Race: lower incidence in African-Americans, Native Americans, and Asians

Sex: equal

Precipitating factors: bacterial infections, especially streptococcal infection (guttate psoriasis), trauma (Koebner phenomenon), stress, genetic predisposition, and medication use (most commonly lithium, beta blockers and antimalarials). Rapid corticosteroid taper may induce pustular psoriasis.

PATHOGENESIS

Polygenic disease with a 41% risk for a child to develop psoriasis if both parents are affected. The primary pathophysiology involves hyperproliferation and abnormal differentiation of epidermal keratinocytes as well as abnormal cellular immune response.

PHYSICAL EXAMINATION

Plaque variant with well-demarcated pink to erythematous papules and plaques with overlying silvery-white scale (Figs. 50.1-50.2). Pinpoint bleeding observed with scale removal (Auspitz sign). Guttate variant with teardrop-shaped

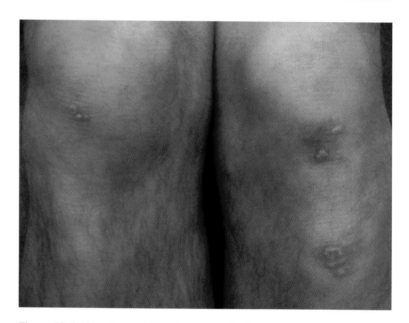

Figure 50.1 *Classic psoriatic plaques on the knees*

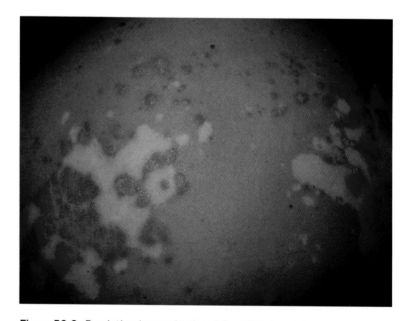

Figure 50.2 *Psoriatic plaques koebnerizing vitiligo patches.*

lesions. Erythematous generalized pustules seen with pustular psoriasis.

DIFFERENTIAL DIAGNOSES

Tinea corporis, seborrheic dermatitis, eczematous dermatitis, mycosis fungoides, parapsoriasis, lichen simplex chronicus, pityriasis rubra pilaris, Reiter's disease.

LABORATORY DATA

■ Serology

ASO titer for guttate psoriasis.

■ Dermatopathology

Regular psoriasiform epidermal hyperplasia with absent granular cell layer and thinning above the dermal papillae. Other characteristic features include collections of neutrophils in epidermis as well as tortuous blood vessels in the papillary dermis.

COURSE

This disease demonstrates a chronic course with multiple exacerbations and remissions.

MANAGEMENT

There are multiple therapeutic options for treatment of psoriasis. Choosing an appropriate therapy depends on the age, health, and preferences of the patient. It also depends on the extent of the psoriasis. The costs of therapy vary dramatically as well. Alternative therapies are most appropriate in refractory cases. Assessing the side effect profile of treatments is another crucial component of therapy. Combination therapies are generally most effective to decrease inflammation and reduce scale production.

- Topical treatment
  - Corticosteroids, topical and intralesional
  - Calcipotriene
  - Tazarotene
  - Coal tar
  - Anthralin
  - Salicylic acid
- Systemic treatment
  - Methotrexate
  - Retinoids, predominantly acitretin
  - Cyclosporine
  - Biologics such as alefacept, etanercept, efalizumab, and infliximab

- Light treatment
  - Psoralen with ultraviolet A (PUVA)
  - Ultraviolet B (UVB)
  - 311 nm narrow-band UVB (NBUVB)
  - 308 nm UVB excimer laser
    - A novel alternative for treatment of mild to moderate psoriasis.
    - Initial studies have demonstrated that this localized UVB treatment provides much lower cumulative doses of UVB to induce clearance of psoriatic plaques compared to NBUVB therapy.
    - The excimer laser also produces longer remission periods, with minimization of UVB exposure to healthy surrounding skin.
    - Initial doses are usually based on the standard minimal erythema dose (MED) with stepwise incremental increases, administered biweekly. The higher the dose multiples, the faster the clearance. Approximately six to eight treatments are required to clear the majority of lesions at a treatment dose of 4 MED.
    - Small plaques can often be cleared with a single treatment at 6–10 MED with blistering.
    - Treatment time is usually less than 15 min.
    - In combination with air blower device, excimer laser has proved to be effective and safe in treating refractory scalp psoriasis.
    - Studies to determine long-term benefit of excimer laser are not yet available.
    - Drawbacks of excimer laser in psoriasis treatment include limited availability and treatment expense.
- Photodynamic therapy with topical and systemic ALA has been shown to improve psoriasis in some reports. At this time, it is not recommended.
- Pulsed dye laser (Scleroplus 00.45 ms, 7 mm spot, 9 J/cm^2, DCD 40/20; 10 mm spot, 5–6 J/cm^2, DCD 40/20) has been employed to target the vascularity associated with psoriatic lesions with benefit. Improvement is variable (Fig. 50.3).
- Nd:YAG 1320 nm (300 ms, 3–20 Hz, 5–20 J/cm^2, 2–6 W) has been reported to be effective. Scar formation has been noted.

PITFALLS TO AVOID

- Patients should be counseled that psoriasis is a chronic condition with flares and remissions. Laser therapy, such as the excimer laser, is an alternative treatment that should only be considered after a patient has failed multiple other treatment regimens.
- Patients should be aware that any treatment administered may result in spread of the psoriasis (Koebner phenomenon). They should also be aware that surgical treatments performed for any reason may also result in a similar spread.

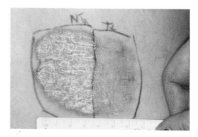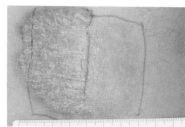
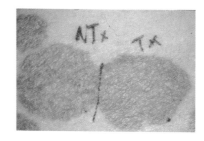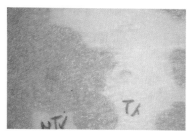

Figure 50.3 *Plaques of psoriasis prior to treatment. Improvement in treated plaque 3 months after pulsed dye laser treatment (585 nm, 10 mm spot size, 5 J/cm2, no cooling, 0.45 ms pulse duration), as compared to the control site (courtesy of Brian Zelickson, MD)*

BIBLIOGRAPHY

Bissonnette R, Tremblay JF, Juzenas P, Boushira M, Lui H. Systemic photodynamic therapy with aminolevulinic acid induces apoptosis in lesional T lymphocytes of psoriatic plaques. *J Invest Dermatol.* July 2002;119(1):77–83.

Boehncke WH, Elshorst-Schmidt T, Kaufmann R. Systemic photodynamic therapy is a safe and effective treatment for psoriasis. *Arch Dermatol.* February 2000;136(2):271–272.

Gerber W, Arheilger B, Ha TA, Hermann J, Ockenfels HM. Ultraviolet B 308-nm excimer laser treatment of psoriasis: a new phototherapeutic approach. *Br J Dermatol.* December 2003;149(6):1250–1258.

Ros AM, Garden JM, Hedblad MA. Psoriasis response to the pulsed dye laser. *Lasers Surg Med.* 1996;19:331–335.

Ruiz-Esperanza J. Clinical response of proriasis to low energy irradiance with the Nd:YAG laser at 1320 nm. Report of an observation in 3 patients. *Dermatol Surg.* 1999;25:403–407.

Stringer MR, Collins P, Robinson DJ, Stables GI, Sheehan-Dare RA. The accumulation of protoporphyrin IX in plaque psoriasis after topical application of 5-aminolevulinic acid indicates a potential for superficial photodynamic therapy. *J Invest Dermatol.* July 1996;107(1):76–81.

Taylor CR, Racette AL. A 308-nm excimer laser for the treatment of scalp psoriasis. *Lasers Surg Med.* 2004;34(2):136–140.

SECTION
TEN

Adipose Tissue Alterations

CHAPTER 51 Gynecomastia

Gynecomastia is the increased presence of benign glandular tissue, in the form of a firm mass, around the nipple in males. It is accompanied by an increased fat deposition. In contrast, increased fat deposition alone, in the absence of glandular proliferation, is known as pseudogynecomastia. It can be bilateral or unilateral. It is common at birth, puberty, in middle-aged and elderly adults. Many cases are idiopathic. Multiple precipitating factors exist including hormonal abnormalities, medication, cirrhosis, hypogonadism, testicular tumors, hyperthyroidism, and chronic renal insufficiency. For this reason, in the appropriate clinical setting, the appearance of gynecomastia demands a medical workup.

EPIDEMIOLOGY

Incidence: most common in newborns but also common in puberty and older males

Age: birth (0–3 weeks), puberty (10–17), middle-aged and elderly age groups (50–80)

Race: none

Sex: males

Precipitating factors: hormonal imbalances, hormonal therapy for prostate cancer, drugs, e.g., finasteride, cirrhosis, hypogonadism, testicular tumors, hyperthyroidism, chronic renal insufficiency. About one-quarter of the cases are idiopathic.

PATHOGENESIS

In cases of hormonal imbalances, the fundamental defect is a decrease in androgen levels with a concomitant increase in estrogen levels.

PHYSICAL LESIONS

A firm subcutaneous nodule extends concentrically from the nipple. It may be unilateral or bilateral.

DIFFERENTIAL DIAGNOSIS

Breast cancer, pseudogynecomastia, breast hypertrophy.

LABORATORY EXAMINATION

Serum hCG, LH, testosterone, and estradiol levels should be investigated in the setting of pain, tenderness, or recent onset or clinical suspicion of endocrine abnormalities.

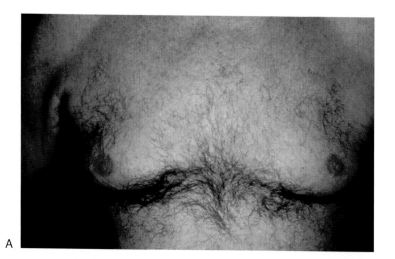

A

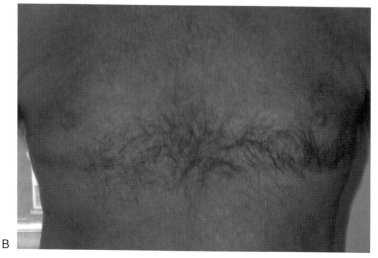

B

Figure 51.1 **(A)** *Gynecomastia in a middle-aged male.* **(B)** *Improvement of gynecomastia after liposuction*

COURSE

This depends on the etiology. Newborn gynecomastia persists for a few weeks. In teenagers, it may last a few years. Discontinuance of medication will ameliorate the symptoms in drug-induced cases. In cases of hormonal imbalance, kidney disease and hyperthyroidism, correction of the underlying illness will produce improvement.

KEY CONSULTATIVE QUESTIONS

- Age of onset
- Medication history
- Hormonal changes
- Renal or thyroid disease
- Hormonal therapy for prostate cancer
- Associated symptoms

MANAGEMENT

Most gynecomastia is temporary and will resolve without therapy. If it is related to puberty, clinical observation and follow-up will likely be all that is needed. Discontinuation of an offending medication is typically all that is required to treat drug-induced gynecomastia. Unilateral gynecomastia requires a mammogram with an appropriate follow-up as needed. Medical and surgical options are available for patients who have persistent gynecomastia into late puberty producing emotional distress, pain, or tenderness.

TREATMENT

■ Oral Medications

Medical therapy for gynecomastia is beyond the scope of this textbook. It is best performed by a physician trained in internal medicine or endocrinology. Medications include androgens, antiestrogens, and aromatase inhibitors.

■ Prophylaxis in Prostate Cancer

Breast radiation can be performed prophylactically in patients undergoing antiandrogen therapy or orchiectomy for prostate cancer. Concomitant tamoxifen administration with finasteride/flutamide therapy can also be prophylactic for gynecomastia.

■ Surgery

In the event of medical treatment failure, surgical therapy is the next option. It is reserved for patients with refractory gynecomastia. The treatments depend on the extent of gynecomastia.

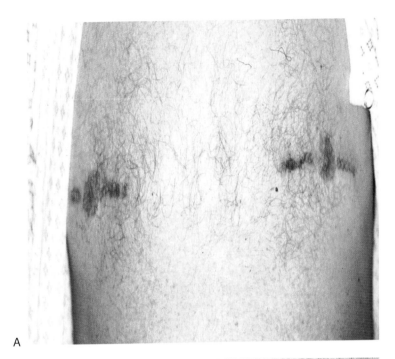

A

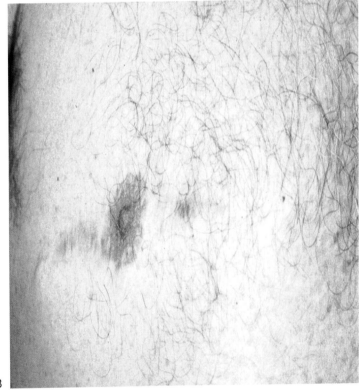

B

Figure 51.2 (A) *Periareolar hypertrophic scars following breast reduction surgery in a male.* **(B)** *Improvement after five treatments with a 595 nm pulsed dye laser at a fluence of 5 J/cm², a pulse duration of 1.5 ms, and a 7 mm spot size.*

- Surgical excision includes standard elliptical excision as well as subcutaneous mastectomy.
- Conventional and ultrasound-assisted liposuction, i.e., localized removal of glandular tissue and/or excess fat (Fig. 51.1). This is particularly successful in early-stage and limited gynecomastia.
  - Liposuction is performed through small incisions in the axilla and sternum to minimize scarring.
  - Liposuction is less effective in longstanding and substantial gynecomastia.
  - In prostate cancer patients, earlier intervention is more efficacious.
  - Residual periareolar fat may be noted post-liposuction which can be improved with localized dissection of fat via a small periareolar incision.
  - Postprocedure skin laxity may be noted.
- Combination surgical excision and tumescent liposuction. This involves liposuction, open excision, and skin reduction for laxity. Liposuction has also been combined with subcutaneous mastectomy.
- Surgical excision with plastic surgical repair, particularly in the event of breast tissue sagging (Fig. 51.2). Excessive fat, glandular tissue, and loose skin is excised via elliptical excision including the nipple and areola. The nipple/areola complex is then placed in the appropriate anatomic position as a full-thickness skin graft after the excess glandular tissue is removed.

PITFALLS TO AVOID/COMPLICATIONS/ MANAGEMENT/OUTCOME EXPECTATIONS

- It is important to recognize that gynecomastia has multiple etiologies before attempting to treat it.
- In most cases, watchful waiting is the best therapy.
- In cases of an underlying systemic cause, referral to the appropriate specialist is mandated.
- In cases of drug-induced gynecomastia, discontinuation of the medication is the best management.
- In cases refractory to medical management, there are several surgical options. Complications from these procedures include a poor cosmetic result, postoperative scarring, incomplete removal, postprocedure skin laxity, permanent numbness in the area, and hematoma formation.

BIBLIOGRAPHY

Aslan G, Tuncali D, Terzioglu A, Bingul F. Periareolar-transareolar-perithelial incision for the surgical treatment of gynecomastia. *Ann Plast Surg*. 2005;54(2):130–134.

Bembo SA, Carlson HE. Gynecomastia: its features, and when and how to treat it. *Cleve Clin J Med*. 2004;71(6): 511–517.

Gabra HO, Morabito A, Bianchi A, Bowen J. Gynaecomastia in the adolescent: a surgically relevant condition. *Eur J Pediatr Surg.* 2004;14(1):3–6.

Gasperoni C, Salgarello M, Gasperoni P. Technical refinements in the surgical treatment of gynecomastia. *Ann Plast Surg.* 2000;44(4):455–458.

Iwuagwu OC, Calvey TA, Ilsley D, Drew PJ. Ultrasound guided minimally invasive breast surgery (UMIBS): a superior technique for gynecomastia. *Ann Plast Surg.* 2004;52(2):131–133.

Rohrich RJ, Ha RY, Kenkel JM, Adams WP Jr. Classification and management of gynecomastia: defining the role of ultrasound-assisted liposuction. *Plast Reconstr Surg.* 2003;111(2):909–923.

Graf R, Auersvald A, Dama Sio RC, Rippel R, et al. Ultrasound-assisted liposuction: an analysis of 348 cases. *Aesthetic Plast Surg.* 2003; 27(2):146–153.

CHAPTER 52 Cellulite

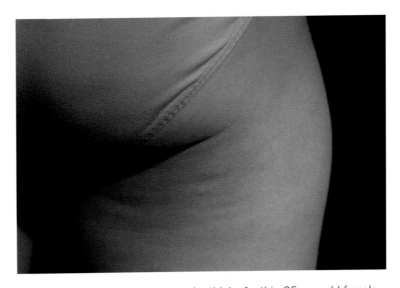

Figure 52.1 *Cellulite on the posterior thigh of a thin 35-year-old female*

Cellulite describes an orange peel type dimpling of skin in the upper posterior thighs and buttocks. The term derives from the French medical literature of 150 years ago. Although there is no associated morbidity or mortality, it is among the most common cosmetic complaints of female patients. It is present in nearly all postpubertal females, regardless of weight.

EPIDEMIOLOGY

Incidence: 85–98% of postpubertal females; far less common in males

Age: begins in females after puberty

Race: more common in Caucasians

Sex: far more common in females

Precipitating factors: female gender, androgen deficiency in males (rare)

PATHOGENESIS

Unknown.

PHYSICAL LESIONS

There is an orange peel or cottage cheese type dimpling of the upper and outer thighs and buttocks (Fig. 52.1). Other common locations include the breasts, lower abdomen, upper arms, and nape of neck.

DIFFERENTIAL DIAGNOSIS

None.

LABORATORY EXAMINATION

None indicated as the clinical appearance is classic.

COURSE

Begins in puberty in females and persists throughout life. In males with androgen deficiencies, the clinical appearance worsens as the androgen deficiency becomes more severe. It may present de novo in males undergoing hormonal therapy for prostate cancer.

KEY CONSULTATIVE QUESTIONS

In males, inquire as to possibility of any endocrine abnormalities. There is a rare association with endocrine abnormalities in males.

MANAGEMENT

There is no medical indication to treat cellulite. Still, many patients request therapy. Currently, there are numerous purported therapies, none of which have proven to be very effective. Interestingly, despite the lack of scientific evidence of improvement, many patients report subjective improvement and satisfaction with therapy.

TREATMENTS

■ Diet

- There is no data to show that diet and exercise are effective treatments.
- Still, weight loss diminishes cellulite's clinical appearance.
- Weight gain worsens its appearance.

■ Topical Treatments

- Aminophylline, retinoids, lactic acid, xanthines, and many others have all been used with little evidence of efficacy.
- Some creams may produce more harm than benefit.
- In fact, one study indicated 25% of the cellulite creams examined contained known allergens.

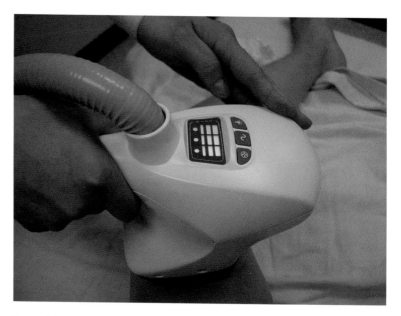

Figure 52.2 *VelaSmooth (Syneron Medical Ltd., Yokneam Illit, Isreal) laser treatment of thigh of a young female*

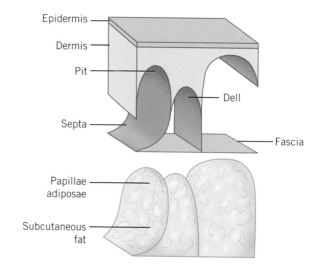

Figure 52.3 *The clinical appearance of cellulite is most likely produced by herniations of subcutaneous fat into the dermis creating the "pits" and "dells" associated with cellulite*

■ Interventional Treatments

Liposuction

- There are a few reports of improvement; however, typically it does not improve cellulite.
- In some cases, it can accentuate the appearance of cellulite.
- Prior to performing a liposuction procedure, it is useful to inform patients that their cellulite will not resolve and may, in fact, worsen. This will protect against postprocedure disappointment.

Endermologie

- Endermologie is an FDA approved device to improve the appearance of cellulite.
- Skin is kneaded by a handheld machine.
- It is rolled over affected areas of the body that are covered by a nylon suit.
- It purports to improve blood and lymphatic flow as well as skin architecture.
- Twice weekly treatments of 10–45 min each are recommended.
- There is little evidence to support its efficacy.

Subcision

- Requires local anesthesia.
- Using a scalpel or special 16-gauge needle, the fat septae are cut in the deep subcutaneous fat.
- Side effects include pain, bruising, scar, and puckering.
- Little data to support efficacy.

Mesotherapy

Phosphatidylcholine injections: not a recommended therapy.

- Injection into subcutaneous fat.
- Deoxycholate is the active ingredient.
- No data to show efficacy.

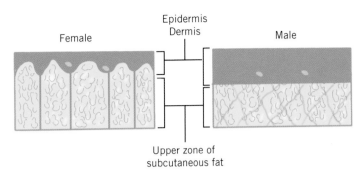

Figure 52.4 *In contrast to female fat architecture, male fat is made up of relatively small fat lobules with septae oriented in an oblique fashion to the dermis. This prevents fat herniations and the appearance of cellulite*

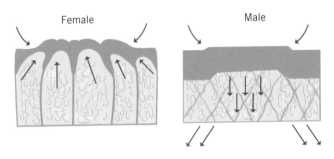

Figure 52.5 *The ability to pinch female fat and replicate the findings of cellulite is termed the "mattress phenomenon." It is present on the posterior thighs in nearly all females and reflects the underlying fat architecture. Male fat architecture, however, prevents this clinical finding*

TABLE 52.1 ■ **Cellulite Light Therapies**

TriActive	VelaSmooth
FDA approved device Low intensity (810 nm)	FDA approved device 700–2000 nm infrared light, continuous-wave radiofrequency
Suction massage	Mechanical suction

Light Therapy (Table 52.1)

- VelaSmooth system (Syneron Medical Ltd., Yokneam Illit, Isreal) combines near-infrared light at a wavelength of 700–2000 nm, continuous-wave radiofrequency and mechanical suction (Fig. 52.1).
  - Twice weekly treatments for a total of eight to ten sessions have been recommended.

– There are no long-term data to support its efficacy in patients.

- The TriActive Laserdermology system (Cynosure, Inc., Chelmsford, Massachusetts) combines six near-infrared diode lasers at a wavelength of 810 nm, localized cooling, and mechanical massage.

  – Three weekly treatments for 2 weeks and then biweekly treatments for 5 weeks are suggested.

  – There are no long-term data to support its efficacy in patients.

- There are currently many investigations into possible laser treatment for cellulite.

PITFALLS TO AVOID/ COMPLICATIONS/ MANAGEMENT/OUTCOME EXPECTATIONS

- Patients should be informed that there are no completely effective treatments for cellulite.

- Most of the positive results relating to cellulite treatment are anecdotal or reported in small, unscientific studies. Many of the therapies are expensive, especially given their lack of efficacy.

- Some may even produce more harm than benefit.

- There may be a more promising future for laser and light source treatments.

BIBLIOGRAPHY

Avram MM. Cellulite: a review of its physiology and treatment. *J Cosmet Laser Ther.* 2004;6:181–185.

Draelos Z, Marenus KD. Cellulite etiology and purported treatment. *Dermatol Surg.* 1997;23:1179–1181.

Kinney BM. Cellulite treatment: a myth or reality: a prospective randomized, controlled trial of two therapies, endermologie and aminophylline cream. *Plast Reconstr Surg.* 1999;104:1115–1117.

Lis-Balchin M. Parallel-placebo-controlled clinical study of a mixture of herbs sold as a remedy for cellulite. *Phytother Res.* 1999;13:627–629.

Pierard-Franchimont C, Pierard GE, Henry F, Vroome V, G Cauwenbergh. A randomized, placebo-controlled trial of topical retinol in the treatment of cellulite. *Am J Clin Dermatol.* 2000;1:369–374.

Rossi AR, Vergnanini, AL. Cellulite: a review. *J Eur Acad Dermatol Venereol.* 2000;14:251–262.

Van Vliet M, Ortiz A, Avram M, Yamauchi P. An assessment of traditional and novel therapies for cellulite. *J Cosmet Laser Ther.* 2005;7:7–10.

CHAPTER 53 HIV Lipodystrophy/Facial Lipoatrophy

HIV lipodystrophy describes a constellation of changes in subcutaneous and visceral fat distribution in patients on antiretroviral therapy. The findings include subcutaneous fat loss in the malar and buccal fat pads, i.e., facial lipoatrophy (Fig. 53.1), as well as on the extremities. It also features fat accumulation on the dorsocervical fat pad, i.e., buffalo hump, breasts, and intraabdominal cavity. Its characteristic appearance is significant in that it reduces patient compliance with antiretroviral therapy and deprives patients of HIV status privacy, particularly in communities where HIV rates are high.

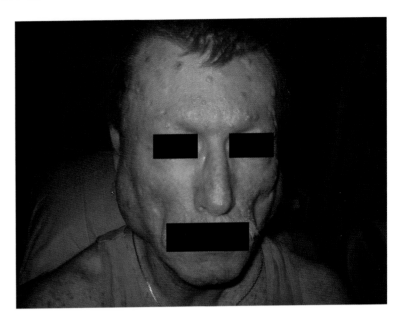

Figure 53.1 *Marked facial atrophy in a patient with HIV infection. Notice the molluscum contagiosum on his face, a chacteristic finding in HIV disease.*

EPIDEMIOLOGY

Incidence: 25–83% of patients treated with antiretrovirals depending on the criteria used

Age: all ages, but older age is predictive of severity

Race: none

Sex: equal, severe findings more frequent in females

Precipitating factors: protease inhibitors are most commonly implicated but this condition is associated with all antiretrovirals. It also presents infrequently in patients naive to HIV therapy. Typically, patients are on combination therapies

PATHOGENESIS

Unknown, but likely multifactorial.

DERMATOPATHOLOGY

Complete or near complete loss of fat. Juxtaposition of the dermis and fascia may be seen. Adipocytes are markedly reduced in number and size.

PHYSICAL LESIONS

Lipodystrophies display fat accumulation and fat loss.

- Fat accumulation
  - Dorsocervical fat pad, i.e., buffalo hump
  - Breasts
  - Intrabdominal cavity, i.e., Crix belly
- Fat loss
  - Malar and buccal fat pads
  - Extremities and buttocks

DIFFERENTIAL DIAGNOSIS

Other lipodystrophies, HIV wasting syndrome, Cushing's disease, malnutrition states, anorexia nervosa, metabolic X syndrome, cachexia secondary to cancer, malabsorption syndromes, thyrotoxicosis, and multiple symmetric lipomatosis.

LABORATORY EXAMINATION

The clinical findings and history are sufficient to make a diagnosis. Laboratory workup should include assessment of blood glucose, lipids, and triglycerides. If Cushing's disease is clinically suspected, laboratory examination should be performed.

COURSE

HIV lipodystrophy does not spontaneously regress in the absence of treatment or medication change.

KEY CONSULTATIVE QUESTIONS

- Medication history
- HIV status
- Duration
- Associated hyperglycemia, hyperlipidemia, hypertriglyceridemia

MANAGEMENT

Cosmetic improvement can be essential to promoting a patient's adherence to their HIV medication regimen. There are several means by which the cosmetic appearance of HIV lipodystrophy can be improved. These include medication changes, filler substances, and liposuction. Diet and exercise can be helpful both for cosmesis and metabolic derangements.

TREATMENTS

There are several treatments that can improve the cosmetically striking appearance of these disorders. They can be divided into two categories: treatment of lipoatrophy and treatment of fat accumulation. Additionally, changes in medications can be pursued. This is best entrusted to a physician who specializes in the care of HIV patients.

■ Oral Medications

All changes to an antiretroviral regimen are best handled by physicians who specialize in HIV treatment. These changes can improve the appearance of HIV lipodystrophy and are beyond the scope of this textbook.

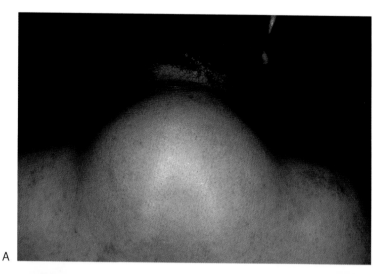

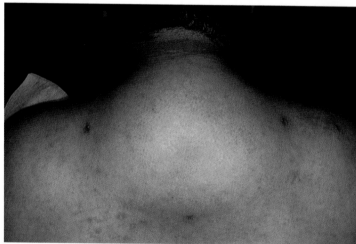

Figure 53.2 (A) *"Buffalo hump" in dorsocervical back of a HIV-infected male.* **(B)** *Substantial reduction in the size of buffalo hump after liposuction procedure*

▪ Treatment of Facial Lipoatrophy

Temporary fillers

• Poly-L-lactic acid, Sculptra, (Sanofi Aventis, Paris, France) is FDA approved for the treatment of HIV facial lipoatrophy (Fig. 53.3)

  – Synthetic, biodegradable polymer, i.e., the material used in Vicryl sutures

  – Multiple treatments required, depending on the severity of lipoatrophy

  – 18–24 month duration of filler material

  – No need for allergy testing

• Radiesse (Bioform Medical Inc., San Mateo, CA): consists of calcium hydroxylapatite microsperes. It has also been used to treat HIV lipoatrophy

Permanent fillers

• Silicone: Not FDA approved

  – A highly purified 1000-cSt silicone oil has been examined in 77 patients

  – The data showed that the number of treatments and the amount of silicone required for full treatment was correlated to the initial severity of facial lipoatrophy

  – The investigators noted no adverse events but cautioned that long-term efficacy and safety are yet to be determined

▪ Treatment of Fat Accumulation

Liposuction/lipectomy

• Localized liposuction/lipectomy uses tumescent local anesthesia rather than general anesthesia

• Ultrasound-assisted liposuction has also been employed

• It is effective in removing excess fat in the dorsocervical region, (Fig. 53.2)

• Recurrence is a risk

PITFALLS TO AVOID/COMPLICATIONS/ MANAGEMENT/OUTCOME EXPECTATIONS

• It is important to make certain that the multiple medical issues in these patients are being monitored appropriately.

• Fillers can be very effective for improving facial lipoatrophy.

• A temporary filler, such as Sculptra, (Sanofi Aventis, Paris, France) has FDA approval. Furthermore, its non-permanent nature allows for temporary side effects in the event of poor results or granuloma formation. Unfortunately, temporary fillers require indefinite treatment sessions and expense.

• Permanent fillers, such as silicone have promising initial data, but further studies are needed to assess long-term efficacy and safety concerns. Granuloma formation and

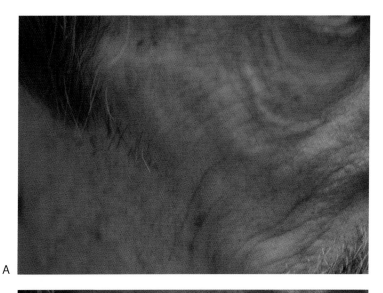

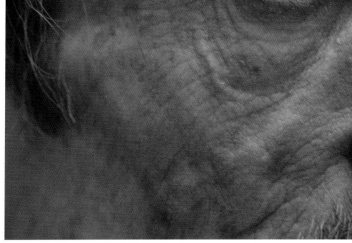

Figure 53.3 (A) *HIV lipoatrophy before Radiesse (Bioform Medical, Inc., San Mateo, CA) injection.* **(B)** *HIV lipoatrophy following Radiesse injection*

other permanent adverse side effects are serious potential hazards. There is the potential of granuloma formation many years after initial treatment.

- Silicone is not FDA approved for the treatment of HIV lipodystrophy.
- Liposuction can be very effective in patients with buffalo humps. Localized liposuction/lipectomy uses tumescent localized anesthesia rather than general anesthesia, which decreases the possibility of serious adverse events. Still, liposuction can be expensive and results vary according to the experience of the practitioner.

BIBLIOGRAPHY

Boix V. Polylactic acid implants. A new smile for lipoatrophic faces? *AIDS.* 2003;17(17):2533–2535.

Connolly N, Manders E, Riddler S. Short communication: suction-assisted lipectomy for lipodystrophy. *AIDS Res Hum Retroviruses.* 2004;20(8):813–815.

Hadigan C, Yawetz S, Thomas A, Havers F, Sax PE, Grinspoon S. Metabolic effects of rosiglitazone in HIV lipodystrophy; a randomized, controlled trial. *Ann Intern Med.* 2004;140(10):786–794.

Jones DH, Carruthers A, Orentreich D, Brody HJ, Lai MY, Azen S, Van Dyke GS. Highly purified 1000 cSt silicone oil for treatment of human immunodeficiency virus-associated facial lipoatrophy: an open pilot trial. *Dermatol Surg.* 2004; 30(10):1279–1286.

Koutkia P, Canavan B, Breu J, Torriani M, Kissko J, Grinspoon S. Growth hormone-releasing hormone in HIV-infected men with lipodystrophy: a randomized controlled trial. *JAMA.* 2004;292(2):210–218.

Pilero PJ, Hubbard M, King J, Faragon JJ. Use of ultrasonography-assisted liposuction for the treatment of human immunodeficiency virus-associated enlargement of the dorsocervical fat pad. *Clin Infect Dis.* 2003;37: 1374–1377.

Vleggaar D, Bauer U. Facial enhancement and the European experience with Sculptra (poly-L-lactic acid). *J Drugs Dermatol.* 2004;3(5):542–547.

CHAPTER 54 Lipodystrophy

Lipodystrophies are a diverse group of congenital and acquired disorders that feature partial or complete loss of fat. Each condition features development of cadaveric facies and a distinctive pseudo-muscular body habitus. These disorders are extremely rare. There are four categories of lipodystrophy: acquired partial lipodystrophy (APL), acquired generalized lipodystrophy (AGL), congenital generalized lipodystrophy (CGL), and familial partial lipodystrophy (FPL). Treatments vary according to the clinical findings.

EPIDEMIOLOGY

Incidence: very rare; acquired lipodystrophies are more common than congenital lipodystrophies

Age: congenital, childhood, or puberty depending on the disorder

Race: none

Sex: females > males

Precipitating factors: inheritance and genetic defects play an important role in several lipodystrophies such as CGL, FPL, and APL. In AGL, there may be an association with bacterial or viral illnesses

PATHOGENESIS

Unknown.

DERMATOPATHOLOGY

Complete or near complete loss of fat is a feature of each of the lipodystrophies. Juxtaposition of the dermis and fascia may be seen. Adipocytes are markedly reduced in number and size.

PHYSICAL LESIONS

Each of the lipodystrophies feature generalized, partial, or localized fat loss. They also feature, to varying degrees, cadaveric facies and a distinctive pseudo-muscular body habitus. Superficial veins appear prominent. In FPL, there may be an increased muscle mass. APL characteristically presents with fat loss above the waist only, but in some cases, there is a compensatory fat hypertrophy of the legs creating a striking appearance (Fig. 54.1).

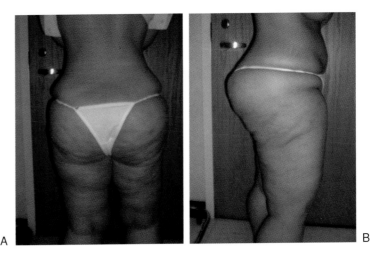

A   B

Figure 54.1 *A young woman demonstrating striking appearance of Barraquer–Simons lipodystrophy prior to liposuction*

DIFFERENTIAL DIAGNOSIS

HIV/HAART lipodystrophy, malnutrition states, metabolic X syndrome, cachexia secondary to cancer, malabsorption syndromes, thyrotoxicosis, Cushing's syndrome, and multiple symmetric lipomatosis.

LABORATORY EXAMINATION

The clinical findings are sufficient to make a diagnosis. Laboratory workup should include assessment of blood glucose, lipids, and triglycerides. In APL, laboratories should be sent for C3 nephritic factor.

COURSE

The course varies according to the disorder. Presentation can be rapid over a few weeks or insidious over months to years. Once lipodystrophy presents, fat loss does not recover.

KEY CONSULTATIVE QUESTIONS

- Family history
- Duration
- Has the fat loss ceased?
- Associated hyperglycemia, hyperlipidemia, hypertriglyceridemia
- Hematuria

MANAGEMENT

There are three primary goals of therapy: improving cosmesis, treating metabolic derangements, and treating systemic manifestations. It is essential that any management begin with a complete endocrine, cardiac, and gastrointestinal workup with referral to appropriate specialists. Improving the cosmetic appearance is often difficult. It is most successful in local or partial lipodystrophies rather than generalized lipodystrophies.

TREATMENTS

There are several treatments that can improve the cosmetically striking appearance of these rare disorders. It is recommended that no treatment should proceed prior to the resolution of active fat loss.

■ Temporary Fillers

- Collagen or Restylane (Med. as Aesthetics, Inc., Scottsdale Arizona) (hyaluronic acid)

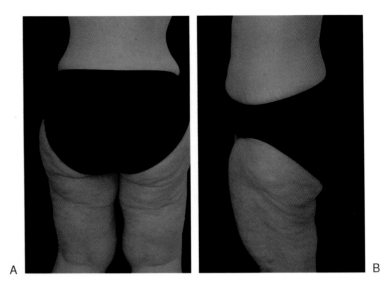

Figure 54.2 *Dramatic improvement in fat contour following liposuction treatment of same patient with Barraquer-Simons lipodystrophy*

- Sculptra (Sanofi Aventis, Paris, France), an injectable form of poly-L-lactic acid
  - Same material used in Vicryl sutures
  - FDA approved for the treatment of HIV facial lipoatrophy
  - Duration of 18–24 months
- Autologous fat transfer from the abdomen, buttocks, or hip has had variable success
  - Autotransplanation into areas of fat loss results in loss of transplanted fat
- Fillers can be very effective for improving facial lipoatrophy. Temporary fillers have the advantage of FDA approval. Furthermore, their nonpermanent nature allows for temporary side effects in the event of poor results or granuloma formation. Unfortunately, temporary fillers require (repeat) treatment sessions and expense.

■ Permanent Fillers

- Medical-grade silicone
- Permanent fillers are attractive in these patients precisely because their disorders are permanent. After a series of injections, they do not require indefinite retreatments. Unfortunately, poor technique and granuloma formation are hazards. Granuloma formation may occur years after treatment. Silicone is not FDA approved for the treatment of lipodystrophies.

■ Liposuction/Lipectomy (Fig. 54.2)

- This can be effective for removing excess fat, particularly in APL patients who exhibit compensatory fat accumulation in the legs and FPL patients with excess dorsocervical and visceral fat.
- Localized liposuction/lipectomy uses tumescent localized anesthesia rather than general anesthesia.

■ Plastic Surgery

- Facial lipoatrophy can be corrected with symmetrical rotation of the temporalis muscle into the face.
- Surgical implantation of abdominal muscles or bilateral transfer of anterolateral thigh flaps has also been used for augmentation of facial lipoatrophy.

PITFALLS TO AVOID/COMPLICATIONS/ MANAGEMENT/OUTCOME EXPECTATIONS

- Make certain that the multiple medical issues in these patients are being monitored appropriately before considering cosmetic treatment.

- Make certain that fat loss has ceased prior to treatment.
- Limited efficacy of cosmetic treatments for generalized or extensive partial lipodystrophies.
- Localized liposuction can be very effective in lipodystrophy patients with fat hypertrophy, but can be expensive. Results vary according to the experience of the physician.
- Facial plastic surgical procedures can be effective, but require major invasive surgery with its attendant risks of morbidity.

BIBLIOGRAPHY

Coessens BC, Van Geertruyden JP. Simultaneous bilateral facial reconstruction of a Barraquer–Simons lipodystrophy with free TRAM flaps. *Plast Reconstr Surg*. 1995; 95:911–915.

Garg A. Acquired and inherited lipodystrophies. *N Engl J Med*. 2004;350(12):1220–1234.

Goossens S, Coessens B. Facial contour restoration in Barraquer–Simons syndrome using two free tram flaps: presentation of two case reports and long-term follow-up. *Microsurgery*. 2002;22:211–218.

Guelinckx PJ, Sinsel NK. Facial contour restoration in Barraquer–Simons syndrome using two anterolateral thigh flaps. *Plast Reconstr Surg*. 2000;105:1730–1736.

Hurwitz PJ, Sarel R. Facial reconstruction in partial lipodystrophy. *Ann Plast Surg*. 1982;8:253–257.

Serra JM, Ballesteros A, Mesa F, Bazan A, Paloma V, Sanz J. Use of the temporalis muscle flap in Barraquer–Simons progressive lipodystrophy. *Ann Plast Surg*. 1993;30: 180–182.

Zafarulla MYM. Lipodystrophy: a case report of partial lipodystrophy. *Br J Oral Maxillofac Surg*. 1985;23:53–57.

CHAPTER 55 Striae Distensae

Striae distensae, more commonly known as "stretch marks," are atrophic linear bands of skin that appear after certain precipitating factors such as pregnancy, steroid use, and dramatic changes in weight or muscle mass (Fig. 55.1). At presentation, they feature a purple or pink color (striae rubra) that fades to a paler white (striae alba) over time. They are most common in adult women.

EPIDEMIOLOGY

Incidence: common

Age: puberty, pregnancy

Race: more common in Caucasians

Sex: females > males (associated with puberty and pregnancy)

Precipitating factors: topical and oral steroid use, Cushing's syndrome, pregnancy, breast-feeding, puberty, genetic collagen defects, and dramatic changes in weight, height, or muscle mass

PATHOGENESIS

There are changes in the extracellular dermal matrix including fibrillin, elastin, and collagen, resulting from prolonged stretching of the skin.

PATHOLOGY

There are scar-like features. Typically, there is an atrophic epidermis with narrow collagen bundles arranged parallel to the skin surface. The rete ridges are effaced. In early striae, there is a superficial, deep, and interstitial lymphocytic perivascular infiltrate and occasional eosinophils. The infiltrate fades in older lesions.

PHYSICAL LESIONS

Multiple symmetric linear band-like plaques of atrophic skin that present most commonly in the outer thighs, breasts, and buttocks of women along the lines of cleavage. They present with a pink/purple hue (striae rubra) and become paler with fine wrinkling over time (striae alba). Striae are largest and most abundant in patients with Cushing's disease. In pregnancy, striae are most abundant on the abdomen. In weight lifters, they are most prominent on the shoulders. Topical corticosteroid use most commonly produces striae on the face, genitalia, flexural areas, and body folds.

DIFFERENTIAL DIAGNOSIS

Linear focal elastosis.

LABORATORY EXAMINATION

The characteristic clinical appearance of striae negates any need for skin biopsy. Additional laboratory workup to rule out Cushing's disease is indicated in the appropriate clinical setting.

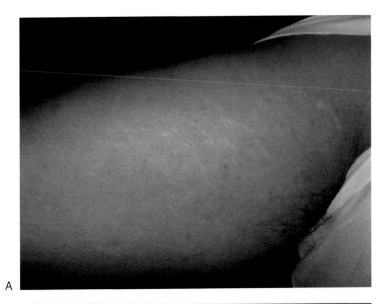

A

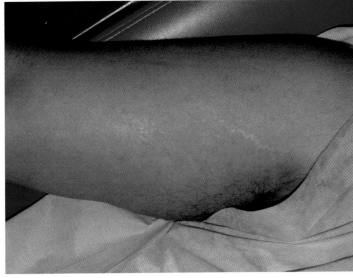

B

Figure 55.1 **(A)** *Striae alba at baseline.* **(B)** *Striae alba at 11 months follow-up after four treatments with a 1450-nm diode laser (Smoothbeam, Candela Corp., Wayland, MA) at energy settings of 13–14 J/cm², using a 6 mm spot size with a pulse duration of 30 ms. Treatment was performed at intervals of 2–3 months*

COURSE

Striae begin as pink or purple atrophic lesions that become paler and less obvious over time.

KEY CONSULTATIVE QUESTIONS

- Duration
- Skin phototype
- Pregnancy
- Assess for symptoms of Cushing's disease
- Use of corticosteroids
- History of weight change
- History of weight lifting

MANAGEMENT

There is no medical indication to treat striae. Still, many individuals are significantly bothered by their appearance and request treatment. There are numerous options to treat striae. Unfortunately, none of the treatments is completely successful. Prior to treatment, patients' expectations need to be tempered. Combination treatment involving laser and topical regimens such as tretinoin is often the best method of treatment. Fortunately, the appearance, particularly the color of striae, improves with time. Patients with skin phototypes I–III respond better than those with types IV–VI to laser therapy. Test sites prior to therapy are recommended. There is little data to show that treatments significantly improve striae over nonintervention.

TREATMENT (Fig. 55.2)

- The pulsed dye laser (585 nm) with a 7 or 10 mm spot size and 2–4 J/cm^2 fluence has been shown to improve the erythema of striae, but is associated with the risk of hyperpigmentation in darker skin phototypes.

  - Best for striae rubra.

  - Improvement can be seen even in cases of poor initial response 6 months after treatment.

  - Studies recommend against treating skin phototypes V and VI.

  - Some data casts doubt on the effectiveness of pulsed dye laser.

    - Multiple treatments produced only minor subjective improvement of "mature" striae but not significant photographic or histologic improvement.

- Short-pulsed erbium:YAG and CO$_2$ lasers can be modestly effective but are no longer commonly used due to such side effects as prolonged, difficult healing and pigmentary alteration. They are not recommended.

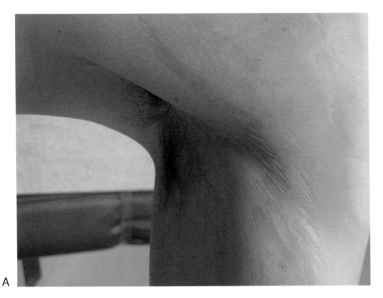

A

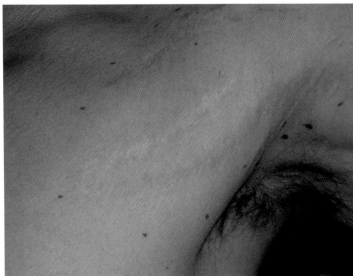

B

Figure 55.2 (A) *White striae, axilla. Prominent atrophy, textural changes, and depigmentation are observed.* **(B)** *White striae, axilla, following three fractional resurfacing laser treatments. Mild improvement of the atrophy and textural changes are noted. Mild post-inflammatory hyperpigmentation is observed, which resolved 3 weeks after the last laser treatment*

- The excimer laser (308 nm) has been examined for treatment of striae alba and scars in 31 adults. Treatments began at the MED minus 50 mJ/cm^2 to affected areas and were performed biweekly for 10 weeks. An improvement in coloration, by visual inspection (60–70%) and colorimetric analysis (100%), was noted and correlated strongly with the number of treatments performed. The pigment correction, however, returned close to baseline after a 6-month follow-up. No blistering or pigmentary disturbances were noted.

TOPICAL TREATMENT

- Early striae
  - Treninoin (0.1%) cream can improve the appearance of striae, particularly early striae, while decreasing their length and width.
- Mature striae
  - Tretinoin (0.05%) and 20% glycolic acid can improve striae.
  - Glycolic acid (20%) and 10% L-ascorbic acid can improve striae.

MICRODERMABRASION

Microdermabrasion can produce small improvement after 6–10 treatments. Microdermabrasion can also be used in association with laser therapy given its fairly benign side effect profile.

PITFALLS TO AVOID/OUTCOME EXPECTATIONS/COMPLICATIONS/ MANAGEMENT

- Patients should be informed that complete resolution is not realistic. Rather, significant cosmetic improvement in appearance is the goal.
- Laser therapy must be used with caution in dark skin phototypes given the risk of hyperpigmentation.
- Topical tretinoin can produce skin irritation.

BIBLIOGRAPHY

Alexiades-Armenakas MR, Bernstein LJ, Friedman PM, Geronemus RG. The safety and efficacy of the 308-nm excimer laser for pigment correction of hypopigmented scars and striae alba. *Arch Dermatol.* 2004;140(8): 955–960.

Ash K, Lord J, Zukowski M, McDaniel DH. Comparison of topical therapy for striae alba (20% glycolic acid/0.05% tretinoin versus 20% glycolic acid/10% L-ascorbic acid). *Dermatol Surg.* August 1998;24(8):849–856.

Goldberg DJ, Sarradet D, Hussain M. 308-nm Excimer laser treatment of mature hypopigmented striae. *Dermatol Surg.* 2003;29(6):596–598. Discussion 598–599.

Jimenez GP, Flores F, Berman B, Gunja-Smith Z. Treatment of striae rubra and striae alba with the 585-nm pulsed-dye laser. *Dermatol Surg.* 2003;29(4):362–365.

McDaniel DH, Ash K, Zukowski M. Treatment of stretch marks with the 585-nm flashlamp-pumped pulsed dye laser. *Dermatol Surg.* 1996;22(4):332–337.

Nehal KS, Lichtenstein DA, Kamino H, Levine VJ, Ashinoff R. Treatment of mature striae with the pulsed dye laser. *J Cutan Laser Ther.* 1999;1(1):41–44.

Nouri K, Romagosa R, Chartier T, Bowes L, Spencer JM. Comparison of the 585 nm pulse dye laser and the short pulsed CO_2 laser in the treatment of striae distensae in skin types IV and VI. *Dermatol Surg.* 1999;25(5):368–370.

SECTION
ELEVEN

Wound Healing Alterations

CHAPTER 56 Hypertrophic Scars, Keloids, and Acne Scars

INTRODUCTION

Hypertrophic scars and keloids are both characterized by excess fibrous tissue at a site of injury in the skin. Hypertrophic scars are confined to the original wound site, whereas keloids, by contrast, extend beyond the original wound site (Table 56.1). Both are common and frequently disturb patients greatly, both as an unsightly scar as well as a reminder of previous trauma or surgery. Acne scars result from the loss of underlying collagen and elastic tissue from dermal inflammation associated with acne, particularly cystic acne. Acne scars are also very common and a source of distress to the patient, both for their obvious appearance on the face as well as a reminder of previous acne.

HYPERTROPHIC SCARS AND KELOIDS: PHYSICAL EXAMINATION

Hypertrophic scars present as thick, firm linear plaques at the site of trauma. Initially they may be erythematous but often become skin-colored with time. Keloids are firm, fibrous plaques that extend outside the site of injury with claw-like projections.

DIFFERENTIAL DIAGNOSIS

Dermatofibroma, scar sarcoid, dermatofibrosar coma protuberans, granuloma.

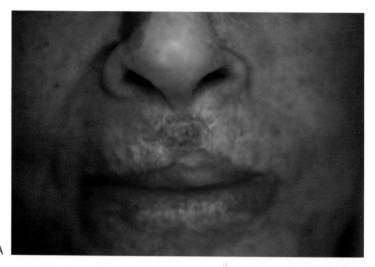

A

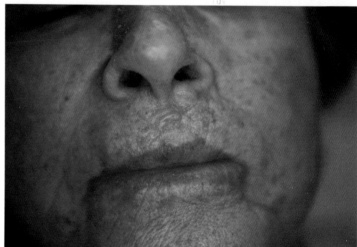

B

Figure 56.1 (A) *Erythematous hypertrophic scar at surgical site.* **(B)** *Improvement in erythema after several treatments with a 595 nm pulsed dye laser*

TABLE 56.1 ▪ Hypertrophic Scars Versus Keloids

	Keloid	Hypertrophic scar
Definition	Excess fibrous tissue formation in a wound that extends *beyond* the original wound site	Excess fibrous tissue formation in a wound that remains *within* the original wound site
Course	Does not spontaneously regress	Spontaneous regression within 6 months is frequent
	May arise weeks or months after injury	Usually arise within weeks of injury
Precipitating factors	Family history, surgery, trauma, burn acne, earlobe piercing; most common in skin types IV–VI, but may arise in all skin types and all ages	Family history, surgery, trauma, burn, acne; may arise in any patient at any all ages
,		
Incidence	Common; Males = females	Common; Males = females
	Sternum: most common location	Sternum: most common location

LABORATORY EXAMINATION

None. If, however, a keloid is unresponsive to multiple therapies, skin biopsy to rule out dermatofibrosarcoma protuberans is indicated.

MANAGEMENT

There are multiple therapies that are effective for decreasing the unsightly appearance of keloids and hypertrophic scars. None is completely satisfactory and none can be designated as a treatment of choice. Patients should be educated as to the refractory nature of keloids and hypertrophic scars and that multiple treatments over months are typically required for efficacy.

These treatment options include intralesional triamcinolone acetonide, intralesional 5-fluorouracil (5-FU), silicone sheeting, imiquimod, radiation, elliptical excision, and pulsed dye laser (595 nm). These treatments provide different benefits. Some reduce erythema, others flatten lesions, and some perform both the functions. Most often, intralesional steroids are a good initial therapy. Treatments can be broadly divided into laser and nonlaser therapies (Table 56.2).

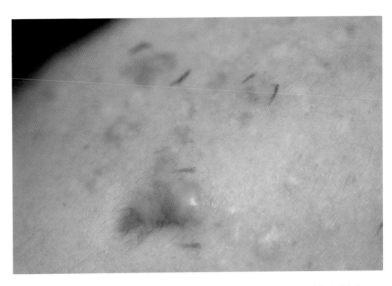

Figure 56.2 *Mild purpura after pulsed dye laser treatment of keloidal acne on back of a teenager. Intralesional kenalog was also used to produce eventual clinical improvement after a series of treatments*

TABLE 56.2 ■ **Nonlaser Treatment Options**

	Dose	Interval of time	Hypertrophic scar	Keloids	Comments
Intralesional 1 triamcinolone acetonide	5–40 mg/mL (site dependent)	Every 2–6 weeks	For most scars, moderate to dramatic improvement	Most successful with early intervention; variable success	Effective, safe, inexpensive; care to avoid atrophy
Intralesional 5-fluorouracil	50 mg/mL	1–3 times weekly for the first 1–2 weeks; then every 2–5 weeks	Can be effective; second-line therapy	Not effective	No clear advantage over triamcinolone acetonide
Silicone sheeting		12 h per day for 12 weeks	Variable improvement	Variable improvement	Safe, no good long-term studies
Imiquimod	Induces tumor necrosis factor alpha and interferon alpha and gamma	Nightly application for 6–8 weeks starting the day of surgery	Not studied	Study showed no recurrences up to 6 months; risk hyperpigmentation in scar. Further study needed to confirm these results	No long-term studies for recurrence rates
Excision surgical			Mostly unsuccessful, not recommended without adjuvant therapy	Very high recurrence rate without adjunct therapy. All patients must be aware recurrent keloid may be worse than original	Immediate gratification but increased risk of recurrence

LASER

Pulsed dye laser (595 nm), i.e., PDL, has emerged as an important adjuvant for treatment of keloids and hypertrophic scars (Figs. 56.1-56.2). Given its selective targeting of superficial blood vessels, PDL can dramatically improve the erythema associated with hypertrophic scars and keloids. It has also been shown help to flatten lesions as well (Table 56.3). CO_2 laser treatment of these lesions, while reported successful in some of the literature, is not recommended due to a high rate of recurrence. Intralesional corticosteroids are a helpful adjuvant to laser therapy to help flatten lesions and reduce pruritus (Fig. 56.3).

STUDIES

* One study examined the effect of a flashlamp pumped PDL at 585 nm or a flashlamp PDL at 510 nm on 15 patients with red hypertrophic scars. After an average of nearly two treatments, 77% improvement was noted. After three treatments, 7 of the 15 patients had complete resolution.

* Another study using the 585 nm PDL treated one half of median sternotomy hypertrophic scars/keloids in 16 patients and left the other side untreated. Patients received two treatments every 6–8 weeks and were examined after 6 months. Blinded observers and photography revealed "significant improvement" in redness, scar height, skin surface texture, and pruritis in laser-treated scar areas after 6 months.

TABLE 56.3 ■ **Pulsed Dye Laser for Hypertrophic Scars/Keloids**

Mechanism of action	Unknown
Expectation	Improves erythema, thickness, and pliability by up to 30–90%
PDL settings	3–7 J/cm², 7 or 10 mm spot, 0.45 or 1.5 ms pulse duration
Average number of treatments	—Four to six; but may require far more

A

B

Figure 56.3 (A) *Earlobe keloid. Keloid located on posterior ear lobule.* **(B)** *Earlobe repair. Immediate postprocedure appearance after excision and repair of posterior ear lobule keloid. Subsequent injections with intralesional kenalog prevented recurrence (photographs courtesy of Tomi Pandolfino, MD)*

CLINICAL EXPERIENCE

* Avoid elective surgery in patients with a history of keloids/hypertrophic scarring.

* Consider beginning therapy at the time of surgery or at suture removal.

* Keloids are more difficult to treat and more unpredictable in their response than hypertrophic scars.

* Hypertrophic scars often improve with no treatment in 6 months.

ACNE SCARS

Acne scarring is a common sequela of severe inflammatory or cystic acne. It can present in a mild or cosmetically disfiguring form. The best prevention of acne scarring is aggressive treatment of acne vulgaris at the time of presentation, including, when appropriate, isotretinoin. Acne scars have several varieties including atrophic, ice-pick, rolling, and boxcar scars. Treatments vary according to the type of scar being treated. They also vary in terms of duration of efficacy and expense. Prior to surgical or ablative therapy, it is important to elicit any recent history of Accutane use within the previous 6 months as well as a history of hypertrophic or keloidal scarring to avoid poor wound healing and scarring after therapy.

▣ Physical Lesions

- Atrophic scars are depressed from the skin surface and result from local loss of tissue from inflammation, intralesional steroids, skin surgery, weight loss, or rapid growth (Table 56.4).
- Ice-pick scars are narrow, deep, vertical, cylindrical depressions at the site of the infundibulum. Given their depth, they are more resistant to therapy (Table 56.5).
- Rolling scars are shallow depressions that are best appreciated with a change in surface lighting. They can vary in size and often coalesce with neighboring rolling scars. They are wider than ice-pick scars. Their depressed appearance reflects an underlying fibrosis of the dermis and subcutaneous fat.
- Boxcar scars are wider than ice-pick scars but less deep. They have a well-defined circular or oval shape (Table 56.5).

▣ Key Points in Treating Acne Scars

- Emphasize improvement rather than complete resolution as an obtainable result.
- Discuss all treatment options. All options have advantages and disadvantages.
- Many patients will benefit from a combination of therapy.
- Obtain complete medical history and medication use, i.e., Accutane before doing any surgical/ablative treatment.
- Make sure acne is being or has been treated to prevent future scars.

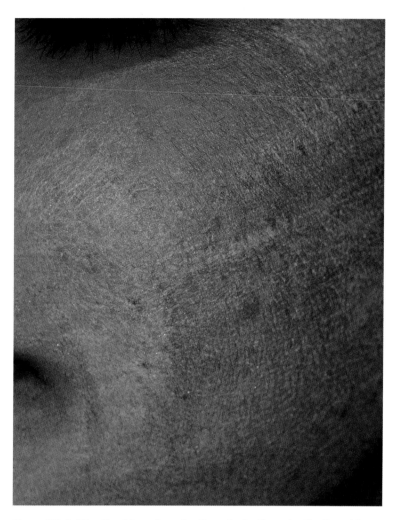

Figure 56.4 *"Frosting" is a sign of self-neutralization of salicylic acid peel. Here it is being applied for acne scars in a patient with type IV skin. This superficial peel is relatively safe in darker skin phototypes*

TABLE 56.4 ■ **Treatment Options for Atrophic Scars**

Therapy	Type of therapy	Course	Comments
Topical	Tretinoin 0.05–1% nightly	Slight improvement after 6–12 months	Slight improvement as monotherapy. Most effective as an adjunct with other modalities. If initial irritation, apply every other night until better tolerated
Laser	1450-nm diode: 12–13 J/cm^2, 6 mm spot size 33–36 ms cryogen cooling spray, three to four treatments over 4–6 months; treats active acne as well	10–30% improvement	Mild to moderate improvement
	Fractional resurfacing: four to six treatments, 12–20 mJ/cm^2, density of 1000–2000 MTZ/cm^2, density setting of 125 MTZ/cm^2, intervals of 1–4 weeks	Moderate improvement	Safe in all skin types Risk of transitory hyperpigmentation; post-laser erythema weeks to months; may cause acne flare Side effects include temporary erythema, edema, crusting, and mild pain
	Ultrapulsed pulse carbon dioxide laser	40–60% improvement; more effective than nonablative laser	Some may develop bronzing and mild flaking at 5–7 days Long-term data lacking More downtime and side effects than nonablative laser Post-laser erythema lasting weeks to months; risk of hyperpigmentation, infection and permanent hypopigmentation Best for shallow, wide scars such as boxcar scars Antivirals for patients with history of HSV
Fillers	Restylane (hyaluronic acid)	Dramatic improvement 4–8 months	Temporary Low risk allergy, granuloma Adverse effects last longer than that in the case of bovine/human collagen
Fillers	Autologous fat	Dramatic improvement and longer duration than other fillers	Longer duration No risk of allergy, granuloma More difficult to master effective technique
Fillers	Bovine collagen: Zyderm I, Zyderm II, Zyplast	Good, temporary improvement for 2–3 months	Requires test site for allergy Higher risk of allergy (i.e., 1–3%) Overcorrect scars Easier procedure for inexperienced practitioners than other fillers Adverse effects: shorter duration
Fillers	Human collagen	Good, temporary improvement for 2–3 months	
Mechanical/chemical	Microdermabrasion, glycolic and salicylic acid peels (Fig. 56.4) TCA peels; dermabrasion	Mild improvement	Microdermabrasion/glycolic acid peels are safe; salicylic acid peels safe in skin types IV–VI; dermabrasion should not be performed except in extremely experienced hands
Surgical	Subcision (incision into dermis with mechanical trauma inducing fibrosis)	Mild improvement	Safe
Surgical	Punch excision, punch grafting, punch autografting, punch elevation	Good improvement	Time consuming Multiple treatments Better for ice-pick scars

BIBLIOGRAPHY

Alster T. Laser scar revision: comparison study of 585 nm pulsed dye laser with and without intralesional corticosteroids. *Dermatol Surg.* 2003;29(1):25–29.

Alster TS, Williams CM. Treatment of keloid sternotomy scars with 585 nm flashlamp-pumped pulsed-dye laser. *Lancet.* 1995;345(8959):1198–1200.

Berman B, Kaufman J. Pilot study of the effect of postoperative imiquimod 5% cream on the recurrence rate of excised keloids. *J Am Acad Dermatol.* October 2002; 47(suppl 4):S209–S211.

Berman B, Viall A. Imiquimod 5% cream for keloid management. *Dermatol Surg.* 2003;29(10):1050–1051.

Chua SH, et al. Nonablative 1450 nm diode laser in treatment of facial atrophic acne scars in type IV Asian skin. *Dermatol Surg.* 2004;(10):1287–1291.

Dierickx C, Goldman MP, Fitzpatrick RE. Laser treatment of erythematous/hypertrophic and pigmented scars in 26 patients. *Plast Reconstr Surg.* January 1995;95(1):84–90.

Fitzpatrick RE. Treatment of inflamed hypertrophic scars using intralesional 5-FU. Dermatol Surg. 1999;25(3): 224–32.

Jacob CI, Dover JS, Kaminer MS. Acne scarring: a classification system and review of treatment options. *J Am Acad Dermatol.* 2001;45(1):109–118.

Nouri K, et al. 585 nm pulsed dye laser in treatment of surgical scars starting on suture removal day. *Dermatol Surg.* 2003;29(1):65–73.

TABLE 56.5 ■ Ice-pick/Boxcar Scar

	Advantage	Disdvantage
Punch harvesting and suture or punch harvest and implant full-thickness graft	Low cost, potential dramatic improvement; best for narrow, deep scars such as ice-pick scars or deep boxcar scars	Unpredictable, risk of making cosmetic appearance worse; time consuming
Ablative CO_2/Erbium:YAG	Potential 40–60% long-term improvement; best for shallow boxcar scars	Post-laser erythema weeks to months; risk of hyperpigmentation, infection and permanent hypopigmentation
	Immediate improvement	
		Antivirals for patients with history of HSV
Fillers, i.e., Restylane, collagen, etc. (see Table 56.4)		No permanent improvement
	Low risk	Need to repeat at least twice annually
	Lasts 4–8 months	
Nonablative laser	Low risk of serious side effects	Improvement 10–30%
1450 nm diode	No downtime	
12–13 J/cm^2	Treats any active acne	
33–36 ms cryogen cooling spray three to four treatments over 4–6 months		

SECTION TWELVE

Exogenous Cutaneous Alterations

CHAPTER 57 Ear Piercing

Ear piercing is performed to facilitate an individual's desire to wear earrings. By having the procedure performed in a medical facility by a physician, the patient is reassured that the procedure is being performed in a safe, controlled environment.

KEY CONSULTATIVE QUESTIONS

• Contact allergens to metals
• History of keloids or hypertrophic scarring

MANAGEMENT

There are two common methods for ear piercing. It can be performed by hand or with the help of an automatic ear-piercing gun (Fig. 57.1). Before performing either procedure, it is important to make certain that the correct location for piercing has been selected. Symmetry with the contra-lateral ear is essential for a good cosmetic appearance. The patient should review the sites using a mirror prior to treatment.

TREATMENT

• Sterilize all instruments.
• Sterilize and anesthetize the ear lobule.
• Using slow pressure, advance a 14–18 gauge needle through the posterior lobule into the anterior lobule.
• If an automatic ear-piercing gun is used, the gun is advanced from the anterior lobule towards the posterior lobule.
• Use a sterilized earring with a stainless steel post.
• The post of the earring is advanced with the needle and the tip is pulled back through the ear.
• The clasp is put on the posterior post.
• Leave the earring in place for 14 days.
• Clean the site with hydrogen peroxide and topical antibiotic ointment.

PITFALLS TO AVOID/COMPLICATIONS/ MANAGEMENT/OUTCOME EXPECTATIONS

• A good clean sterile technique can avoid post-procedure infections.
• It is important to elicit any history of hypertrophic scars or keloids in these patients (Fig. 57.2). Ear piercing should not be performed on these patients.

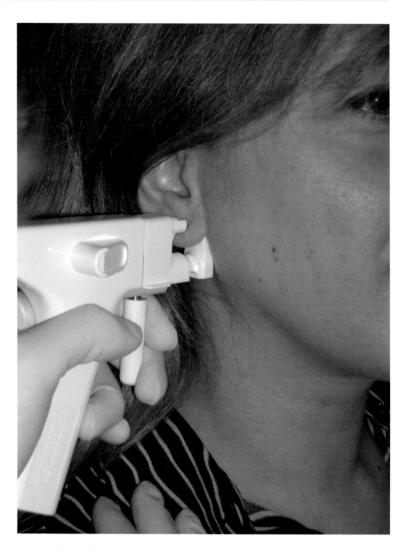

Figure. 57.1 *Ear-piercing gun being used on earlobe of a young female*

- Any history of nickel or other metal allergens should be elicited prior to any procedure as well.

- In the event of contact dermatitis or allergy, topical steroids are the mainstay of treatment.

BIBLIOGRAPHY

Atkin DH, Lask GP. Ear piercing and surgical repair of the earlobe. In: Lask GP, Moy RL, eds. *Principles and Techniques of Cutaneous Surgery*. New York: McGraw-Hill, Inc; 1996.

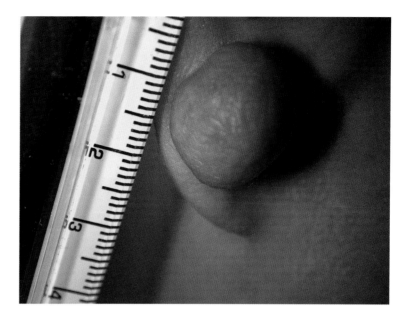

Figure 57.2 *Keloid on posterior earlobe secondary to ear piercing (courtesy of Tomi Pandolfino, MD)*

CHAPTER 58 Tattoo Removal

More than 10 million Americans have tattoos. Over time, many decide that they want the tattoo to be removed. Quality-switched (Q-switched) lasers are effective in removing most tattoo pigments safely (Figs. 58.1-58.3). The appropriate laser wavelength is determined by the tattoo ink's absorption spectrum. It is believed that laser pulses in the nanosecond range target tattoo pigments and break them into smaller particles, thereby facilitating removal of the pigment transepidermally or via macrophages and local scavenger cells. In order to treat multicolored tattoos, several Q-switched laser wavelengths must be employed.

KEY CONSULTATIVE QUESTIONS

- Was the tattoo placed by an amateur or a professional tattoo artist?
- Was the tattoo placed for the purpose of radiation therapy?
- Is the tattoo the result of trauma or injury?
- Tattoo colors (Table 58.1)
- Previous treatments
- Use of isotretinoin within past year
- History of keloids/hypertrophic scars

• Duration of tattoo
• Skin phototype
• History of HSV at site of treatment
• History of allergic or granulomatous reaction to tattoo pigment
• Is the tattoo placed over or covering another tattoo?
• History of gold ingestion

MANAGEMENT

It is important to ask the patient who placed the tattoo. Professional tattoo pigments are denser and placed deeper in the dermis than most amateur tattoos. This renders these tattoos more refractory to treatment, particular those that are multicolored and contain metallic pigments. It is important to inform the patient prior to treatment that complete resolution is not always feasible. It is also important to counsel that multiple treatments over 1–2 years may be required for maximal improvement.

PRETREATMENT ASSESSMENT

• Patients with darker skin types are more likely to suffer pigmentary changes.
• Professional tattoos require more treatments than amateur tattoos.
• Older tattoos respond more favorably than new tattoos.
• Black and dark blue tattoos respond more effectively than yellow tattoos.
• Assess for suntan. If patient is tanned, delay treatment until tan resolves unless the 1064 nm Q-switched Nd:YAG is being used.

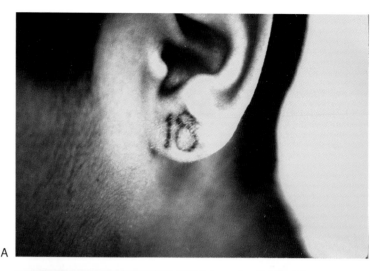

A

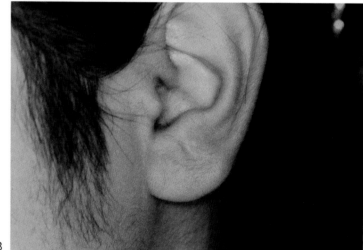

B

Figure 58.1 **(A)** *Tattoo on left earlobe prior to therapy.* **(B)** *Resolution after six treatments with 1064 nm Q-switched Nd:YAG laser.*

TABLE 58.1 ■ **Laser Therapy by Tattoo Color**

Tattoo pigment	Light spectrum	Most effective lasers	Comment
Red	Green	Frequency-doubled Q-switched Nd:YAG (532 nm)	May cause pigment alteration in darker skin Least painful of Q-switched lasers
Yellow	Green	Frequency-doubled Q-switched Nd:YAG (532 nm)	Not very effective
Green	Red/near infrared	Q-switched ruby (694 nm) Q-switched alexandrite (755 nm)	May cause hypopigmentation in darker skin
Light blue	Red/near infrared	Q-switched ruby (694 nm) Q-switched alexandrite (755 nm)	May cause hypopigmentation in darker skin
Dark blue & Black	Red/near infrared	Q-switched ruby (694 nm): light skin types only Q-switched alexandrite (755 nm): light skin types only Q-switched Nd:YAG (1064 nm): all skin types	Q-switched Nd:YAG (1064 nm) safe in all skin types. Less pigment loss

- Assess for scarring within the tattoo. If present, show the patient and document prior to treating.

NUMBER OF TREATMENTS

- Professional tattoos require about 6–12 treatments prior to removal; occasionally, more than 12 treatments are needed for maximal improvement.
- Amateur tattoos utilize less dense pigment and require about four to six treatments.
- Radiation tattoos and traumatic tattoos are more superficial and less dense than professional tattoos, requiring only a few treatments for resolution (Fig. 58.4).
- In general, radiation tattoos can be removed in—one to two treatments. Sometimes, they require additional treatments.
- Lower extremity tattoos typically require more treatments.
- Lower fluences and larger spot sizes can be as effective as smaller spot sizes and increased fluences.
- Test spot may be appropriate in darker skin phototypes if concerning.

TATTOO TREATMENT

- Photograph of tattoo prior to treatment.
- Topical anesthesia or 1% lidocaine, in the form of local injection or nerve block, will make the treatment more comfortable for the patient.
- Treat the affected areas with the appropriate Q-switched laser allowing for up to a 10% overlap (Table 58.2).
- The clinical endpoint is immediate tissue whitening. For the 1064-nm Q-switched Nd:YAG, in addition to tissue whitening there may be a small amount of pinpoint bleeding at the site of treatment (Figs. 58.5-58.6).
- Tissue splatter may produce scarring. If this occurs, decrease the fluence.
- If the tattoo is multicolored, treat the red pigment first. Erythema and inflammation from other treated sites may obscure visualization of red tattoo pigment.
- Apply topical antibiotics and a nonadherent dressing after completing the treatment.
- Counsel sunscreen and sun avoidance to the treatment area.

POST-TREATMENT CARE

- Sun avoidance, sunscreens
- Telfa dressing and antibiotic ointment with paper tape
- Return for treatment in 6–8 weeks

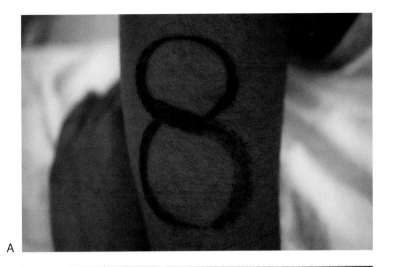

A

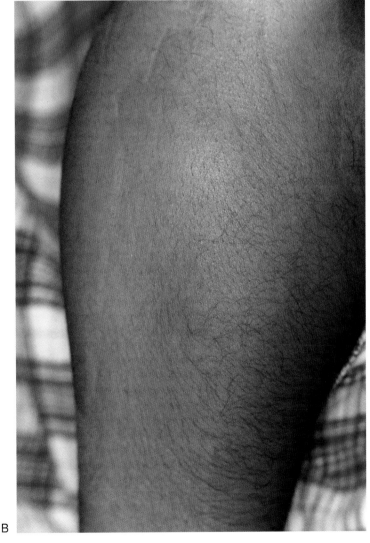

B

Figure 58.2 (A) *Tattoo on forearm prior to therapy.* **(B)** *Significant improvement after five treatments with 1064 nm Q-switched Nd:YAG laser*

ADVERSE EFFECTS/PRECAUTIONS

- Pigmentary alteration

- Blistering (especially, Q-switched alexandrite and ruby) (Fig. 58.7)

- Scarring (Fig. 58.8)

- In a patient with an allergic reaction to tattoo ink in the past (Fig. 58.9), there is the possibility of a recurrence secondary to the release of tattoo ink following laser therapy. Allergic precautions should be taken. Systemic allergic reactions can occur with Q-switched lasers (unlike destructive modalities—dermabrasion, etc.)

- Rust-colored tattoos should be treated carefully as well as red and flesh-colored cosmetic tattoos, e.g., lip liner (Fig. 58.10).

  - The tattoo may darken as a result of oxidation of iron or titanium oxide pigment within the tattoo

  - A test site can be performed 4–8 weeks prior to treatment for possible darkening

  - This darkening can sometimes be treated with lasers or may require excision.

  - They respond slowly to laser therapy.

- Practice caution in treating patients with history of gold salt ingestion. Chrysiasis, manifested as dark-blue pigmentation, can result from treatment with Q-switched lasers (Fig. 58.11)

PITFALLS TO AVOID/COMPLICATIONS/ MANAGEMENT/OUTCOME EXPECTATIONS

- Response to tattoo treatment is dependent upon the depth of pigment, the color of pigment, and the size of pigment particles.

- Effective treatment for a professional tattoo may require up to a dozen or more treatment sessions over a period of 1–2 years. Furthermore, complete removal is often not feasible.

- A successful treatment often leaves some residual tattoo pigment.

- Physicians should counsel patients that significant lightening may be the best clinical endpoint.

- Tattoo treatment can produce hyper and hypopigmentation in any patient, especially those with darker skin types.

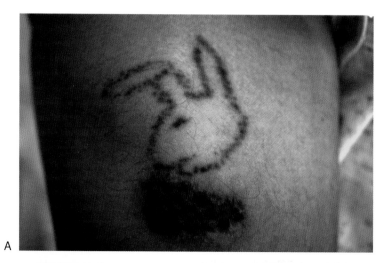

A

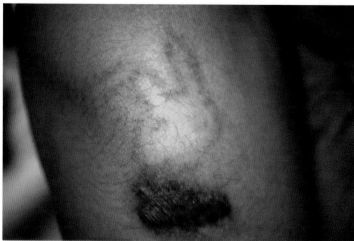

B

Figure 58.3 **(A)** *Left shoulder tattoo with inferior scar resulting from prior treatment with dermabrasion.* **(B)** *Improvement after six treatments with 1064 nm Q-switched Nd:YAG laser. While improvement is not complete, the cosmetic result is far superior to that of dermabrasion*

TABLE 58.2 ■ **Laser Therapy by Quality-Switched Lasers**

Laser	Initial settings	Effective against these tattoo inks
Frequency doubled Q-switched Nd:YAG (532 nm)	1.5–4.0 J, 4.0–8.0 mm spot size	Red, orange, yellow
Q-switched ruby (694 nm)	4.0–6.0 J, 6.5 mm spot size	Green, blue, black
Q-switched alexandrite (755 nm)	5.0–6.5 J, 2.0–4.0 mm spot size	Green, blue, black
Q-switched Nd:YAG (1064 nm)	3.0–10.0 J, 2.0–8.0 mm spot size	Blue, black (safest in dark skin types)

- The frequency-doubled Q-switched Nd:YAG, Q-switched ruby, and Q-switched alexandrite lasers are more likely to cause durable pigmentary changes than the Q-switched Nd:YAG (1064 nm).
- Most frequently, pigment alteration is temporary.
- Lower fluences and additional time between treatments should be employed in darker skin phototypes.

BIBLIOGRAPHY

Alster T. Q-switched alexandrite laser (755 nm) treatment of professional and amateur tattoos. *J Am Acad Dermatol.* 1995;33:69–73.

Ferguson JE, August PJ. Evaluation of the Nd/YAG laser for treatment of amateur and professional tattoos. *Br J Dermatol.* 1996;135(4):586–591.

Fitzpatrick RE, Goldman MP. tattoo removal using the alexandrite laser. *Arch Dermatol.* 1994;130:1508–1514.

Grevelink JM, Anderson RR, et al. Laser treatment of tattoos in darkly pigmented patients: efficacy and side effects. *J Am Acad Dermatol.* 1996;34:653–656.

Kilmer SL, Anderson RR. Clinical use of the Q-switched ruby and the Q-switched Nd:YAG (1064 nm and 532 nm) lasers for treatment of tattoos. *J Dermatol Surg Oncol.* 1993;19(4):330–338.

Levine VJ, Geronemus RG. Tattoo removal with the Q-switched ruby laser and the Q-switched Nd: YAG laser: a comparative study. *Cutis.* 1995;55:291–296.

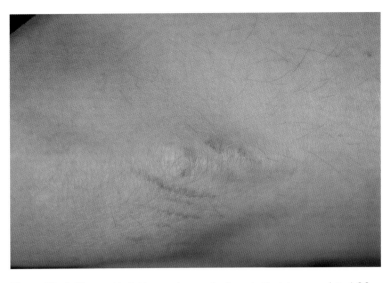

Figure 58.4 *Traumatic tattoo on knee of a female that has persisted 30 years after childhood bicycle fall. Q-switched 1064 nm Nd:YAG cleared the tattoo in three treatments*

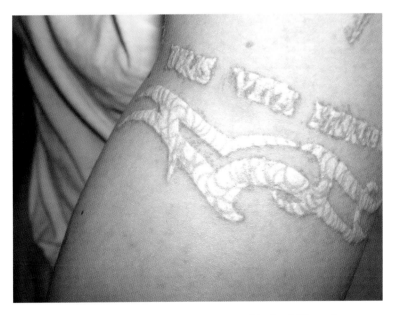

Figure 58.5 *Tissue whitening after treatment with the 532 nm frequency-doubled Q-switched Nd:YAG. Tissue whitening is the appropriate end-point when treating tattoos with Q-switched lasers*

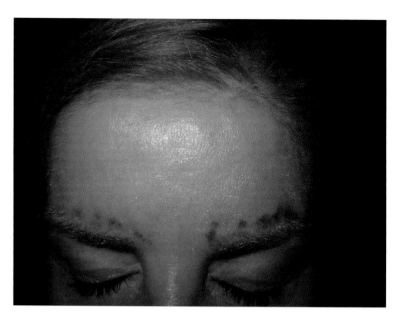

Figure 58.6 *Purpura immediately after treatment of an eyebrow tattoo with a Q-switched Nd:YAG laser.*

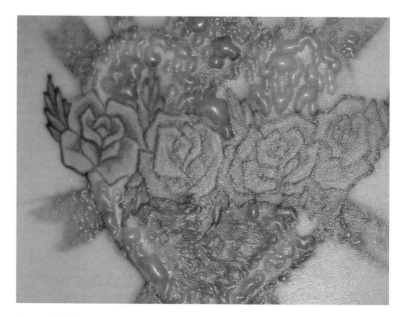

Figure 58.7 *Exuberant blistering reaction in red tattoo pigment. The reaction occurred with each treatment and predictably resolved completely within a few days with routine topical skin care (photograph courtesy of Teresa Soriano, MD)*

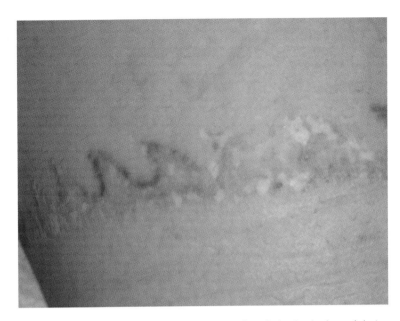

Figure 58.8 *Scarring after treatment with a Q-switched ruby laser (photograph courtesy of Teresa Soriano, MD)*

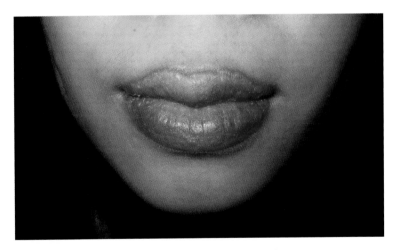

Figure 58.9 *Allergic hypersensetivity reaction to red tattoo*

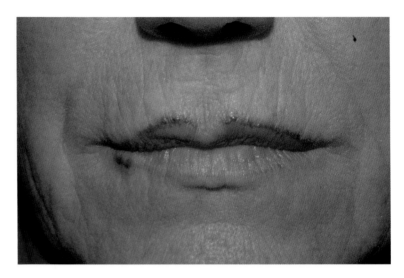

Figure 58.10 *Treatment of cosmetic tattoo with a 532 nm Q-switched Nd:YAG laser produces dramatic darkening*

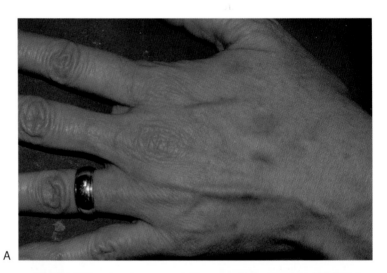

A

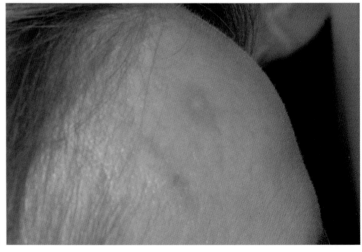

B

Figure 58.11 *Two examples of chrysiasis, a rare but well-described complication of Q-switched laser therapy in patients with a history of ingesting gold salts. In both of these patients, the characteristic dark-blue pigmentation was produced after Q-switched laser treatments of lentigines on the (A) dorsal hand and (B) forehead, respectively*

CHAPTER 59 Torn Earlobe

Torn earlobe is a common consequence of wearing heavy earrings for a prolonged period of time (Fig. 59.1). It may also arise as the result of a congenital defect or trauma.

KEY CONSULTATIVE QUESTIONS

* Precipitating event of earlobe tear
* History of keloids or hypertrophic scarring

MANAGEMENT

There are several surgical methods to repair torn earlobes. Different techniques are suited for different tears.

TREATMENTS (Figs. 59.1-59.3)

Most commonly, the Z-plasty repair or Interlocking Ls repair produce the best result.

* Sterile preparation and technique
* Local anesthesia should be injected into the repair site
* The epidermis of the opposing edges of the tear wound should be excised
  – Scalpel
  – Scissors
* Interrupted 6-0 epidermal sutures approximate and evert the wound edges of the anterior and posterior lobe
  – Be certain to approximate the wound edges of the inferior rim of the ear carefully to avoid distortion or misalignment
  – The wound edges should be under minimal tension
* No subcutaneous sutures are used
* Z-plasty repair (Fig. 59.2) or Interlocking Ls repair on the rim will produce tissue approximation while preventing the dimpling of the inferior rim of the earlobe
* Patients should be counseled to refrain from wearing earrings for 3 months following the repair

PITFALLS TO AVOID/COMPLICATIONS/ MANAGEMENT/OUTCOME EXPECTATIONS

* Meticulous attention to approximating the wound edges and the inferior rim of the ear are essential for a satisfactory result.
* Caution in a patient with a history of keloids or hypertrophic scars.

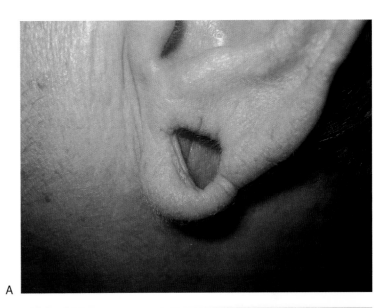

A

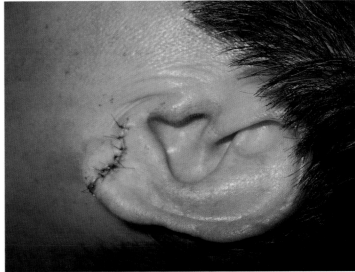

B

Figure 59.1 (A) *A young female with large tear defect of earlobe at the site of heavy earring.* **(B)** *Torn earlobe reconstructed by primary repair (courtesy of Dan Behroozan, MD)*

- Patient should not wear earrings for 3 months after surgery.
- Wound strength is less than the original strength of the lobe. Avoid wearing heavy earrings to prevent recurrence.

BIBLIOGRAPHY

Tipton JB. A simple technique for reduction of the earlobe. *Plast Reconstr Surg.* 1980;66:630–632.

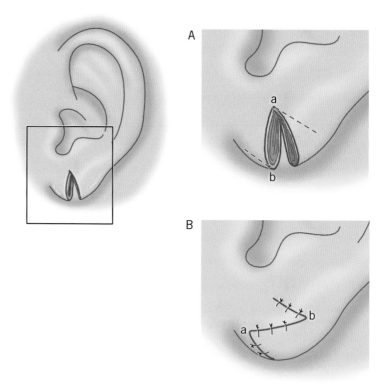

Figure 59.2 *Repair of complete earlobe tear utilizing a Z-plasty to prevent dimpling of the inferior aspect of earlobe*

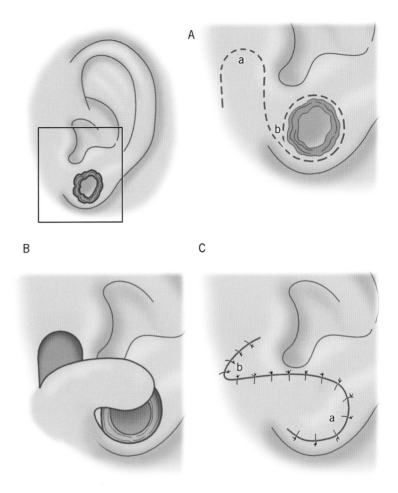

Figure 59.3 *One stage preauricular flap to repair earlobe deformities*

INDEX

In this index, the letters "f" and "t" denote figures and tables, respectively.